THE PAPERLESS MEDICAL OFFICE FOR BILLERS AND CODERS

Using Optum™ PM and Physician EMR

Virginia Busey Ferrari

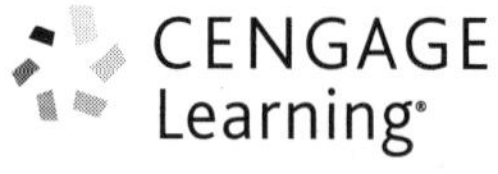

Australia • Brazil • Mexico • Singapore • United Kingdom • United States

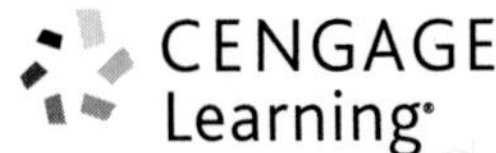

The Paperless Medical Office for Billers and Coders: Using Optum™ PM and Physician EMR
Virginia Busey Ferrari

General Manager: Dawn Gerrain

Product Team Manager: Stephen Smith

Senior Director, Development: Marah Bellegarde

Product Development Manager: Juliet Steiner

Content Developer: Lauren Whalen

Product Assistant: Courtney Cozzy

Marketing Director: Michele McTighe

Marketing Manager: Erica Glisson

Senior Production Director: Wendy Troeger

Production Manager: Andrew Crouth

Content Project Manager: Thomas Heffernan

Senior Art Director: Jack Pendleton

Cover Image(s): iStock.com/traffic_analyzer

Library of Congress Control Number: 2014931294

ISBN-13: 978-1-1332-7901-3

Cengage Learning
200 First Stamford Place, 4th Floor
Stamford, CT 06902
USA

Cengage Learning is a leading provider of customized learning solutions with office locations around the globe, including Singapore, the United Kingdom, Australia, Mexico, Brazil, and Japan. Locate your local office at: **www.cengage.com/global**

Cengage Learning products are represented in Canada by Nelson Education, Ltd.

To learn more about Cengage Learning, visit **www.cengage.com**
Purchase any of our products at your local college store or at our preferred online store **www.cengagebrain.com**

Printed in United States of America
Print Number: 02 Print Year: 2014

CONTENTS

PREFACE

Electronic technology is the major means through which workers communicate in today's health care environment. *The Paperless Medical Office for Billers and Coders: Using Optum™ PM and Physician EMR* is an electronic health record solution that integrates instructional theory with state-of-the-art practice management and electronic medical record software.

Optum™ PM and Physician EMR is one of the most advanced web-based practice management systems (PM) and electronic medical records (EMR) in the industry. The product is certified through the Certification Commission for Health Information Technology (CCHIT®) and is used by thousands of providers throughout the country. The Optum™ product provides state-of-the-art features and user-friendly software and is compliant with governmental mandates.

The PM side of Optum™ is a sophisticated practice management system that automates time-consuming administrative tasks such as eligibility checks, scheduling, reminders, patient visit documentation, claims submission, and related billing and coding functions. Its features include:

- Interactive dashboards that prioritize work lists automatically
- A rules-based, front-end clinical editing tool that scrubs outgoing claims prior to submission
- An online code lookup software that boosts coding accuracy

The EMR side of Optum™ monitors and measures all clinical data and prioritizes anything that needs attention. Some of the outstanding features of Optum™ EMR include:

- Automatic refill requests
- Chart management
- Lab management
- Medication history
- Prescription (Rx) writing
- Report management

Purpose of the Text

The Paperless Medical Office for Billers and Coders was written to fill a void in today's EHR training market and provide training specifically for financial functions and those PM and EMR activities that affect billing and coding. Many EHR training solutions are available but this workbook provides 8–10 hours of step-by-step training activities that simulate typical workflows in ambulatory health organizations related to the billing and coding functions. This workbook takes students through critical information on integrating EHR software into the medical practice, and then offers step-by-step guidance on how those principles can be applied using the Optum™ PM and Physician EMR software.

Chapters 1 and 2 include introductory activities in the Optum™ PM and Physician EMR software. Chapters 3 through 9 contain step-by-step front- and back-office functions related to billing and coding activities for students to complete. At the end of each activity, students will be asked to print a screenshot or report that captures the work they have completed. Students are encouraged to keep this documentation in an "assignments" folder, to submit to their instructor.

Features

The *Help* system within the Optum™ software includes a plethora of educational materials and training tutorials that provide tips for using Optum™ PM and Physician EMR. In addition to text materials, the Optum™ *Help* system provides training videos that walk users through each function within the system. Because this product is a live program, updated training materials containing the most recent information for Meaningful Use, ICD-10, and HIPAA are available.

The 8–10 hours of hands-on, step-by-step training activities include Professionalism Connections and Manager Challenge components. Students will learn how to use the different functions of the Optum™ software to meet billing and coding needs critical to the financial health of the practice.

Chapter Elements

Learning Objectives. The Learning Objectives state chapter goals and outcomes.

Sustainability Icon. The Sustainability icon appears throughout the workbook to highlight chapter material that addresses the responsible use of resources. Each "print prompt" throughout the text is accompanied by the Sustainability icon to encourage electronic submission of activities.

Manager Challenge. Each chapter begins with the Manager Challenge feature, which introduces students to the chapter material and challenges them to think critically about how best to complete the tasks they have been assigned in a competent and professional manner.

Professionalism Connection Box. The Professionalism Connection boxes provide helpful information on how students can best present themselves in a professional manner. This includes showing proficiency in assigned tasks as well as communicating and interacting effectively with patients and staff.

Tip Box. The Tip boxes provide helpful hints for using Optum™ PM and Physician EMR.

FYI Box. FYI boxes provide details on functions of Optum™ PM and Physician EMR that are available in real-world settings but are not available in your student version of Optum™.

Alert Box. Alert boxes present critical information to know when completing activities in Optum™ PM and Physician EMR.

Spotlight Box. Spotlight boxes highlight important material included throughout the text. It is critical that users of EHR software are familiar with this information. Different types of Spotlight boxes are included in the text, depending on the information being presented. These types include Administrative Spotlight, PM Spotlight, and Clinical Spotlight.

Activities. The Step-by-Step Activities give instructions on how to complete front- and back-office functions in Optum™ PM and Physician EMR. They feature detailed information on steps to be performed as well as full-color screenshots that illustrate key steps.

Mini-Case Studies. The Mini-Case Studies provide additional opportunity for students to test their ability to complete key chapter activities without the benefit of step-by-step instructions.

DISCLAIMER

Due to the evolving nature and continuous upgrades of real-world EMRs such as this one, as you log in and work in your student version of Optum™ there may be a slightly different look to your live screen from the screenshots provided in the workbook.

Keep in mind that you will be asked to work in "current dates" when completing activities, so your appointment and encounter dates will not match those used in the workbook screenshots.

When prompted, follow the instructions given in the workbook to complete the activities.

Organization of the Workbook

The Paperless Medical Office for Billers and Coders is organized to match the daily flow of an office. The first two chapters serve as an introduction to the Optum™ PM and Physician EMR software and how to navigate it. Beginning with Chapter 3: Patient Demographics, and continuing throughout the workbook, students follow the logical sequence of what occurs from the time the patient registers and schedules an appointment through to processing the insurance claim form generated from the patient's visit and any related collection activities.

The following breakdown summarizes what is included in each chapter:

Chapter 1: Introduction to the Paperless Medical Office

This chapter briefly discusses the process of converting paper health records to electronic health records and illustrates what occurs in an electronic health network. Students are also instructed on how to update their browser settings to be compatible with the Optum™ software.

Chapter 2: Introduction to Optum™ PM and Physician EMR

Students learn how to log in to Optum™ in this chapter and use the *Help* system. Basic navigation functions of the *Main Menu, Home,* and *Dashboard* are presented here as well as the discussion of administrative features available within Optum™ PM. Students will gain a firm understanding of using an electronic messaging system and will demonstrate their knowledge by performing messaging activities.

Chapter 3: Patient Demographics

In this chapter, students learn the fundamentals of entering patient demographics, registering new patients, and viewing and performing eligibility checks.

Chapter 4: Appointment Scheduling

Scheduling is the central theme of this chapter. Students will learn how to book appointments and how to check in patients, create a batch, accept payments, print patient receipts, run a journal, and post the batch.

Chapter 5: Preliminary Duties in the EHR and Patient Workup

This chapter is where the EMR side of Optum™ is introduced. Students will be introduced to the concept of Meaningful Use and receive training in how to activate the care management registries.

Students then learn the major applications of the *Clinical Today* module—the clinical or EMR side of Optum™. Because this workbook focuses on billing and coding, only minimal clinical-related activities will be performed. Student activities include basic check-in duties and transferring patients throughout the visit. In addition, students will learn how to read the tasks menu and complete related tasks associated with billing and coding activities. As students continue learning EMR-related functions, they will complete portions of the encounter and progress note that are required to capture the visit for billing.

Chapter 6: Completing the Visit

This chapter focuses on what occurs following the patient's examination. Students will learn how to complete the visit, resolve open encounters, and sign the progress note. In order to generate claims, charges must be captured for the patient's appointment. Students will enter procedure and diagnostic codes for billing purposes.

Chapter 7: Billing

Students switch back to administrative tasks in this chapter. Once the visit is completed, the financial activities begin. Creating a batch for financial activities, manually entering charges, and editing an unposted charge are just a few of the activities in this chapter. Users will also learn how to generate electronic and paper claims and perform activities related to electronic remittance.

Chapter 8: ClaimsManager and Collections

In this chapter users will learn the functions of the *ClaimsManager* feature in Optum™ and will check the status of unpaid or inactive claims. Students will learn how to generate patient statements, create custom collections letters, and navigate the collections process.

Chapter 9: Applied Learning for the Paperless Medical Office

This chapter is the finale of the workbook. It includes a comprehensive case study that tests users' knowledge and understanding of the material presented throughout the workbook without providing step-by-step instructions. Students build both competence and confidence from performing the activity in this chapter.

About the Author

Virginia Ferrari is an adjunct faculty member at Solano Community College in the Career Technical Education/ Business division, where she has taught medical front office, medical coding, and small business courses. In addition, she has been a contributing author for other Cengage Learning textbooks, including the Seventh Edition of *Medical Assisting: Administrative and Clinical Competencies*. Prior to joining Solano Community College, Virginia served as the manager of extended services for one of the fastest-growing physicians networks in the San Francisco Bay area. In addition to overseeing the conversion and implementation of electronic medical records, she served on the Best Practice Committee, Customer Satisfaction Committee, Pilot Project for Risk Adjust Coding, and Team Up for Health, a national collaborative for Diabetes Self-Management Education. Virginia holds dual bachelor degrees in sociology and family and consumer studies from Central Washington University and a master's degree in health administration from the University of Phoenix. Virginia also holds certification from the National Healthcareer Association as a Certified Electronic Health Record Specialist (CEHRS).

System Requirements for Optum™ PM and Physican EMR

Minimum Requirements

- Pentium 4, 2 GHZ or greater
- Operating System: Windows 8, Windows 7, Windows Vista, iPad IOS6
- Windows XP: 1 GB or greater; Windows Vista, Windows 7, & Windows 8: 1.5 GB
- Microsoft Internet Explorer 8, 9, or 10
- Microsoft Word 2003, 2007, 2010, or 2013
- Acrobat Reader
- 1024 × 768 resolution

Third-Party Software

Third-party software (such as Yahoo! and Google toolbars, or Norton and McAfee, etc.) does not follow the rules set up in Internet options; therefore, it tends to block Optum™ PM and Physician EMR functionality with respect to pop-ups. If this does happen, then you need to add training.caretracker.com, rapidrelease.caretracker.com, and optum.webex.com to the allowed or safe sites lists of those programs. Follow the instructions in the next section, Internet Settings (Add as Trusted Site).

Internet Settings (Add as Trusted Site)

1. Open Internet Explorer browser window.
2. On the menu bar, click Tools and then select Internet Options from the menu. Internet Explorer displays the Internet Options dialog box.
3. Click the Security tab, and then click Trusted Sites.
4. Click Sites. Internet Explorer displays the Trusted Sites dialog box.
5. In the Add this website to the zone box, type: training.caretracker.com.
6. Click Add. Internet Explorer adds the address to trusted sites.
7. Repeat steps 5 and 6 for rapidrelease.caretracker.com and optum.webex.com.
8. Deselect the Require server verification (https:) for all sites in this zone checkbox.
9. Click Close to close the Trusted Sites box.
10. Click OK on the Internet Options box to save your changes.

Bandwidth Recommendations

If there are multiple workstations utilizing Optum™ PM and Physician EMR, then each will require a minimum of 300 kb of bandwidth per active workstation with a DSL or cable connection. For a T1 or Dedicated connection, a minimum of 60 kb per workstation is required.

Recommended Screen Resolution

The recommended screen resolution is 1024 × 768.

Supported Browser

Optum™ PM and Physician EMR supports only Internet Explorer 8, 9, or 10 for desktop devices. Safari for iPad may also be used. Mozilla Firefox and Google Chrome are not supported.

CHAPTER 1

Introduction to the Paperless Medical Office

LEARNING OBJECTIVES

1. Describe administrative and clinical workflows in Optum™ PM and Physician EMR.
2. List the core functions of electronic health records.
3. Identify the advantages and pitfalls of electronic health records.
4. Receive introduction to online coding processes and EncoderPro.com, the claims software in Optum™ PM and Physician EMR.
5. Set up your computer for optimal functionality when using Optum™ PM and Physician EMR.

Introduction to NAPA Valley Family Health Associates and Optum™ PM and Physician EMR

NVFHA MANAGER CHALLENGE

Welcome to Napa Valley Family Health Associates (NVFHA)! Our practice is located in beautiful Napa Valley in California. The practice consists of four providers, six medical assistants, one X-ray technician, and a medical lab scientist who oversees our laboratory. As a medical assistant with billing and coding responsibilities, you will perform activities related to any of our four providers:

- Amir Raman, DO (Specialty—Internal Medicine)
- Anthony Brockton, MD (Specialty—Family Practice)
- Rebecca Ayerick, MD (Specialty-Pediatrics)
- Gabrielle Torres, NP (Specialty—Family Practice)

We are a busy family health center and take care of patients across the lifespan. To be considered for a job in our practice, you must have a caring attitude, have strong administrative and clinical skills, and get along well with people of all ages and all socioeconomic backgrounds.

(Continues)

NVFHA Manager Challenge *(Continued)*

NVFHA has received the prestigious recognition by the Accreditation Association for Ambulatory Health Care (AAAHC) as a top provider in ambulatory care in the San Francisco Bay area. AAAHC provides an external, independent review of health care delivery organizations and a practice's policies, procedures, processes, and outcomes against nationally accepted standards.

We are a practice that believes in a proactive approach to health care. We look for ways to improve patient outcomes while driving down health care costs. As a matter of fact, we recently applied for NCQA Patient-Centered Medical Home (PCMH) Recognition. Becoming a PCMH is a way of organizing primary care that emphasizes care coordination and communication to transform primary care into "what patients want it to be." Medical homes can lead to higher quality and lower costs and can improve patients' and providers' experience of care. NCQA Patient-Centered Medical Home (PCMH) Recognition is the most widely used way to transform primary care practices into medical homes. We chose Optum™ PM and Physician EMR as our electronic health record system because of its robust functions and reporting capabilities, which are essential to a PCMH model.

My name is Takari Miata, and I am the office manager for NVFHA. I will be challenging you throughout each chapter to perform to the best of your ability. This workbook focuses on billing and coding technical skills, but do not be surprised if you learn a few other skills along the way! Your first challenge is to carefully read and implement all of the directions in this first chapter. Failure to implement the recommended settings may result in an inability to perform some activities. Let's get started!

Core Functions of the EMR/EHR

The electronic record has many features designed to improve patient care and staff efficiency. The type of software that a medical practice selects will depend on many factors, including the type of practice, the goals of the practice, the cost of the software, and the individual preferences of the clinicians and staff.

Advantages of Electronic Medical/Health Records

An EMR system is an electronic platform that facilitates the needs of a medical practice. An advantage of using a fully integrated practice management and EMR such as Optum™ is that it automates the overall workflow to the greatest extent possible to achieve the maximum amount of practice efficiency. Patient care coordination is improved, and there is a demonstrated reduction in errors, which previously resulted from illegible notes or prescriptions.

Pitfalls of the Electronic Health Record

EHRs have many benefits, but there are also a few pitfalls. In an article by the National Center for Biotechnology Information (Menachemi & Collum, 2011), it was noted that despite the growing consensus on benefits of EHR functionalities, there are some potential disadvantages associated with this technology. These include financial issues, changes in workflow, temporary loss of productivity associated with EHR adoption, privacy and security concerns, problems that occur when the system goes down, and other unintended consequences.

Recently, patients and providers have begun expressing concern over privacy issues related to EHRs and the personal information collected by the federal government. The Affordable Care Act (ACA) mandates the Internal Revenue Service (IRS) as the collection and enforcement arm for the federal government, which troubles many Americans. In addition, as the Department of Health and Human Services (HHS) issues more (and new) rules pertaining to the ACA, there is more confusion in the medical industry and intrusion into the patient's private medical files and decision making of personal health concerns.

Administrative and Clinical Workflows in Optum™

Workflow is defined as how tasks are performed throughout the office (usually in a specific order), for example, the patient is checked in, insurance cards are scanned, the patient is taken to the exam room where vital signs are taken/recorded, and so on (Figure 1-1).

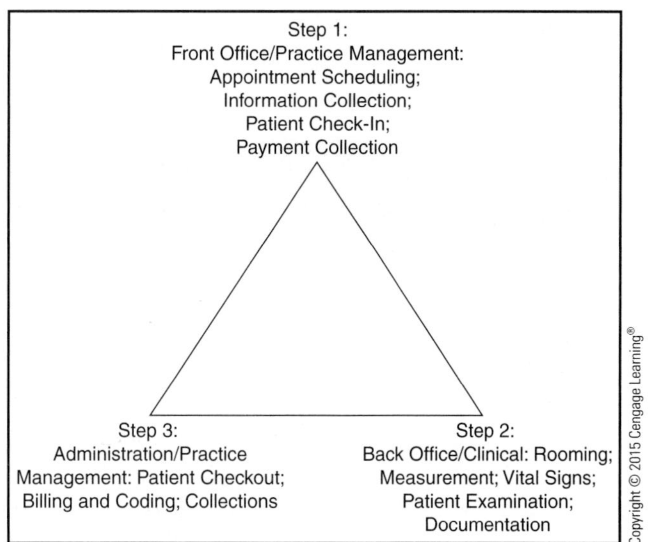

Figure 1-1 Patient Flow

Practice management (PM) software runs the business side of health care, from registering a new patient and scheduling patient visits to coding and billing the patient encounter and generating monthly reports. Optum™ PM software can be customized to user preferences. PM software will maximize provider productivity and meets rigorous scheduling demands. Alert messages, a master index, and insurance profiles help reduce error and administrative expenses during registration and charge entry.

The EMR side of Optum™ focuses on the clinical side, encompassing documentation in the patient's medical record and how use of a certified EMR supports Meaningful Use as defined by the federal government, which sets incentive payments to providers for using an EHR.

Coding Fundamentals

Most EHRs have features that automate the coding process. Although the features of each EHR may vary, the codes are checked for accuracy by a coding specialist or program. Optum's™ automated coding process is the *ClaimsManager* feature, which utilizes *EncoderPro.com*. *EncoderPro.com* is Optum's™ partner for online code verification, which can be run to verify that all procedure, diagnosis, and modifier codes entered for a patient are correct.

To receive reimbursement, every service submitted for payment must be documented in the patient's medical record. Computer-assisted coding works in a variety of ways. Some computer-assisted coding systems assign codes based on keywords, whereas others analyze words/phrases and sentences. The integration of automated coding with the billing system facilitates claims processing.

This billing and coding workbook focuses on medical assistants tasked with responsibilities for collections and the revenue cycle and familiarizes them with coding and compliance, claims scrubber programs, and why it is important for billers and coders to be familiar with and be proficient in using EHRs. Billers and coders will need to be familiar with both ICD-9 and ICD-10 diagnosis coding as the medical industry transitions to ICD-10 effective October 1, 2015. This change in coding is considered to be one of the biggest transformations in medical billing and coding in decades. Medical coders and billers must be up to date on the latest information related to coding, chart auditing, and insurance reimbursement. You must demonstrate familiarity and accuracy of ICD, CPT®, and HCPCS coding and comply with HIPAA standards for billing and insurance.

Readiness Requirements

Welcome to Optum™ PM and Physician EMR, a fully integrated CCHIT® and ONC-ATCB-certified complete Practice Management (PM) and Electronic Health Record (EHR). Optum™ PM is a powerful web-based application that gives medical practices new levels of efficiency, integration, and accountability. In order to use Optum™, you must meet the minimum system requirements and update your browser settings according to the instructions outlined in the "System Requirements" section found on page ix.

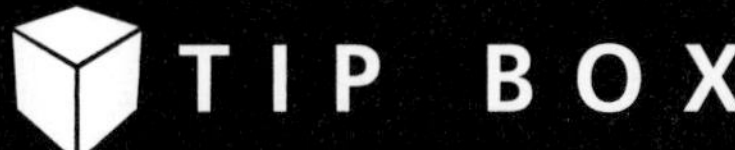

TIP BOX

You will find up-to-date *System Requirements and Recommendations* in the *Help* system of Optum™ at *Home > Getting Started > System Requirements & Recommendations.*

Chapter 2 will introduce you to *Help* and the various content and training available.

To use Optum™ PM and Physician EMR, your computer must have Internet Explorer® version 8 or greater (**Note:** IE® 11 is not yet supported). Other browsing software (outside of Safari® for iPad®) may work differently with the application. See the "System Requirements" section for further technology requirements.

Disable Third-Party Toolbars

Remove all third-party toolbars (Google, Yahoo*!*, Bing, AOL, etc.) from Internet Explorer®. Third-party toolbars cause random performance and functionality issues within Optum™ PM and Physician EMR. Complete Activity 1-1 to disable toolbars.

ACTIVITY 1-1: Disable Toolbars

1. Open an Internet Explorer® browser window.
2. Right-click on the menu bar. The browser displays a list of toolbars. Active toolbars appear with a check mark to the left of the name (Figure 1-2).

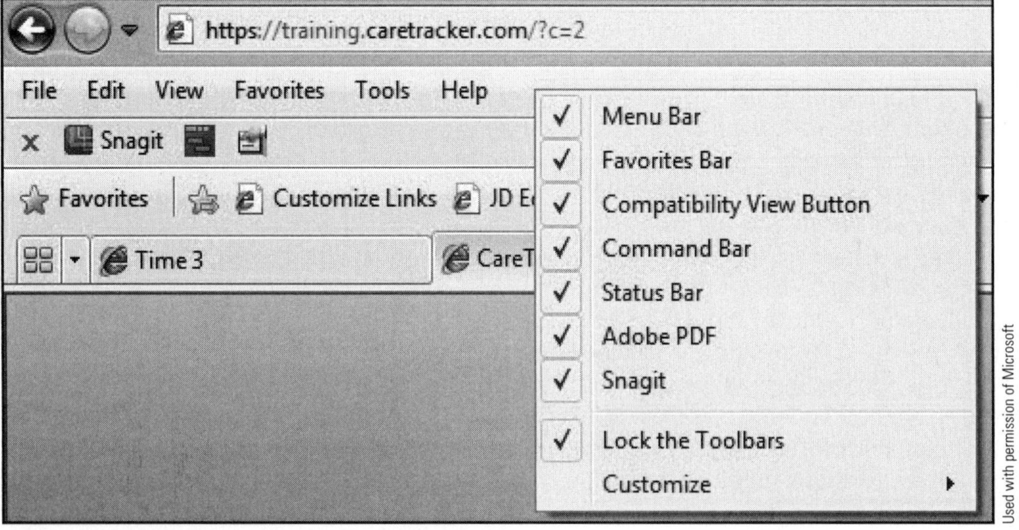

Figure 1-2 Disable Toolbars

3. Click on the toolbars you want to disable (Google, Yahoo*!*, Bing, AOL, etc.). Internet Explorer® disables the toolbar.

Setting Up Tabbed Browsing

Tabbed browsing allows you to open multiple websites in a single browser window. It is very important to set this up to access several patient charts at one time in a single browser. This will make switching between patients much easier and enables you to have multiple items open on the task bar. Complete Activity 1-2 to set up tabbed browsing.

ACTIVITY 1-2: Set Up Tabbed Browsing

1. Open an Internet Explorer® browser window.
2. Select *Tools* > *Internet Options* from the browser menu. The *Internet Options* dialog box displays.
3. In the *Tabs* section, click *Settings*. The *Tabbed Browsing Settings* dialog box displays.
4. Select the following options (Figure 1-3):

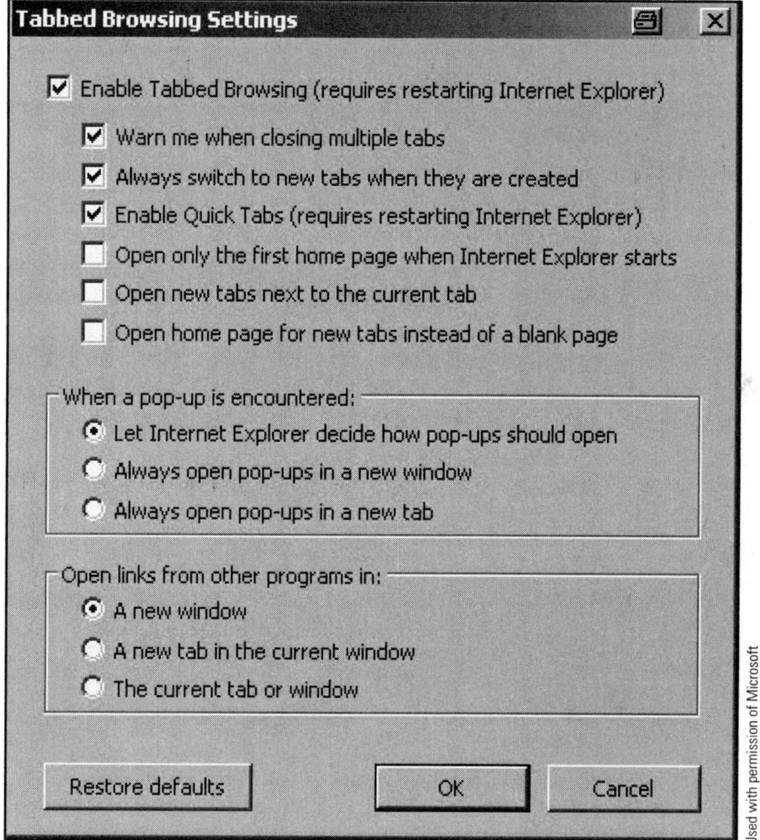

Used with permission of Microsoft

Figure 1-3 Tabbed Browser Settings

5. Click *OK* to close the *Tabbed Browsing Settings* box.
6. Click *OK* on the *Internet Options* box to save your changes.

Disable Pop-Up Blocker

A pop-up window is a small web browser window that appears on top of the website you are viewing. This allows you to avoid having to navigate away from the current window you are viewing. Optum™ PM and Physician EMR uses the pop-up mechanism, enabling an efficient workflow. Many computers have firewall protectors that alleviate nonsense pop-up ads from displaying as you work on a website. However, you must enable pop-ups to use the functionality within Optum™ PM and Physician EMR. Complete Activity 1-3 to turn off pop-up blocker in Internet Explorer® and Safari®.

ACTIVITY 1-3: Turn Off Pop-Up Blocker

1. Open an Internet Explorer® browser window.
2. Select *Tools* > *Pop-up Blocker* > *Turn Off Pop-up Blocker* from the browser menu.

To disable pop-up blocker in Safari® for iPad®:

1. Tap *Settings* from your iPad® home screen.
2. Tap *Safari®* from the *Settings* panes on the left. The *Safari® Pane* displays the browser options.
3. Tap *Block Pop-ups* to turn off pop-up blocker (Figure 1-4).

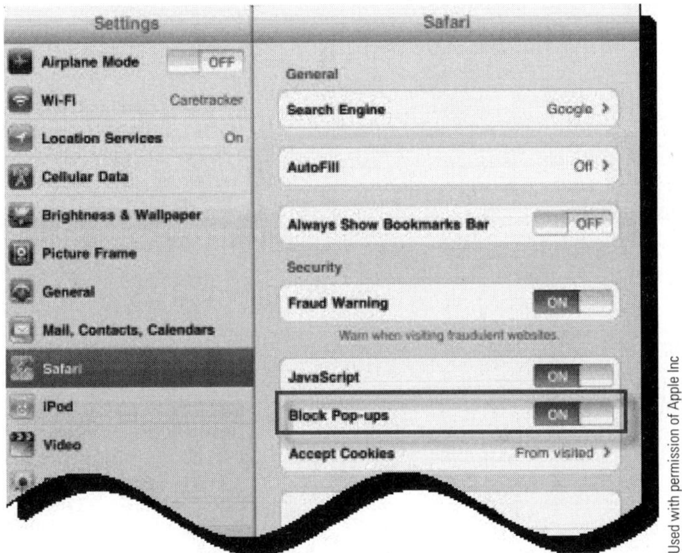

Used with permission of Apple Inc

Figure 1-4 Safari® Pop-Up Blocker

Change the Page Setup

It is important to change the default margin, header, and footer settings to print letters, forms, and claims in Optum™ PM and Physician EMR. Complete Activity 1-4 to change page setup.

ACTIVITY 1-4: Change Page Setup

1. Open an Internet Explorer® browser window.
2. On the browser menu bar, click the arrow next to the printer icon and then click *Page Setup* from the menu. Internet Explorer® launches the *Page Setup* dialog box.
3. Delete the values in the *Header, Footer*, and *Margins* fields. Leaving these fields blank will automatically set their value to zero. For Internet Explorer® 8, select *Empty* in each of the *Header* and *Footer* fields.
4. Click *OK*.

Downloading Plug-Ins

A plug-in is a program that works with Optum™ PM and Physician EMR to give added functionality. Follow each link to download the required plug-in for free.

- Adobe Reader (http://www.adobe.com/products/acrobat/readstep.html)

  To view, navigate, and print PDF files.

- Adobe Flash (http://get.adobe.com/flashplayer/)

  To view animation and interactive content.

- Java (http://www.java.com/)

  To run applications and applets that use Java technology. Java is required to view prerecorded sessions.

Adding Trusted Sites

Add training.caretracker.com, rapidrelease.caretracker.com, and optum.webex.com to the trusted site list (see Figure 1-5). Otherwise some functionality may be blocked, such as running Active X controls and installing browser plug-ins. Adding trusted sites also allows your computer to distinguish between secured sites and harmful sites. Complete Activity 1-5 to add trusted sites.

ACTIVITY 1-5: Add Optum™ to Trusted Sites

1. Open an Internet Explorer® browser window.
2. On the menu bar, click *Tools* and then select *Internet Options* from the menu. Internet Explorer® displays the *Internet Options* dialog box.
3. Click the *Security* tab, and then click *Trusted sites*.
4. Click *Sites*. Internet Explorer® displays the *Trusted sites* dialog box.
5. Deselect the *Require server verification (https:) for all sites in this zone* checkbox.
6. In the *Add this website to the zone* box, type: training.caretracker.com.
7. Click *Add*. Internet Explorer® adds the address to trusted sites.
8. In the *Add this website to the zone* box, type: rapidrelease.caretracker.com.
9. Click *Add*. Internet Explorer® adds the address to trusted sites.
10. In the *Add this website to the zone* box, type: optum.webex.com (Figure 1-5).

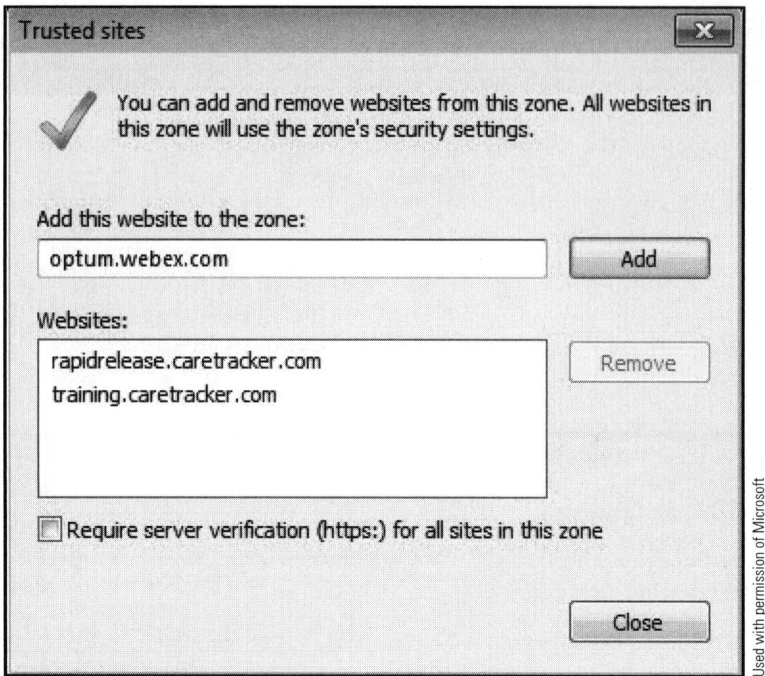

Figure 1-5 Trusted Sites

11. Click *Add*. Internet Explorer® adds the address to trusted sites.
12. Click *Close* to close the *Trusted sites* box.
13. Click *OK* on the *Internet Options* box to save your changes.

Clearing the Cache

The cache is a space in your computer's hard drive and random access memory (RAM) where your browser saves copies of recently visited web pages. Typically these items are stored in the *Temporary Internet Files* folder. It is important to clear your cache on a regular basis and at every release for Optum™ PM and Physician EMR to function more efficiently.

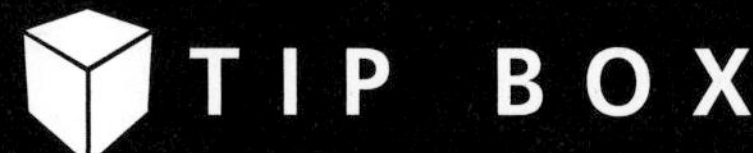

Important!! You must first clear your cache each time you log in to Optum™ PM and Physician EMR. If you are already logged in, log out of Optum™ PM and Physician EMR before clearing your cache.

ACTIVITY 1-6: Clear Your Cache

To clear cache in Internet Explorer® 8 and 9:

1. Open an Internet Explorer® browser window.
2. From the Internet Explorer® *Tools* menu, select *Internet Options*. Windows® displays the *Internet Options* dialog box.
3. On the *General* tab, in the *Browsing history* section, click *Delete*. Windows® displays the *Delete Browsing History* dialog box.
4. Deselect the *Preserve Favorites website data* checkbox.
5. Select the *Temporary Internet files, Cookies,* and *History* checkboxes.
6. Click *Delete*.
7. Click *OK* in the *Internet Options* box when finished.

To clear cache in Safari® for iPad®:

1. Tap *Settings* from your iPad® home screen.
2. Tap *Safari®* from the *Settings* panes on the left. The *Safari® Pane* displays the *Clear History, Clear Cookies,* and *Clear Cache* at the bottom (Figure 1-6).

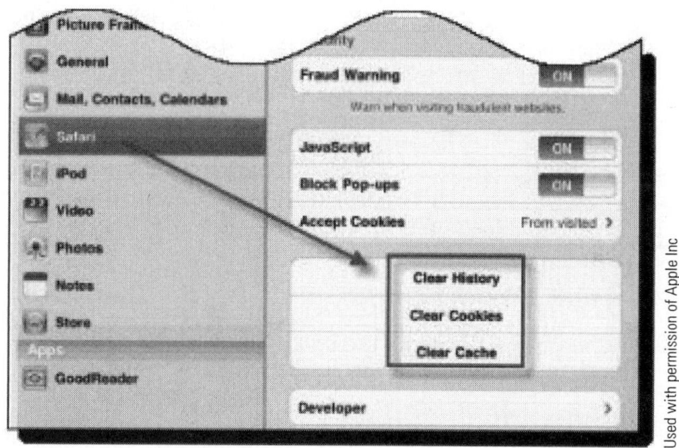

Used with permission of Apple Inc

Figure 1-6 Safari® Clear Settings

3. Tap *Clear History*. iPad® displays a confirmation window.
4. Tap *Clear* in the confirmation window.
5. Tap *Clear Cookies*. iPad® displays a confirmation window.
6. Tap *Clear* in the confirmation window.
7. Tap *Clear Cache*. iPad® displays a confirmation window.
8. Tap *Clear* in the confirmation window.

Setting Your Home Page

Your home page is displayed when Internet Explorer® first opens. You can choose to set Optum™ PM and Physician EMR as your home page if necessary.

ACTIVITY 1-7: Setting Optum™ as Home Page

1. Open an Internet Explorer® browser window.
2. Select *Tools* > *Internet Options* from the browser menu. The *Internet Options* dialog box displays.
3. In the address box of the *Home page* section, type: http://www.cengage.com/optumsimulation (Figure 1-7).

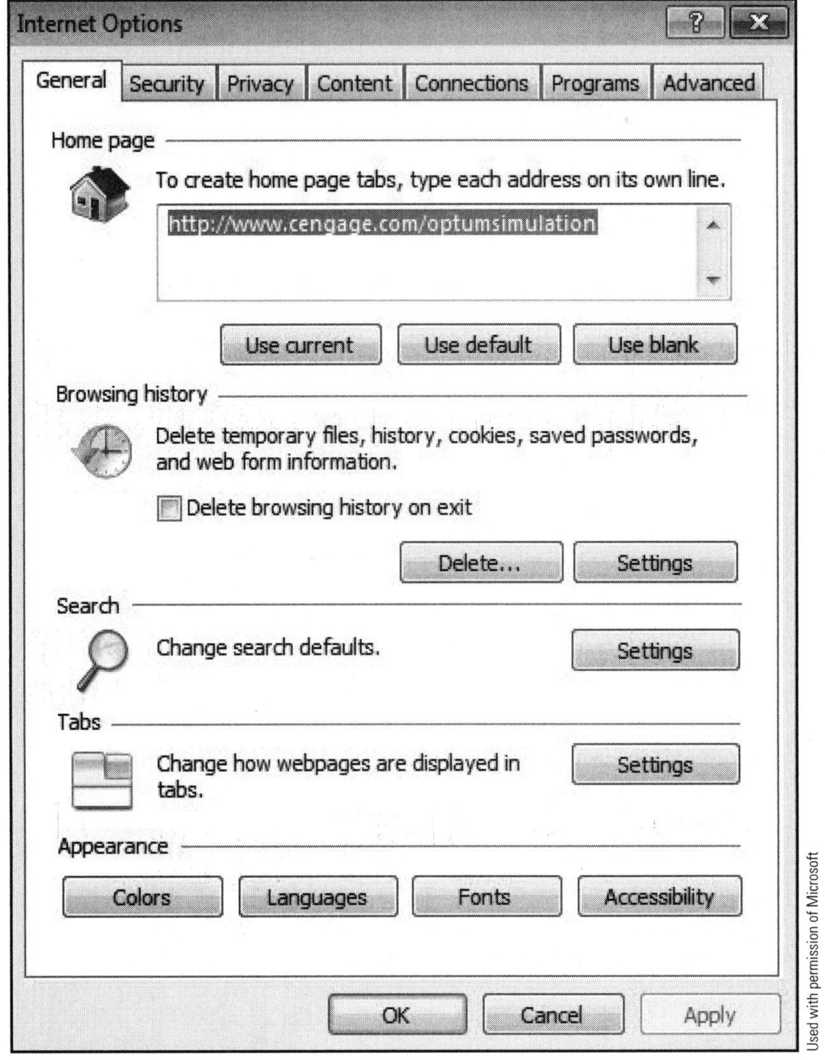

Figure 1-7 Home Page

4. Click *OK*. Optum™ PM and Physician EMR will display as your home page the next time you open Internet Explorer®.

Disable Download Blocking

Complete Activity 1-8 to disable download blocking.

ACTIVITY 1-8: Disable Download Blocking

1. Open an Internet Explorer® browser window.
2. Select *Tools* > *Internet Options* from the browser menu. The browser displays the *Internet Options* dialog box.
3. Click the *Security* tab.
4. Click the *Internet* (globe) link.
5. Click the *Custom level* button.
6. Scroll down to the *Downloads* section.
7. In the *Automatic prompting for file downloads* section, click *Enable.*
8. Click *OK.*
9. Click *OK* in the *Internet Options* box when finished.

Now that you have set your computer to the required settings to work in Optum™ PM and Physician EMR, Chapter 2 will instruct you on how to log in to begin your training.

Resources

The Optum PM and Physician EMR Help home page represents a wealth of information for the electronic health record (https://training.caretracker.com/help/CareTracker_Help.htm).

Centers for Medicare and Medicaid Services. http://www.cms.gov/Regulations-and-Guidance/HIPAA-Administrative-Simplification/Versions5010andD0/index.html

Coding classification standards. (n.d.). Retrieved from http://www.ahima.org/coding/standards.aspx

Health Resources and Services Administration (of the HHS). http://www.hrsa.gov/index.html

Institute of Medicine of the National Academies. (2003, July 31). *Key capabilities of an electronic health record system.* Retrieved from http://www.iom.edu/Reports/2003/Key-Capabilities-of-an-Electronic-Health-Record-System.aspx

Menachemi, N., & Collum, T. H. (2011). Benefits and drawbacks of electronic health record systems. *Risk Management and Healthcare Policy, 4,* 47–55. Published online 2011 May 11. Retrieved from http://www.ncbi.nlm.nih.gov/pmc/articles/PMC3270933/

National Committee for Quality Assurance. (n.d.). Patient-Centered Medical Home Recognition. Retrieved from http://www.ncqa.org/Programs/Recognition/PatientCenteredMedicalHomePCMH.aspx

National Healthcareer Association. (n.d.). *Certified electronic health records specialist (CEHRS™).* Retrieved from http://www.nhanow.com/health-record.aspx

U.S. Department of Health and Human Services, National Institutes of Health. (n.d.). *What health information is protected by the privacy rule?* Retrieved from http://privacyruleandresearch.nih.gov/pr_07.asp

CHAPTER 2

Introduction to Optum™ PM and Physician EMR

LEARNING OBJECTIVES

1. Log in to Optum™ to begin your training.
2. Use the Help system to become familiar with key features of Optum™ PM and Physician EMR and to access step-by-step instructions on using each aspect of the system to quickly and successfully complete required tasks.
3. Become familiar with the Main Menu, Navigation, Home, and Dashboard features.
4. Demonstrate understanding of the Administration features and functions for Practice Management and Electronic Medical Records.
5. Use Message Center components.

NVFHA MANAGER CHALLENGE

Prior to using the computer system in our practice, medical assistants are required to become certified as "Super Users" of the Optum™ PM and Physician EMR software. The training that employees receive to obtain this status is similar to the training you will receive throughout this workbook. This chapter introduces you to the *Help* system, which features a variety of video links and training materials that elaborate on the training outlined in each workbook chapter. Employees who utilize these materials typically perform at a higher level than those who do not. Your challenge is to utilize the *Help* materials to enhance the training process and expand your knowledge.

DISCLAIMER

Due to the evolving nature and continuous upgrades of real-world EMRs such as this one, as you log in and work in your student version of Optum™ there may be a slightly different look to your live screen from the screenshots provided in this workbook.

When prompted, follow the instructions given in the text to complete the activities.

ACTIVITY 2-1: Clear Your Cache

You will be assigned a username and password to log in to Optum™ PM and Physician EMR. Your preassigned username and password can be found on the inside front cover of your workbook. Your password must be changed the first time you log in to Optum™ PM and Physician EMR. You will also be prompted to change your password every 90 days for security reasons. The password must consist of at least eight characters with one capital and one numeric character.

Before beginning the activities, clear your cache. In Chapter 1 you were instructed how to clear your cache for Internet Explorer® 8. Activity 2-1 provides instructions for Internet Explorer® 9.0. If you are using a personal computer (PC), only work in Internet Explorer®. Use Safari® for iPad®. Once the cache has been cleared, you may continue by logging in to your student version of Optum™ (Activity 2-2).

To clear your cache in Microsoft Internet Explorer® 9.0

1. From the Internet Explorer® 9 *Tools* menu, click *Internet Options*. Windows® displays the *Internet Options* dialog box.
2. On the *General* tab, in the *Browsing history* section, click *Delete* (Figure 2-1). Windows® displays the *Delete Browsing History* dialog box.

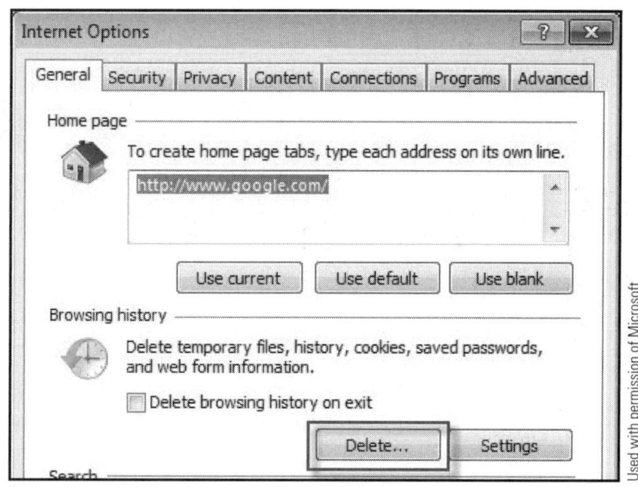

Used with permission of Microsoft

Figure 2-1 IE9 – Delete Browsing History

3. Deselect the *Preserve Favorites website data* checkbox (Figure 2-2).
4. Select the *Temporary Internet files and website files, Cookies and website data,* and *History* checkboxes.
5. Click *Delete.*
6. Click *OK* when deletion is complete.

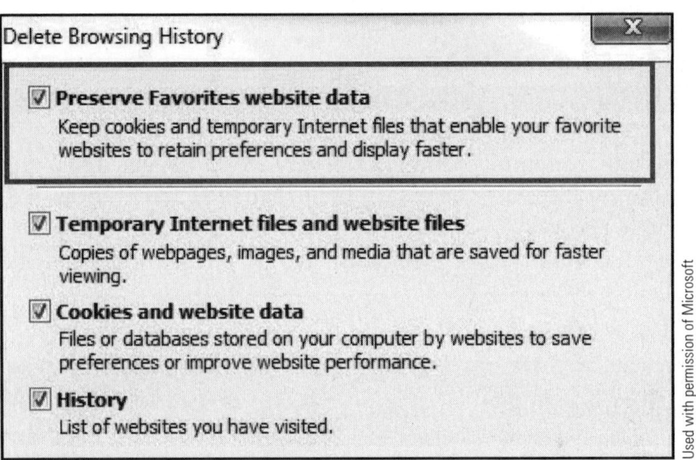

Figure 2-2 Preserve Favorites

Safari® Browser for iPad®: To clear your cache in Safari® for iPad®

1. Tap *Settings* from your iPad® home screen.
2. Tap *Safari®* from the *Settings* panes on the left. The Safari® Pane displays the *Clear History, Clear Cookies,* and *Clear Cache* at the bottom.
3. Tap *Clear History.*
4. Tap *Clear* in the confirmation window.
5. Repeat steps 3 and 4 to clear your cache and cookies (Figure 2-3).

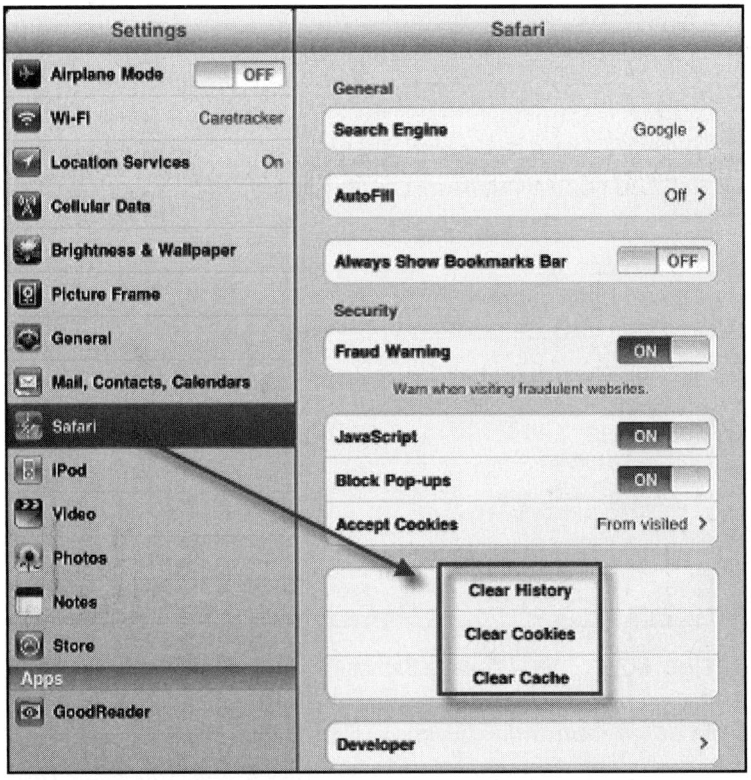

Figure 2-3 Safari Clear Cache

After clearing your cache, begin Activity 2-2 and log in to Optum™.

ACTIVITY 2-2: Log in to Optum™ PM and Physician EMR

1. Go to http://www.cengage.com/optumsimulation. The *Product* list is set to "Cengage Learning Optum PM and Physician EMR" by default (Figure 2-4).

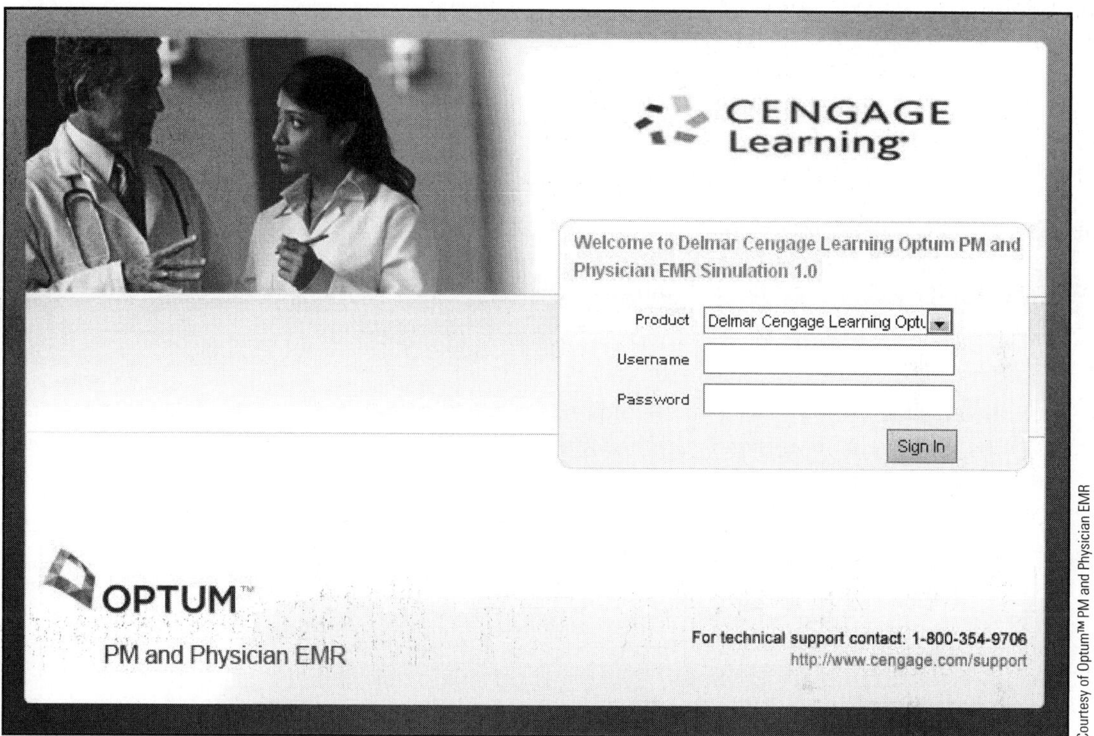

Courtesy of Optum™ PM and Physician EMR

Figure 2-4 Login Screen

2. In the *Username* box, enter the username preassigned to you.
3. In the *Password* box, enter your password. If this is your first time logging in, Optum™ PM and Physician EMR will prompt you to change your temporary password. (**Note:** On subsequent logins, a dialog box called *Operator Encounter Batch Control* will display when you first sign in. Close out of this box by clicking the "X" in the upper-right-hand corner.)

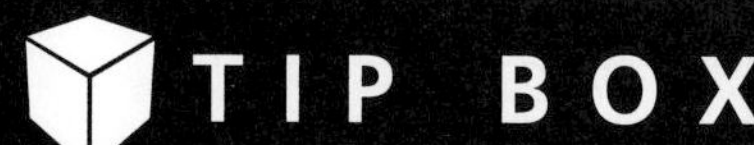

Both the username and password are case sensitive.

Your new password:

- Must differ from your old password by at least one character
- Must consist of at least eight characters
- Must contain at least one capital letter and one number; for example: Password5
- Must be reentered in the *Verify Password* field

4. Click *Save*. A message will display, indicating that Optum™ is creating your account and that you will receive a notification e-mail when the process is complete. Figure 2-5 is an example of the notification e-mail you will receive. (**Note:** You will not be able to log in to Optum™ until you have received the notification e-mail, which may take a few minutes or a few hours. If you do not receive the notification e-mail within 24 hours, please contact technical support.)

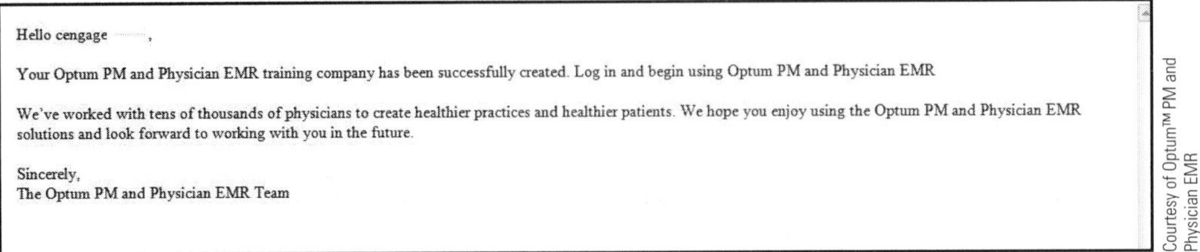

Hello cengage ,

Your Optum PM and Physician EMR training company has been successfully created. Log in and begin using Optum PM and Physician EMR

We've worked with tens of thousands of physicians to create healthier practices and healthier patients. We hope you enjoy using the Optum PM and Physician EMR solutions and look forward to working with you in the future.

Sincerely,
The Optum PM and Physician EMR Team

Courtesy of Optum™ PM and Physician EMR

Figure 2-5 Welcome Login E-mail

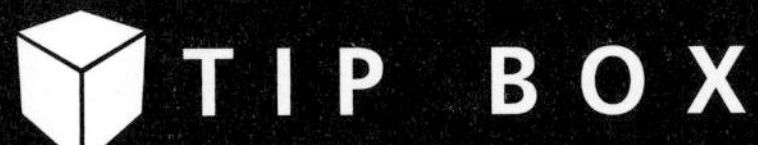

To change your password:

- Click the *Administration* module on the left-hand side of the screen, and then click *Operator Settings* under the *Security* section (Figure 2-6). Optum™ PM and Physician EMR displays the *Password Maintenance* application.

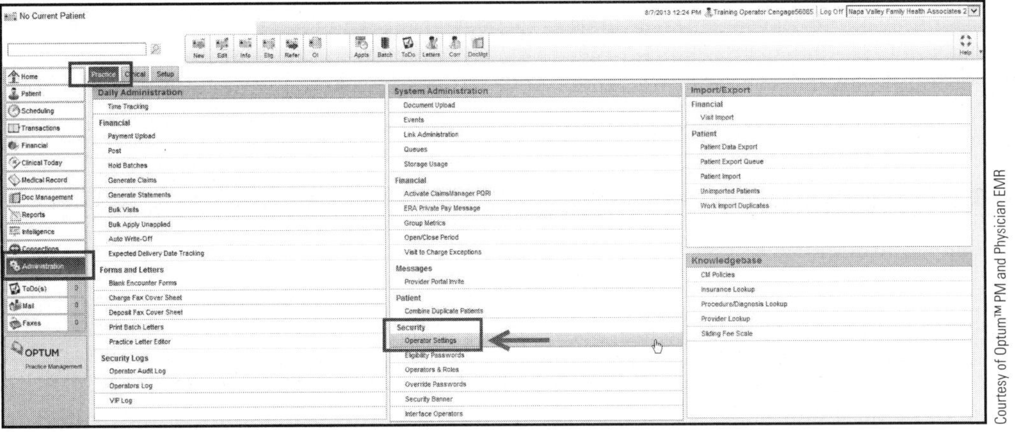

Figure 2-6 Operator Settings

Courtesy of Optum™ PM and Physician EMR

- Enter your current password in the *Old Password* field (Figure 2-7).

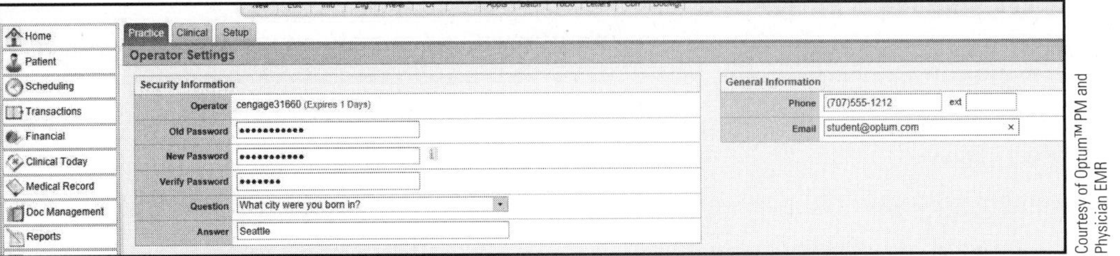

Figure 2-7 Change Password Screen

Courtesy of Optum™ PM and Physician EMR

(Continues)

Tip Box *(Continued)*

- Enter your new password in the *New Password* and *Verify Password* fields.
- Select a security question from the *Question* list.
- Type an answer to the security question in the *Answer* field.
- Click *Save*.
- Record your username and password. You will need this each time you log in to Optum™. Username __________________; Password __________________.

ACTIVITY 2-3: Recorded Training—General Navigation and Help

Optum™ PM and Physician EMR online *Help* integrates product help, recorded training sessions, live webinars, support documentation, and quick reference tools to help you learn about and use Optum™ PM and Physician EMR effectively. The Optum™ PM and Physician EMR *Help* system offers an invaluable one-stop resource for both novice and advanced users. It is designed to familiarize the user with key features of Optum™ PM and Physician EMR, and it provides step-by-step instructions on using each aspect of the system to quickly and successfully complete required tasks.

To learn more about Optum™ and the *Help* features provided, click on the *General Navigation and Help System* training under the *Practice Management Recorded Training* header and view the video. You may also open the associated training documentation PDF and save it to your computer or print for reference. Refer back to the recorded trainings throughout your studies as needed.

1. Click on *Help*.
2. At the top of the screen, click on the *Training* button. (**Note:** The *Training* button is to the left of the *Support* button.)
3. Click on "Learn More" under *Recorded Training*.
4. Scroll down to *Practice Management Recorded Training*.
5. Click on the *General Navigation and Help System* topic (Figure 2-8).

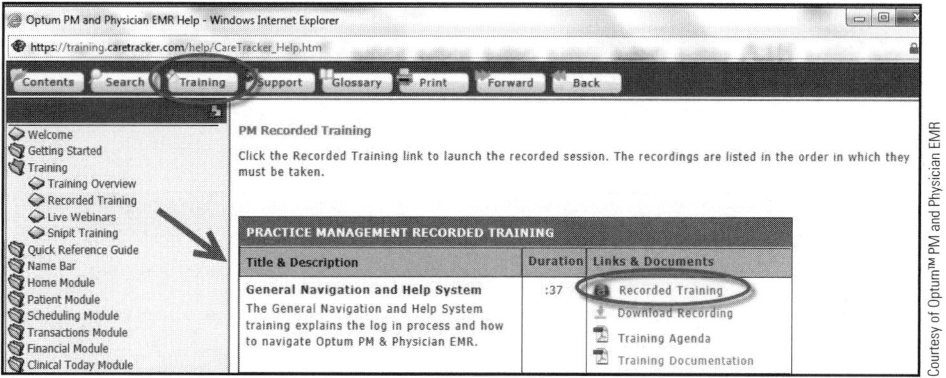

Figure 2-8 General Navigation Help Video

6. Watch the video.

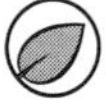

Print a screenshot of the Recorded Training screen, label it "Activity 2-3," and place it in your assignment folder.

ACTIVITY 2-4: Snipit Fiscal Period

A "Snipit" is a short, recorded training that focuses on an individual task or a particular piece of functionality within Optum™ PM and Physician EMR. If you have any questions after watching a Snipit video, you can watch one of the longer recorded training sessions that include the topic. You will view an *Articulate Snipit* in this activity by clicking on *Learn More* under *Snipit Training* (Figure 2-9).

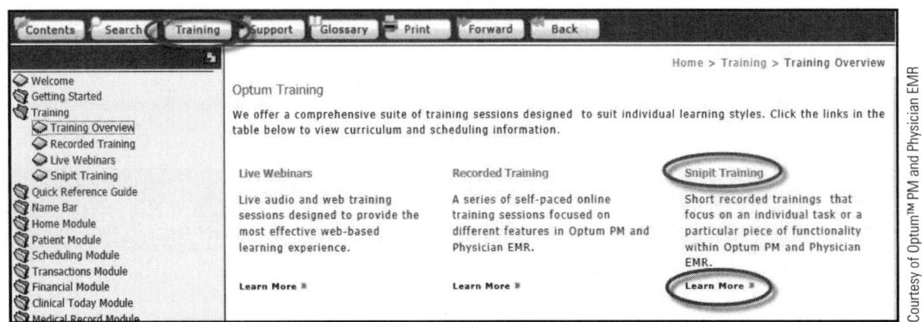

Courtesy of Optum™ PM and Physician EMR

Figure 2-9 Help Snipit-Learn More

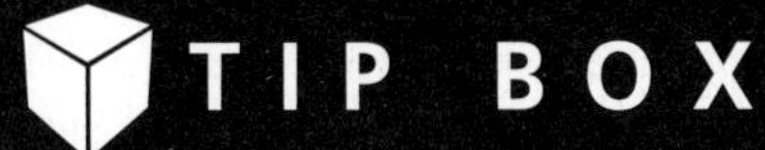

Viewing a Snipit Training

- Click the *Recorded Training* link for the *Snipit* you want to view. The *Articulate* ⓐ recording opens in a new window.
- You must have Adobe Flash Player version 7.0 or later to view an *Articulate* ⓐ recording. The first time you view an articulate recording, you may be prompted to download and install the Adobe Flash Player if you do not already have it installed.
- If you find that the *Recording Training* or *Snipits* are running slow or freezing, you may need to log out, clear your cache, and log back in to begin your activities.

1. Click on *Help*. Click on the *Training* button.
2. Click on "Learn More" under *Snipit Training*.
3. Scroll down to *Snipits Recorded Trainings*, which are listed alphabetically.
4. Click on the "Recorded Training" link next to *Fiscal Period* (Figure 2-10).

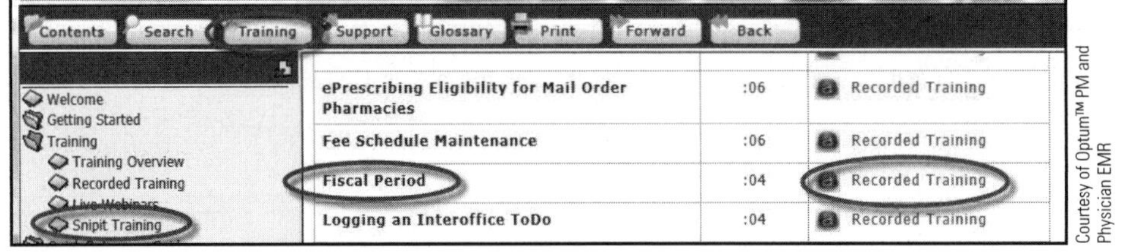

Courtesy of Optum™ PM and Physician EMR

Figure 2-10 Help—Snipit Fiscal Period

5. Watch the video.

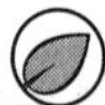

Print a screenshot of the Snipit Fiscal Period screen, label it "Activity 2-4," and place it in your assignment folder.

ACTIVITY 2-5: Open a New Fiscal Year

Working in the correct fiscal period is crucial to the electronic health record. Transactions and entries are permanently linked to a fiscal period and must be accurate. You must define the fiscal periods for your practice before any charges or payments are entered into Optum™ PM and Physician EMR. You can manage the practice's financials by opening and closing each fiscal period. You can post financials to multiple open periods, but you cannot post financials or create a batch for a closed period. The fiscal period and year you are working in displays in all financial transaction applications, such as *Charge, Bulk Charges,* and *Payments on Account*. All reports are linked to the established fiscal periods, not the periods of the calendar year.

Depending on when you begin using this workbook, you may be required to change the fiscal year in addition to opening and closing fiscal periods. This activity instructs you how to open a new fiscal year.

1. Click the *Administration* module. Optum™ PM displays the *Practice* tab.
2. Click the *Open/Close Period* link in the *Financial* section under the *System Administration* header (Figure 2-11). Optum™ PM displays all of your fiscal periods for the current fiscal year.

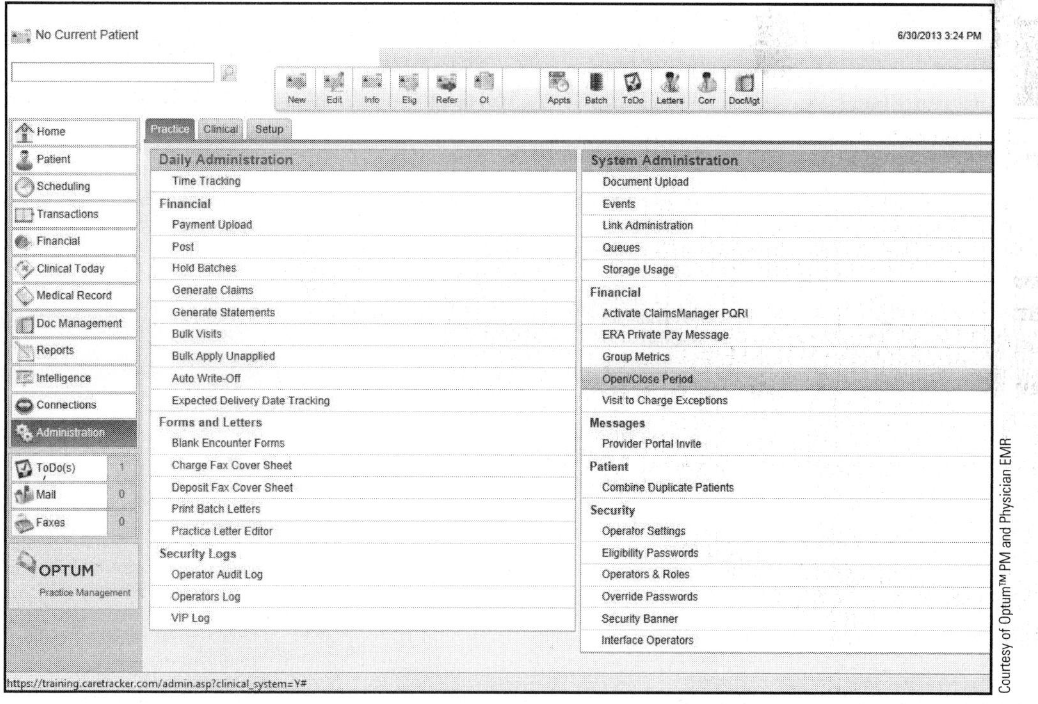

Courtesy of Optum™ PM and Physician EMR

Figure 2-11 Open/Close Period Link

3. To open a fiscal year for all groups within your company, select "Y" from the *All Groups* drop-down menu and then click *Go* (Figure 2-12).

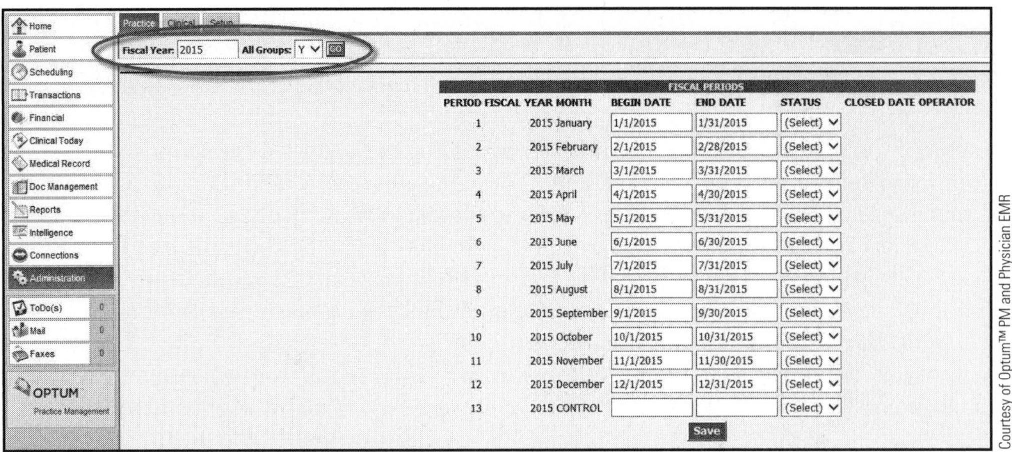

Courtesy of Optum™ PM and Physician EMR

Figure 2-12 Open/Close Fiscal Year

4. By default, the beginning and end date of each period is set to the first and last days of the month. You can change the date range for any month by entering a date in the *Begin Date* and *End Date* boxes for the month.
5. Continue with Activity 2-6 to open a new fiscal period.

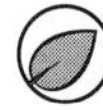 **Print the Open Fiscal Period screen, label it "Activity 2-5," and place it in your assignment folder.**

ACTIVITY 2-6: Open a Fiscal Period

1. Continue from Activity 2-5. If you had already logged out:
   a. Click the *Administration* module. Optum™ PM displays the *Practice* tab.
   b. Under *System Administration/Financial*, click the *Open/Close Period* link. Optum™ PM displays all of your fiscal periods for the current fiscal year.
   c. For multigroup companies, select "Y" from the *All Groups* drop-down list and then click *Go* to open a fiscal period for all groups in the company.
2. From the list in the *Status* column, select "OPEN" for the period you want to open. Select the period (month/year) you are currently working in to open.

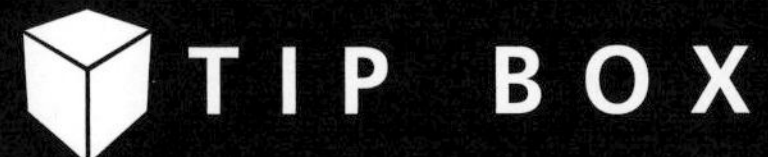

You will have to open/close periods while working throughout the workbook to reflect the current date(s) and activities you are working in.

3. Click *Save*. You can now create batches and post financials for this period (Figure 2-13).

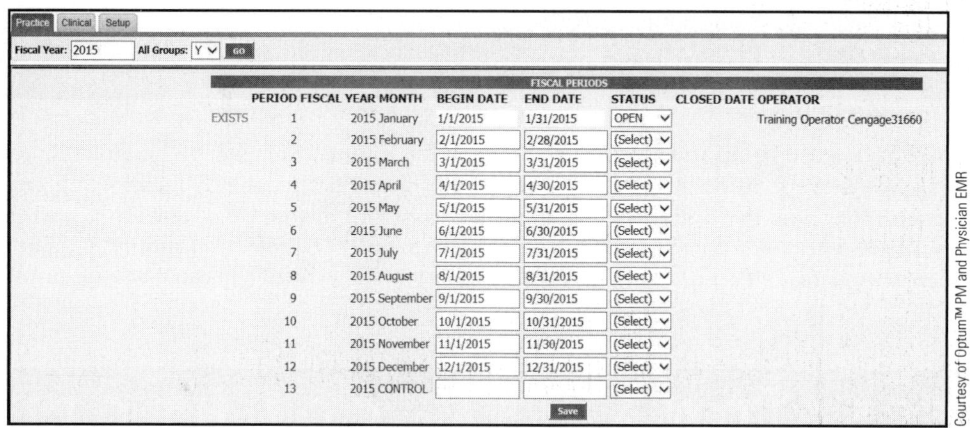

	PERIOD	FISCAL YEAR MONTH	BEGIN DATE	END DATE	STATUS	CLOSED DATE	OPERATOR
EXISTS	1	2015 January	1/1/2015	1/31/2015	OPEN		Training Operator Cengage31660
	2	2015 February	2/1/2015	2/28/2015	(Select)		
	3	2015 March	3/1/2015	3/31/2015	(Select)		
	4	2015 April	4/1/2015	4/30/2015	(Select)		
	5	2015 May	5/1/2015	5/31/2015	(Select)		
	6	2015 June	6/1/2015	6/30/2015	(Select)		
	7	2015 July	7/1/2015	7/31/2015	(Select)		
	8	2015 August	8/1/2015	8/31/2015	(Select)		
	9	2015 September	9/1/2015	9/30/2015	(Select)		
	10	2015 October	10/1/2015	10/31/2015	(Select)		
	11	2015 November	11/1/2015	11/30/2015	(Select)		
	12	2015 December	12/1/2015	12/31/2015	(Select)		
	13	2015 CONTROL			(Select)		

Courtesy of Optum™ PM and Physician EMR

Figure 2-13 Fiscal Period Open

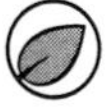
Print the Open Fiscal Period screen, label it "Activity 2-6," and place it in your assignment folder.

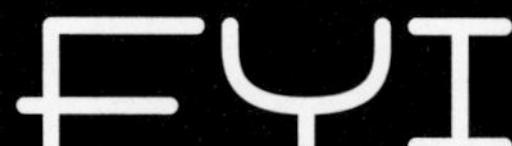

Warning!! Do not close a fiscal period until instructed to do so.

To Close a Fiscal Period

1. Click the *Administration* module. Optum™ PM displays the *Practice* tab.
2. Click the *Open/Close Period* link. Optum™ PM displays all of your fiscal periods for the current fiscal year.
3. For multigroup companies, select "Y" from the *All Groups* list and then click *Go* to close a fiscal period for all groups in the company.
4. From the list in the *Status* column, select "CLOSED" for the period you want to close. You will receive a warning (Figure 2-14) asking, "Are you sure you want to close this period?"

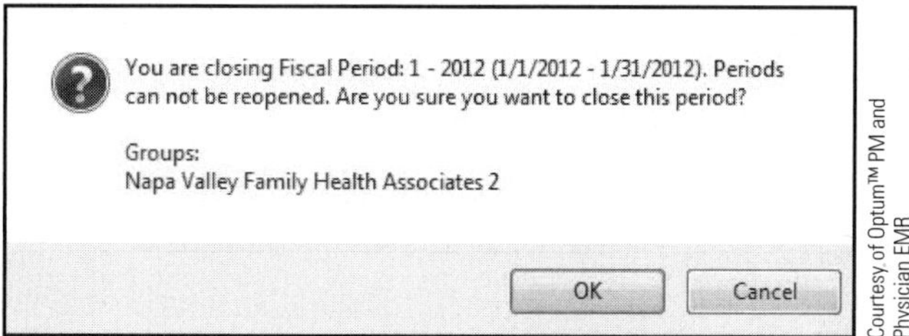

Courtesy of Optum™ PM and Physician EMR

Figure 2-14 Close Period Warning

5. Click *Save*. Your closed period will look like Figure 2-15.

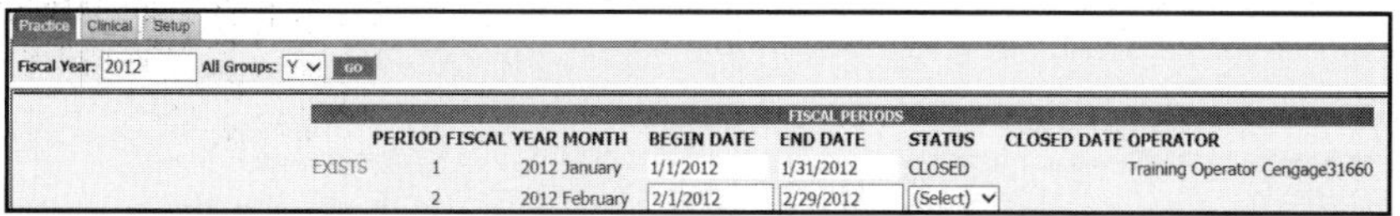

	PERIOD	FISCAL YEAR MONTH	BEGIN DATE	END DATE	STATUS	CLOSED DATE	OPERATOR
EXISTS	1	2012 January	1/1/2012	1/31/2012	CLOSED		Training Operator Cengage31660
	2	2012 February	2/1/2012	2/29/2012	(Select)		

Figure 2-15 Closed Fiscal Period

Courtesy of Optum™ PM and Physician EMR

ACTIVITY 2-7: Change Your Password

Every operator must have a username and a password to log in to Optum™ PM and Physician EMR. You are required to change your password every 90 days. Optum™ PM and Physician EMR reminds users seven days before their password expires and gives you the option of changing the password at that time. If your password expires, you can reset it without having to log a *ToDo* to *Support*. You can also use *Operator Settings* to change your password at any time after you begin using Optum™ PM and Physician EMR, even prior to being required to by the system.

PROFESSIONALISM CONNECTION

The Optum™ PM and Physician EMR software allows management to track where you have been in the system. Never give anyone your password! If someone other than you uses your sign-in to view a patient's record, there is no way to prove that it was not you. If anyone asks for your password, remind him or her that it is against company policy to share passwords.

To Change Your Password

1. Click the *Administration* module. The application displays the *Practice* tab.
2. Click the *Operator Settings* link (Figure 2-16) in the *Security* section. Optum™ PM and Physician EMR launches the *Operator Settings* application.

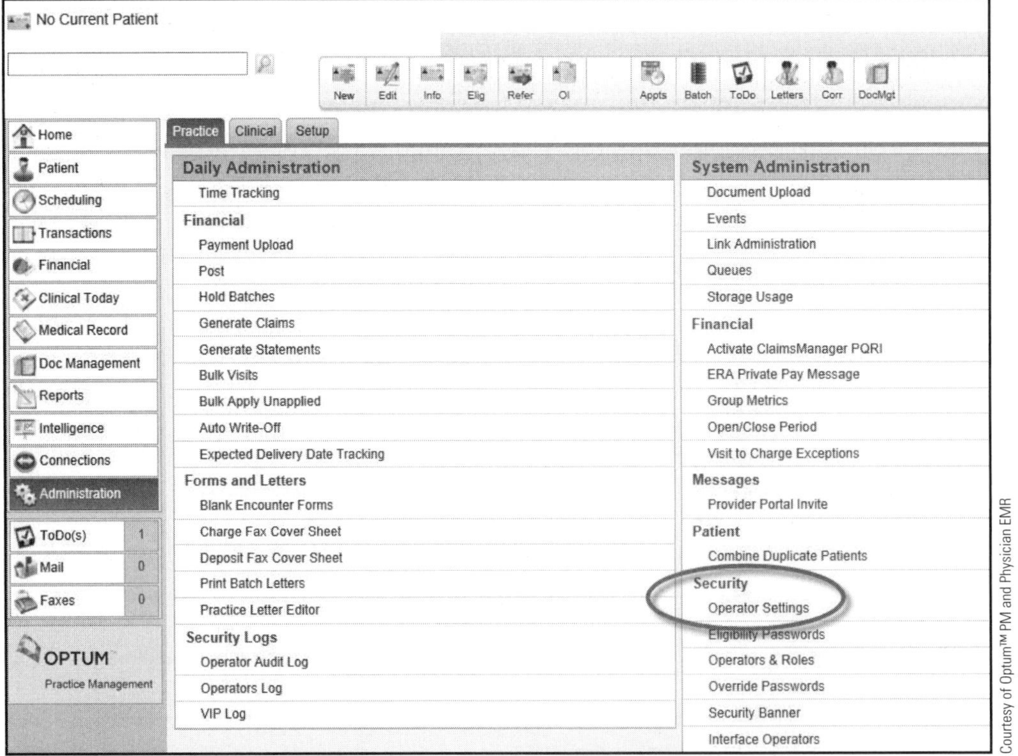

Figure 2-16 Operator Settings Link

3. In the *Old Password* box, enter your current password (the one you created in Activity 2-2).
4. In the *New Password* field, enter your new password (enter a personal password you will remember). Record your username and new password for future reference:

   a. Username ______________________

   b. New Password: ____________________

   The new password must meet the following criteria:

   - The new password must differ from your old password by at least one character.
   - The new password must consist of at least eight characters.
   - At least one of the eight characters must be a capital letter and at least one must be a number; for example: "Password5."

5. In the *Verify Password* box, reenter your new password.
6. From the *Question* list, select a security question.
7. In the *Answer* box, enter the answer to the security question.
8. In the *Phone* and *Email* fields, enter your phone number and e-mail address (see Figure 2-17). It is important to keep this contact information up to date because it is used by *Support* to follow up on support issues or *ToDos*.

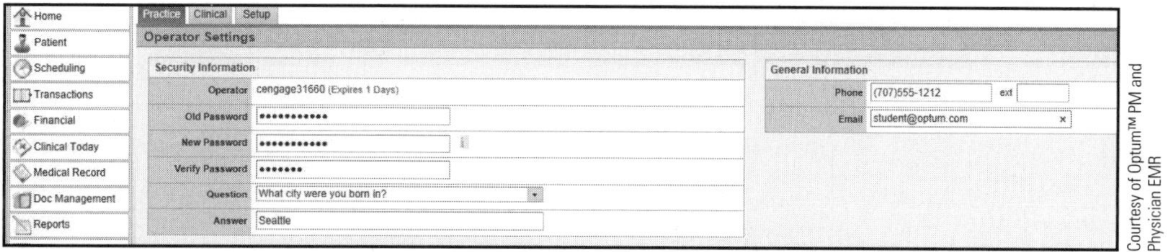

Courtesy of Optum™ PM and Physician EMR

Figure 2-17 Change Password Screen

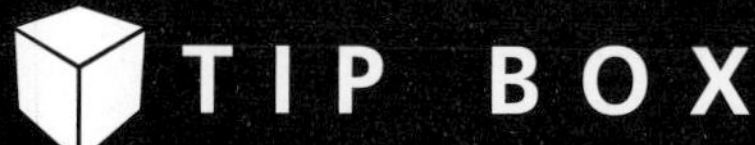

TIP BOX

The application will prompt the operator for an e-mail address if a valid address is not already saved for the operator.

9. Click *Save*. The application redirects you to the login screen where you must log in using your new password. If you do not get an automatic redirect, you may have to log out and log back in again using your new password.

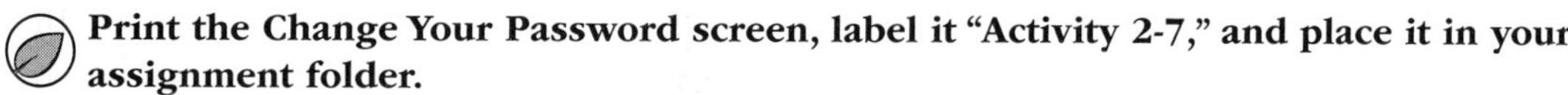

Print the Change Your Password screen, label it "Activity 2-7," and place it in your assignment folder.

ACTIVITY 2-8: Add Item(s) to a Quick Pick List

Throughout Optum™ PM and Physician EMR, drop-down lists are available from which you can select field-specific data to help create a more efficient workflow, known as *Quick Picks*. Options available in a drop-down list are built for each practice and are group specific. Your practice can build drop-down options for locations, employers, insurance companies, and financial transactions.

In order for certain data fields to be available as you work in Optum™ PM and Physician EMR, they need to be added to your "quick picks" list. You can add or remove options from a drop-down list in the *Quick Pick Setup* application.

1. Click the *Administration* module, and then click the *Setup* tab.
2. Click the *Quick Picks* link in the *Financial* section (Figure 2-18). Optum™ PM and Physician EMR launches the *Quick Picks* application.

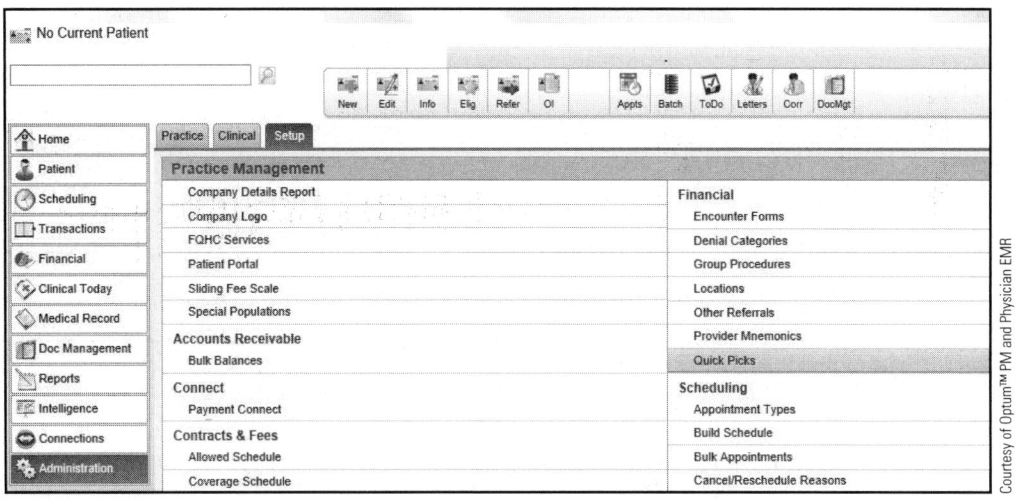

Figure 2-18 Quick Picks Link

3. From the *Screen Type* drop-down list, select the quick pick list to which you want to add an item. The application displays the quick pick list (select "Form Letters").
4. Verify that the item you want to add is not already included in the current quick picks list.
5. Enter the item you want to add in the *Search* box (enter "No") and then click the *Search* icon. The application displays a search window containing a list of possible matches (Figure 2-19). Click on the desired result to select it (select "No Show fee (pat)"). The application closes the search window and adds the data as an option in the list (Figure 2-20).

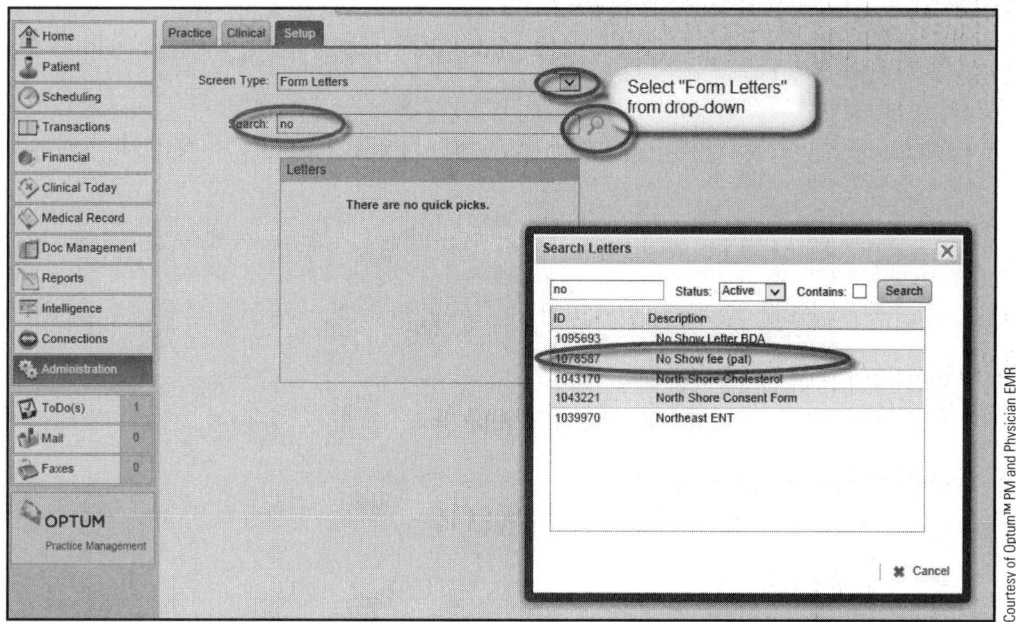

Figure 2-19 No Show Fee Letter

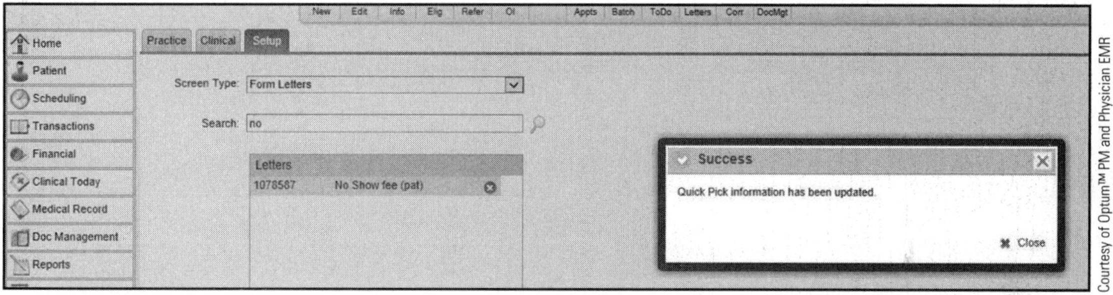

Figure 2-20 Quick Pick Added

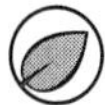 **Print the Quick Pick screen, label it "Activity 2-8," and place it in your assignment folder.**

ACTIVITY 2-9: Create a ToDo

The *ToDo* application is Optum™ PM and Physician EMR's internal messaging system that allows you to assign administrative and patient-related tasks within your practice as well as communicate with the Optum™ PM and Physician EMR support team. You will know you have an open *ToDo* if a number appears next to the *ToDo* link in the left navigation pane. In the *ToDo* application you can review each *ToDo* that has been sent to you, reply to a *ToDo*, transfer a *ToDo*, take ownership of a *ToDo*, or close a *ToDo*. The application is updated in real time.

1. Click the *Home* module, and then click the *Messages* tab. The *Messages* application displays all of your open *ToDo*(s).
2. Click on the *ToDo* icon on the *Name Bar*. The application displays the *New ToDo* window (Figure 2-21).

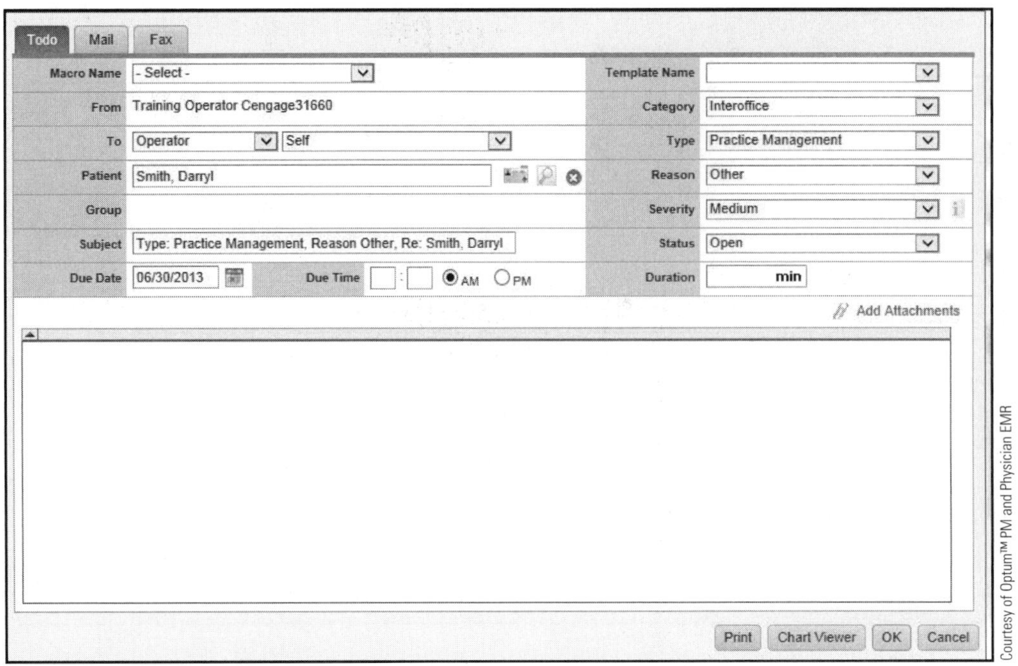

Courtesy of Optum™ PM and Physician EMR

Figure 2-21 New ToDo Dialog Box

3. (FYI only) From the *Macro Name* list, you can select the macro you want to use for the *ToDo*. (A macro is a grouping of one or more templates that you can use to populate the *ToDo* with preformatted content.)
4. By default, the *From* list displays your operator name.
5. In the *To* list, click the required options. The *To* list includes the categories described in Figure 2-22. Select "Operator."

TO LIST OPTIONS	
Field	**Description**
Operator	Enables you to select a Optum PM and Physician EMR user from your company.
Queue	Enables you to select a work queue set up for the practice. This will redirect the ToDo to the queue. For example, you can send a ToDo to the Support queue and an operator in the queue will respond to the ToDo.
Participant	Enables you to select a participant in the ToDo. This can be a person or a queue that participated in the ToDo.

Courtesy of Optum™ PM and Physician EMR

Figure 2-22 List Options for ToDo

6. If you are sending a *ToDo* to a patient, enter his or her full or partial last name in the *Patient* box and then click the *Search* icon. When the *Patient Search* window opens, click on the name of the patient in the search results (search "Wild"; select "Wild, Alison").

Click the *Delete* icon to remove the name from the *Patient* field. Click the *Info* icon to view the patient's contact information in the "At a Glance" *Patient Information* window.

7. By default, the *Subject* box displays information based on the selection in the *Type* and *Reason* lists. However, you can change the subject if necessary.

8. In the *Due Date* and *Due Time* boxes, enter the date and time by which the *ToDo* should be completed. This is important to track overdue items (enter today's date).
9. (FYI only) From the *Template Name* list, select the template you want to use. (You must select a macro before selecting a template.)

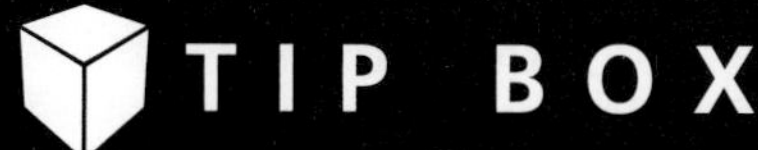

Macros and templates are created in the *Event Manager* application in the *Administration* module.

10. From the *Category* list, select the *ToDo* category (select "Interoffice").
11. In the *Type* list, click the type of the *ToDo* (select "Practice Management").
12. In the *Reason* list, click the reason for the *ToDo* (select "Other").

TIP BOX

If the *ToDo* created is for the Optum™ PM and Physician EMR support department, select "Support Center" from the Category list. This will automatically populate the *To* field with "Queue." Use the drop-down menu from the *Type* and *Reason* lists to identify your issue. Free-text a brief message in the body of the *ToDo* (Figure 2-23), and then click *Save*.

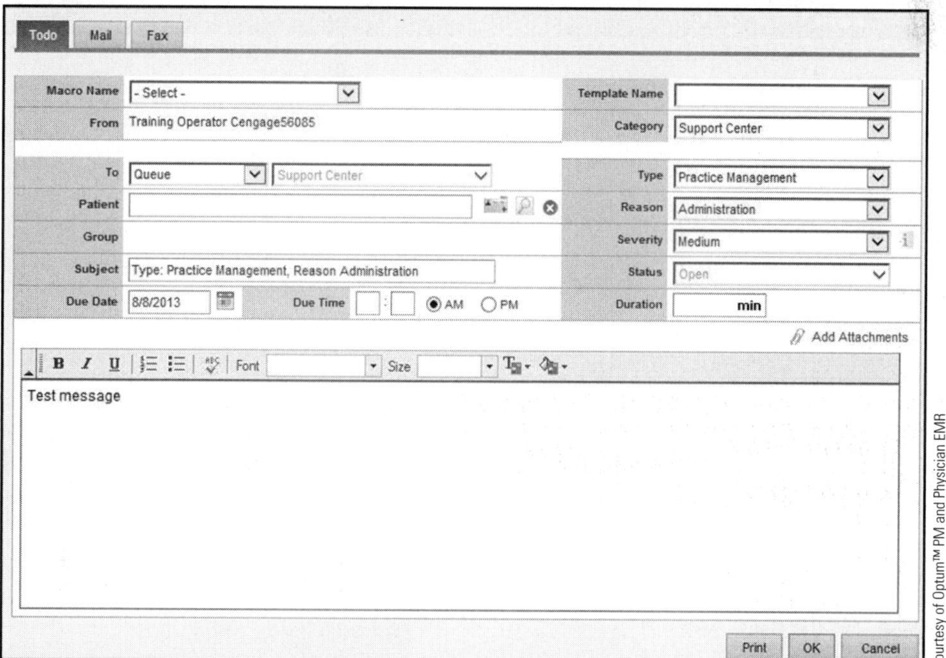

Courtesy of Optum™ PM and Physician EMR

Figure 2-23 Support Center ToDo

13. In the *Severity* list, select the priority level of the *ToDo* (select "Medium").
14. The *Status* list is set to "Open" by default.
15. In the *Duration* box, enter the total time spent working on the *ToDo*.
16. (FYI only) The content box is not functional in your student version of Optum™. However, in the live version you would use it to enter your *ToDo* information. You could format and spell-check the note if needed. If you selected a template, this field would be automatically populated with the content in the template. (**Note:** Although this field is not active in your student version of Optum™, by following the prior steps in this activity you will have created a *ToDo* that will appear in your *ToDo* queue).
17. (Optional) Follow instructions in *Help* to attach documents to a *ToDo*.
18. Click *OK*. The *ToDo* will disappear and show in your *Messages Dashboard* (Figure 2-24).

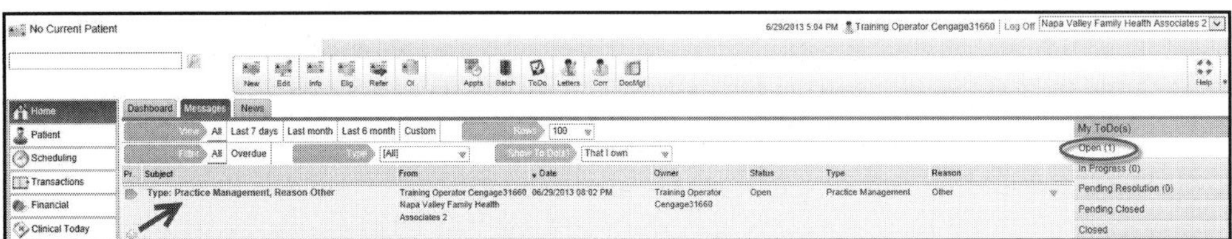

Figure 2-24 Student Created ToDo

Courtesy of Optum™ PM and Physician EMR

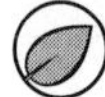

Print the Messages dashboard with the completed ToDo, label it "Activity 2-9," and place it in your assignment folder.

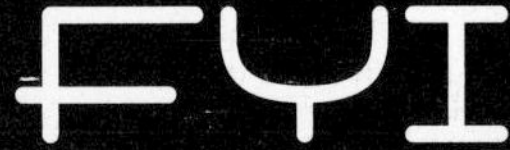

View Queues

Queues are used to organize and group *ToDos*, mail, and faxes in the *Messages Center*. Queues help manage tasks more efficiently by allowing you to route *ToDos* to a group rather than to one individual. At the top of each queue is a set of filters you can use to sort *ToDos*, mail messages, and faxes. Once you are working in Optum™ and sending and receiving messages, you will be able to view the activity in *My Queues*. Follow these instructions to view your *My Queues*:

1. Click the *Home* module, and then click the *Messages* tab. The *My Queues* section at the right side of the window displays all of your queues. The number next to each queue indicates the number of pending *ToDos* in the queue (Figure 2-25).

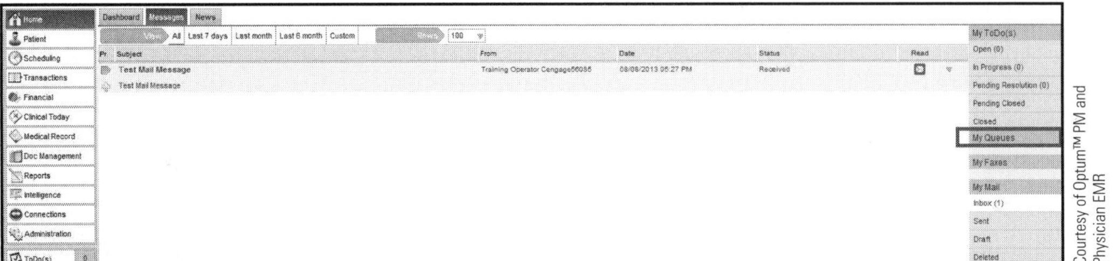

Courtesy of Optum™ PM and Physician EMR

Figure 2-25 My Queues

(Continues)

FYI Box (*Continued*)

2. Click the specific queue you want to access. By default, the queue displays all outstanding *ToDos*.
3. By default, the *Type* list displays *All*. Click a different type, such as questionnaires, refill requests, or phone messages.
4. From the *Status* list, click the status of the *ToDo*. All *ToDos* that match the selected type and status will display. The options in the *Status* list are described in Figure 2-26.

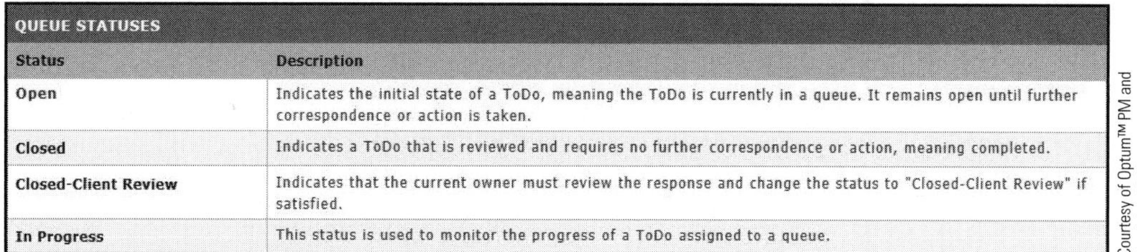

QUEUE STATUSES

Status	Description
Open	Indicates the initial state of a ToDo, meaning the ToDo is currently in a queue. It remains open until further correspondence or action is taken.
Closed	Indicates a ToDo that is reviewed and requires no further correspondence or action, meaning completed.
Closed-Client Review	Indicates that the current owner must review the response and change the status to "Closed-Client Review" if satisfied.
In Progress	This status is used to monitor the progress of a ToDo assigned to a queue.

Courtesy of Optum™ PM and Physician EMR

Figure 2-26 Queue Status List Options

5. Figure 2-27 represents how your *My Queues* would look once you have an activity entered and pending.

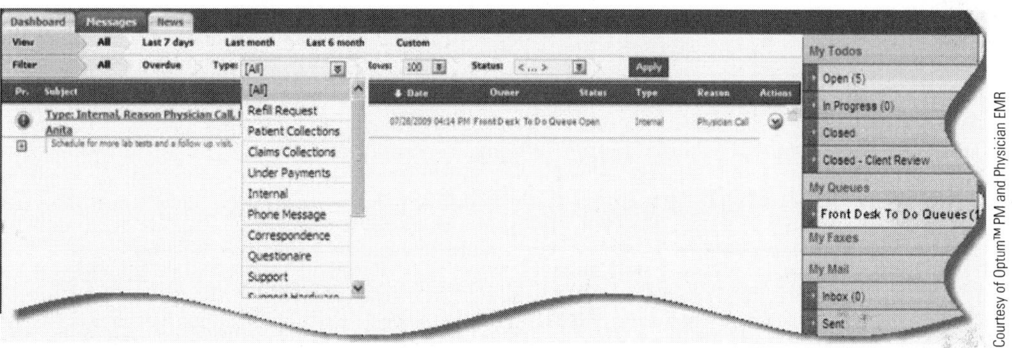

Courtesy of Optum™ PM and Physician EMR

Figure 2-27 Queue Types All

ACTIVITY 2-10: Create a New Mail Message

The *Mail* application allows you to communicate electronically with staff members, providers in your *Provider Portal,* and patients activated in the *Patient Portal*. The mail feature works the same as other e-mail applications, enabling you to open, view, create, send and receive, and delete messages. In addition, you can link attachments such as patient encounter notes, documents, results, referrals and authorization forms, set priorities, and more.

1. Click the *Home* module, and then click the *Messages* tab. The *Messages Center* opens and displays all of your open *ToDos*.
2. Click *Send Mail*, located on the lower right-side *ToDo* pane (Figure 2-28). The application displays the *New Mail* dialog box.
3. (FYI only) From the *Macro Name* list, select the macro you want to use.
4. (FYI only) From the *Template* list, select the template you want to use for the mail message. The application populates the *Notes* field with the content from the template. (You must select a *Macro* before selecting a template.)
5. The *From* list defaults to the operator creating the mail message and cannot be edited.

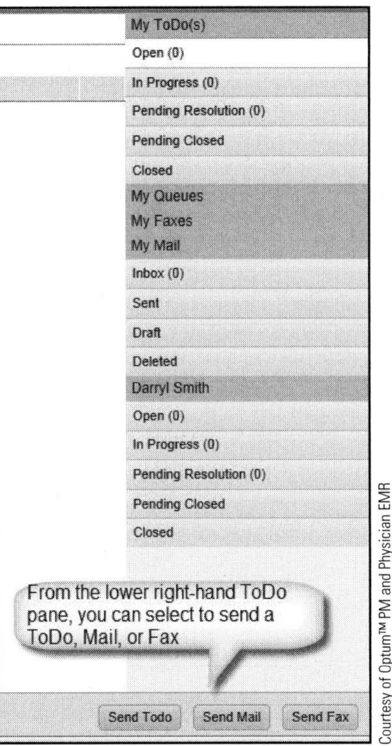

Figure 2-28 Send Mail

6. In the *To* field, click the *Search* icon. Optum™ PM and Physician EMR opens the *Select Operators* dialog box.
7. Place a check mark in the box by your login name (Figure 2-29).

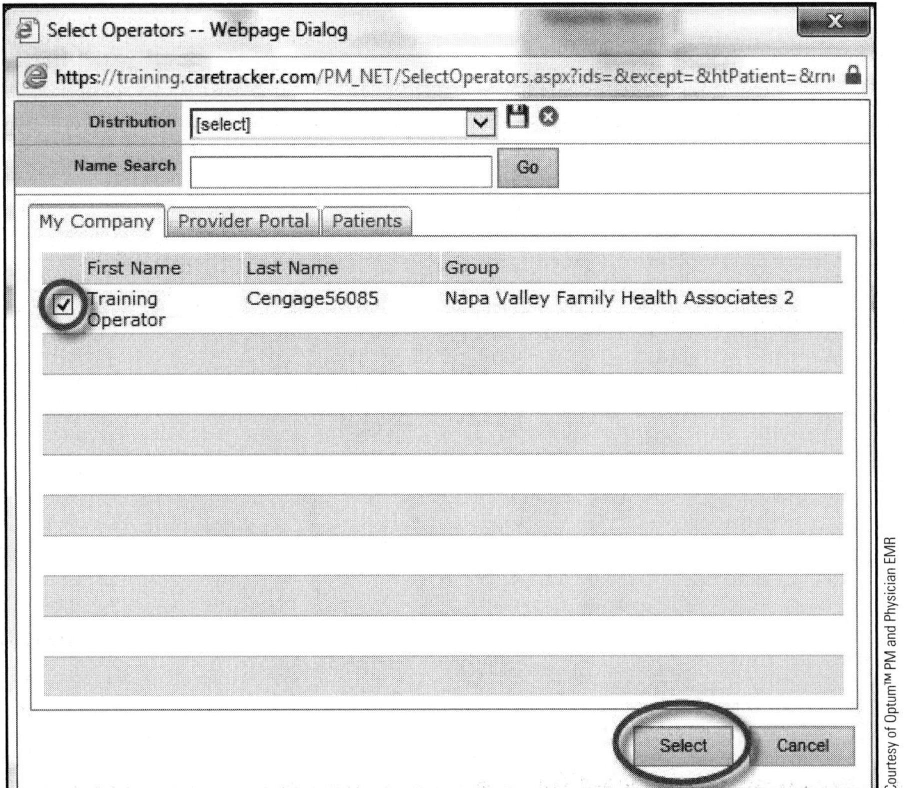

Figure 2-29 Select Operators Dialog Box

8. Click *Select*. The application closes the *Select Operators* dialog box.
9. If a patient is in context, the patient name displays in the *Patient* box. However, you can also send a mail message about a different patient by clicking the *Search* icon. For this activity, you will not select a patient.
10. In the *Subject* box, enter the subject of the mail message (enter "Test Mail Message").
11. By default, the *Severity* list displays "Medium." However, you can change the severity of the mail message if necessary. (Leave as is.)
12. (FYI only) To link a clinical document or chart summary, follow the instructions in *Help*.
13. In the *Notes* box, enter the message and format the information if necessary. Enter "Test Mail Message" (Figure 2-30).

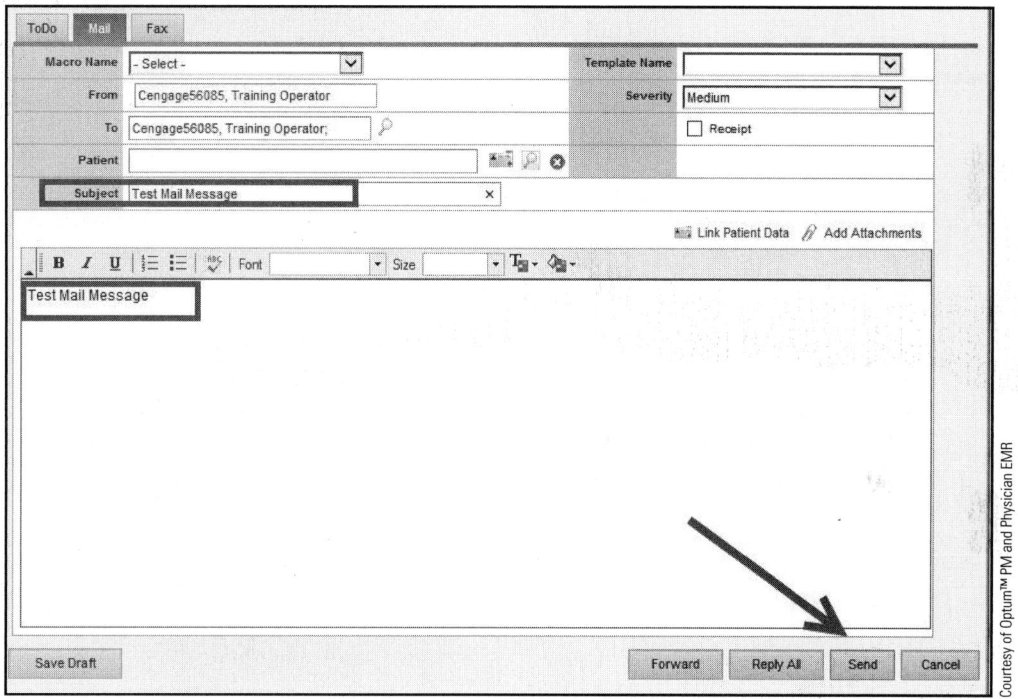

Figure 2-30 Send Test Mail Message

14. You can click *Save Draft* to save the message and send later or click *Send* to send the mail message to the selected operators (click *Send*).

15. To view your sent message, click the *Sent* link on the *My ToDo(s)* pane (Figure 2-31).

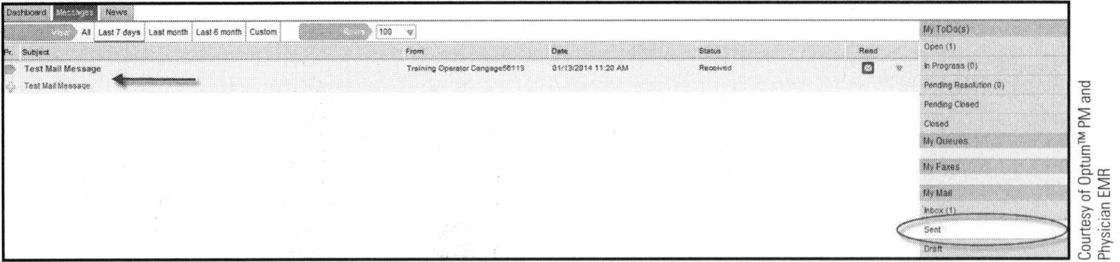

Courtesy of Optum™ PM and Physician EMR

Figure 2-31 Sent Mail Message

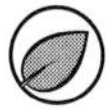 **Print the Sent Message screen, label it "Activity 2-10," and place it in your assignment folder.**

Resource

The Optum™ PM and Physician EMR Help home page represents a wealth of information for the electronic health record (*https://training.caretracker.com/help/CareTracker_Help.htm*).

CHAPTER 3

Patient Demographics

LEARNING OBJECTIVES

1. Identify components of the Name Bar.
2. Demonstrate knowledge of patient Demographics.
3. Search for a patient within Optum™ PM.
4. View and perform Eligibility Checks.

NVFHA MANAGER CHALLENGE

Here at NVFHA, we conduct reference checks on all job applicants who make it to a second interview. Our goal is to hire applicants who have a high capacity for "attention to detail." When entering patient demographic information in the computer it is critical to pay attention to detail because this information impacts so many departments within our practice. If you misspell a patient's name, put in incorrect address information, or omit insurance information, it creates havoc for the clinical team searching for the patient's chart, the billing team that has to send out a second billing statement, and even the insurance company that reviews a claim for the second time. Patients are often impacted as well by these types of errors and lose confidence in the overall practice. These types of errors are costly to the practice because they increase employee hours needed to make corrections and delay reimbursement for services that affect the revenue cycle.

As you go through the activities in this chapter, pay particular attention to your ability to enter information correctly. If you struggle in this area, you may want to slow down a bit and make certain that you are entering the correct information the first time around. Your instructor may have some additional tips. Are you up for the challenge?

ACTIVITY 3-1: Searching for a Patient by Name (currently in the database)

The *Name Bar*, located across the top of the Optum™ window, provides quick access to the most frequently used Optum™ applications (Figure 3-1). A quick reference guide to the various applications launched from the *Name Bar* illustrates each button and a description of the function (Figure 3-2). The *Name Bar* allows you to pull a patient into context to perform specific tasks. A patient is "in context" when his or her information appears in the *Name* list and *ID* box, as illustrated on the *Name Bar* picture.

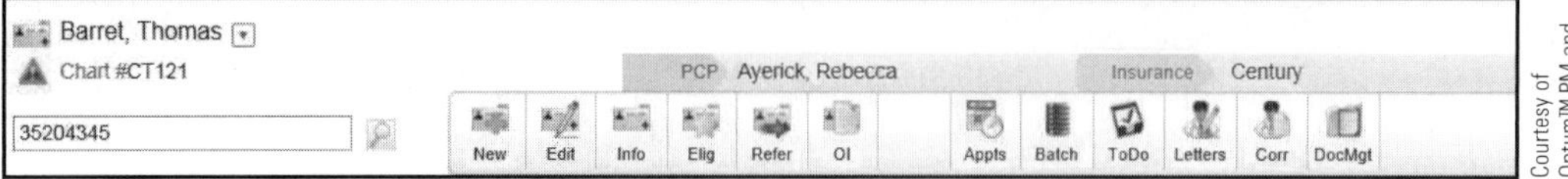

Courtesy of Optum™ PM and Physician EMR

Figure 3-1 Name Bar

NAME BAR	
Button	**Description**
Search	Pulls patients into context by Optum PM and Physician EMR ID number, chart number, claim ID or last name. Enter the patient's first name, last name or at least three letters of each name to display the Advanced Search dialog box that enables you to select a patient.
Alert	Displays the Patient Alerts window. The Patient Alerts window notifies the operator when key information is missing from a patient's demographics or if any problems exist with the patient's account.
Edit	Launches the Demographics application in edit mode for the patient in context.
New	Launches the Demographics application, enabling you to register a new patient in Optum PM and Physician EMR.
Info	Displays a read only summary of the patient's information, including address, contact information, family members, balance information, insurance, etc.
Elig	Displays a history of eligibility checks and enables you to perform an individual electronic eligibility check to ensure that the patient is covered by the insurance company listed as the primary insurance.
Refer	Launches the Referral/Authorization application.
Appts	Displays a list of upcoming patient appointments. In addition, you can view and confirm an appointment, check in/check out a patient, print the encounter form, and perform various other tasks pertaining to the appointment.
OI	Displays information pertaining to dates of service. For example, you can obtain information such as associated procedures, financial transactions and claim activity, and make financial transactions such as payments, adjustments, refunds and more.
Batch	Launches the Batch application, allowing you to create a new batch to enter charges and post payments and adjustments. In addition, you can also set up personal settings when using Optum PM and Physician EMR. For example, the main application to launch when logged on to Optum PM and Physician EMR.
ToDo	Launches the Optum PM and Physician EMR messaging tool, allowing you to communicate with other staff and the Optum PM and Physician EMR Support Department.
Letters	Generates and prints letters to send to a patient.
Corr	Displays a queue of letters generated and enables you to print the letters to send to patients.

Courtesy of Optum™ PM and Physician EMR

Figure 3-2 Description of Name Bar Applications

To Search for Patient Alison Wild by Name

1. In the *ID* search box on the *Name Bar*, enter the first three letters of the patient's last name ["Wil"], and hit [Enter] (Figure 3-3). The pop-up will list any patient matching your search criteria. Click on patient "Alison Wild." You will receive a pop-up asking if you want to navigate away from this page (Figure 3-4). Select *OK* and Optum™ PM will launch the *Patient Demographics* page, displaying the patient's demographics screen.

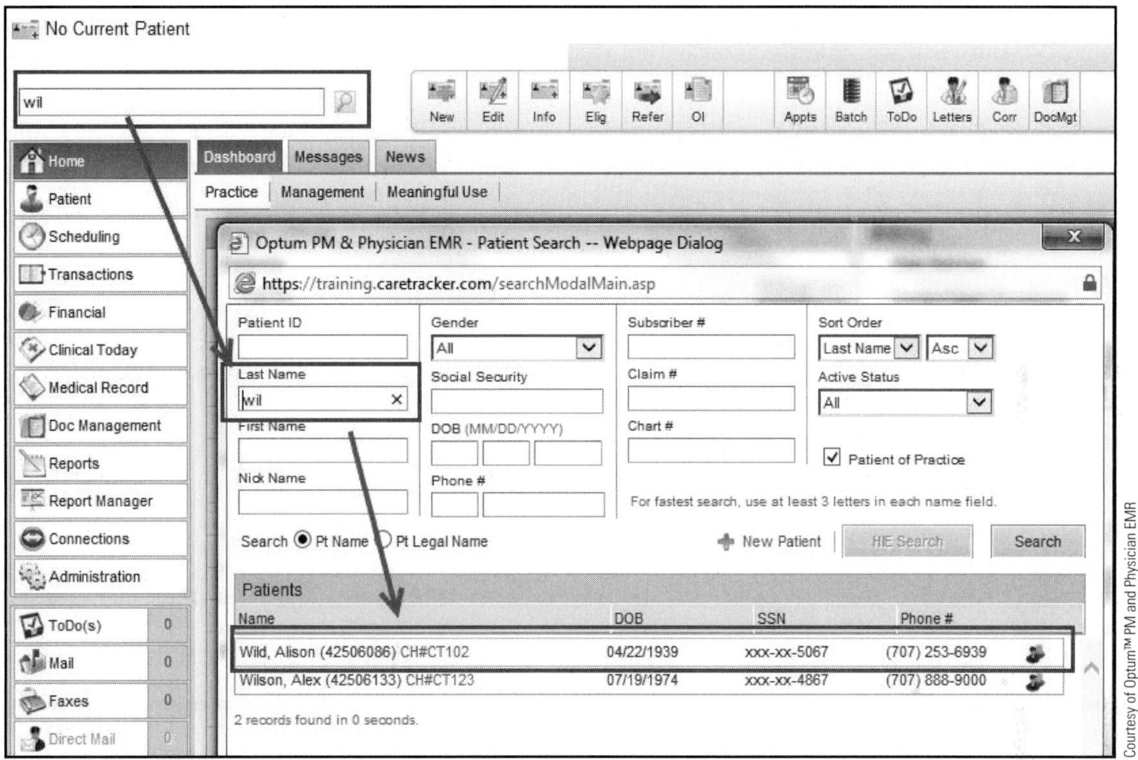

Figure 3-3 Search by First Three Letters of Patient's Last Name

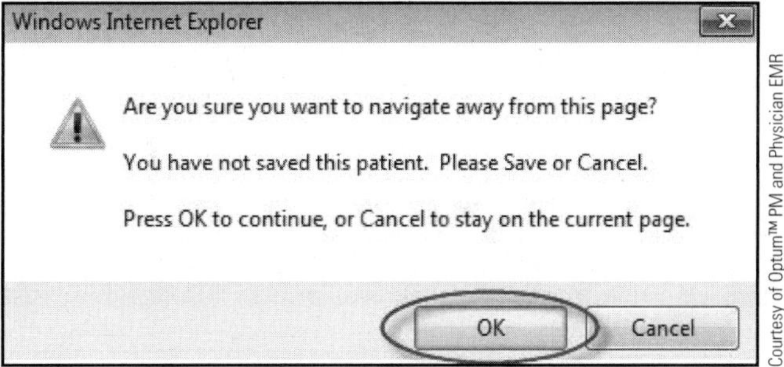

Figure 3-4 Leave This Page Pop-Up Message

2. An alternate method to search for existing patients is:

   a. Remove a patient in context by clicking on the drop-down list at the end of the patient's name (Figure 3-5) and select "None." The name in the patient field will be removed and "No Current Patient" will display.

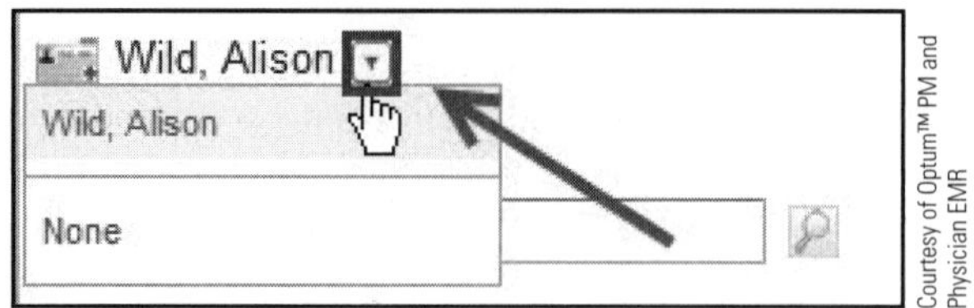

Figure 3-5 Remove Patient from Context Drop-Down

b. With "No Current Patient" in the *ID* search box, click on the *Search* icon, which will bring up the *Patient Search* box.

c. In the *Patient Search* box, enter at least three letters of the patient's last ("Wil") and first name ("Ali"). A previous name such as a maiden name or an alias cannot be used to search for a patient.

d. Click the *Search* button. The *Patient Search* box displays a list of patients that match the information entered (see Figure 3-3), along with the patient ID and chart number.

e. Verify the "second identifier" such as DOB or last four numbers of the Social Security number (see Figure 3-3).

f. Click the *Family* icon to view the patient's family members registered in Optum™ PM and Physician EMR (if applicable).

3. Record the patient's ID number, chart number, and Social Security number for additional activities related to searching for a patient.
4. Click the specific name to launch the patient into context.

Print the Patient Demographics screen displayed, label it "Activity 3-1," and place it in your assignment folder.

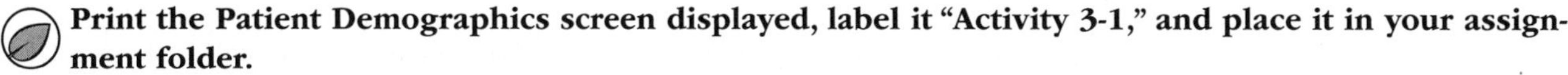

PROFESSIONALISM CONNECTION

Start every conversation with a patient either over the phone or in person by asking for a minimum of two identifiers. Most offices have patients state their first and last names followed by their birth date. This helps to confirm that you are in the correct chart and reduces the risk of documenting in the wrong chart.

ACTIVITY 3-2: Searching for a Patient by ID Number

You now have successfully searched for a patient and know the patient's ID number, chart number, Social Security number, and claim number (if applicable) from the record provided. Using that information, practice searching for the same patient using alternative methods.

1. In the *ID* search box (see Figure 3-3), enter patient Alison Wild's *ID number* (using the *ID number* obtained from the patient search in Activity 3-1). (**Note:** New ID numbers are assigned to patients for each student version of Optum™; therefore, patient ID numbers will vary by student.)
2. Hit [Enter]. The patient with the corresponding *ID number* launches into context.

3. You can also perform a search by patient *ID number* by clicking the *Search* icon. In the *Patient Search* box, enter the *Patient ID* number. A list of patients that match the information entered will pop up.

Print a screenshot of the Search Results screen for Alison Wild, label it "Activity 3-2," and place it in your assignment folder.

ACTIVITY 3-3: Searching for a Patient by Chart Number

You may also search for a patient by chart number. Typically, the chart number and the Optum™ PM and Physician EMR ID are the same. However, if the practice files paper charts by chart number, Optum™ PM and Physician EMR can assign chart numbers based on your medical record number. In your student version, the chart number and ID number are different for existing patients. New patients will have the same chart number and ID number. (**Note:** If your practice has electronically converted patient demographics to Optum™ PM and Physician EMR from another practice management system, the chart number will be the patient's ID number from your legacy practice management system.)

1. With no patient in context, click the *Search* icon; it will take you to the *Patient Search* pop-up box where you will need to enter the patient's *Chart #*.
2. Enter the chart number of patient Alison Wild (CT102) and click *Search* (Figure 3-6).

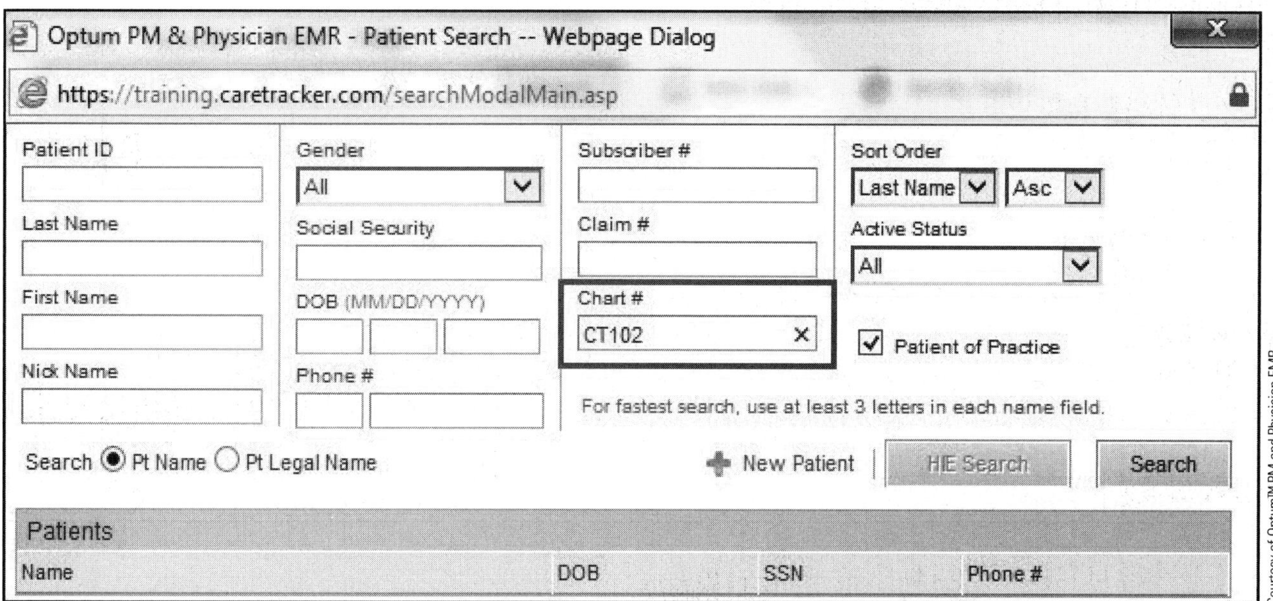

Figure 3-6 Search by Patient Chart Number

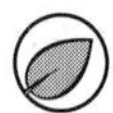 **Print a screenshot of the Search Results screen, label it "Activity 3-3," and place it in your assignment folder.**

3. Click on the patient with the corresponding *Chart #* to launch him or her into context. (**Note:** It may take a few moments for Optum ™ to "search" and populate the patient demographics.)

ACTIVITY 3-4: Searching for a Patient by Social Security Number (SSN)

1. With no patient in context, click the *Search* icon.
2. In the *Patient Search* pop-up box, enter the last four digits of patient Alison Wild's *Social Security* number (5067) obtained in Activity 3-1 (Figure 3-7), and hit [Enter] (or click on the *Search* button).

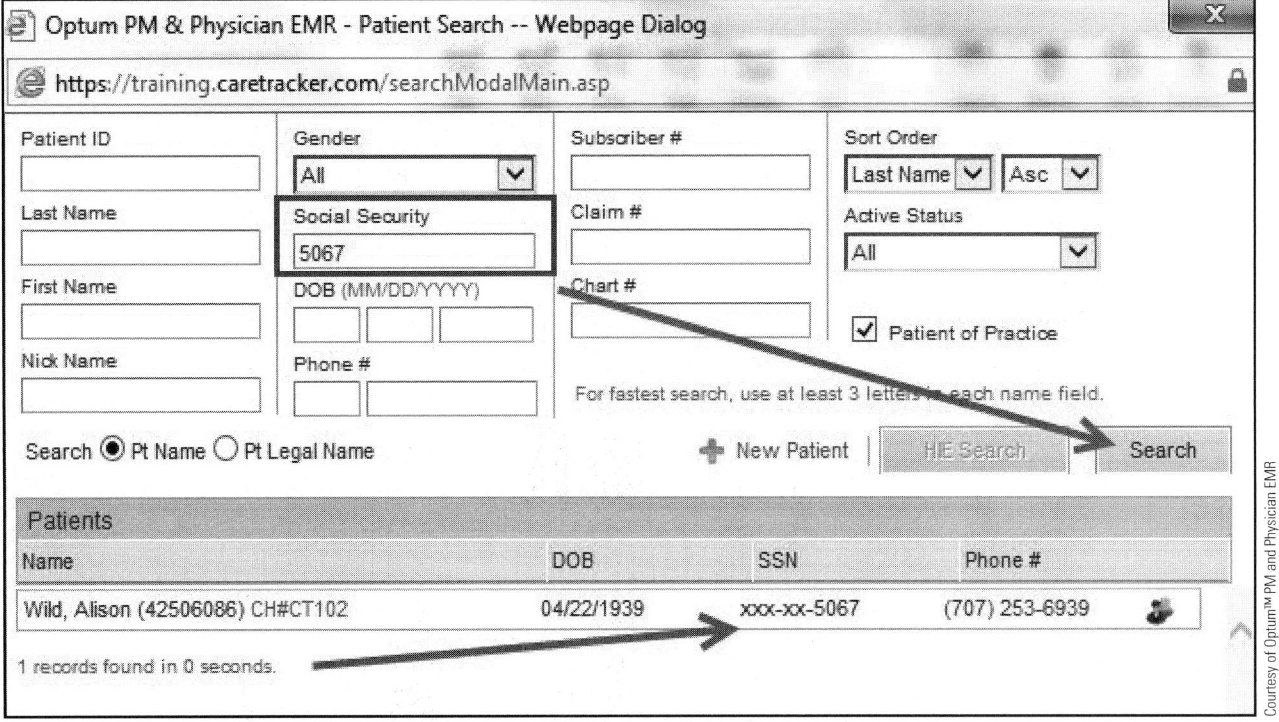

Courtesy of Optum™ PM and Physician EMR

Figure 3-7 Search by Social Security Number

 **Print a screenshot of the Patient Search pop-up screen, label it "Activity 3-4," and place it in your assignment folder.**

3. Click on the corresponding patient (Figure 3-7).
4. The application pulls the patient into context and launches the *Patient Demographics* application.

PROFESSIONALISM CONNECTION

Registration is often the first encounter patients experience during the initial office visit. The medical assistant responsible for this task sets the tone for the remainder of the visit. If the medical assistant is curt and unfriendly, the patient may feel uneasy and may be tempted to leave; however, if the medical assistant is friendly and courteous, the patient will likely feel more at ease and comfortable proceeding with the remainder of the visit. Consider how your role as biller and coder can make a positive impact on patient relations.

ACTIVITY 3-5: Edit Patient Demographics

It is important that all patients in the Optum™ PM and Physician EMR have complete and correct demographic information such as name, contact information, date of birth, insurance and employer information, primary (PCP) and referring provider, and more. This information is required to ensure proper treatment as well as to facilitate billing. If you are registering a new patient, always search the database to be certain that the patient has never been registered. Use two patient identifiers when searching to avoid creating a duplicate account.

It is important to verify accuracy and update information when a patient schedules an appointment or checks in for an appointment. This makes the treatment process faster and avoids unnecessary complications in billing due to outdated information (Figure 3-8).

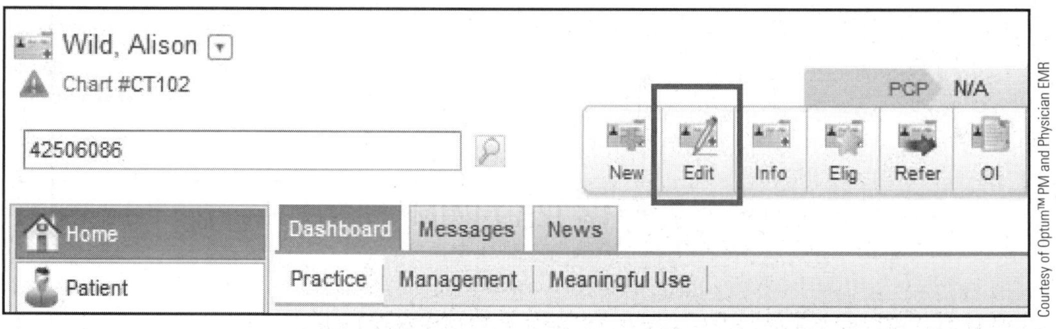

Courtesy of Optum™ PM and Physician EMR

Figure 3-8 Edit Patient Information Tab

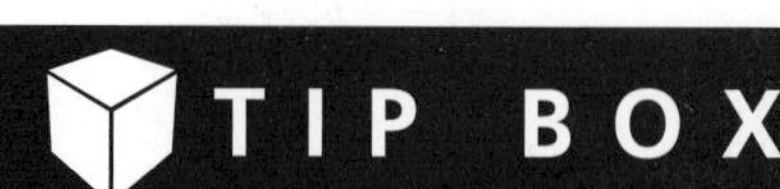

TIP BOX

Navigate through each field by pressing the [Tab] key and Optum™ PM and Physician EMR will automatically format the entry, regardless of the way it is entered. For example, by tabbing through the *First Name* and *Last Name* boxes, Optum™ PM and Physician EMR automatically applies title case to the name, meaning the first letter of each name is capitalized. To navigate back to a field, press [SHIFT+TAB].

Search the existing database to confirm that the patient (Alison Wild) has previously been registered. After confirming she is in the system, review the demographics screen to see if all information is correct and complete. You will notice that the PCP has not yet been entered for Alison. You will edit her demographics to add Dr. Raman as her PCP.

To Edit Patient Demographics

1. With patient Alison Wild in context click on the *Patient* module > *Demographics* tab (Figure 3-9).

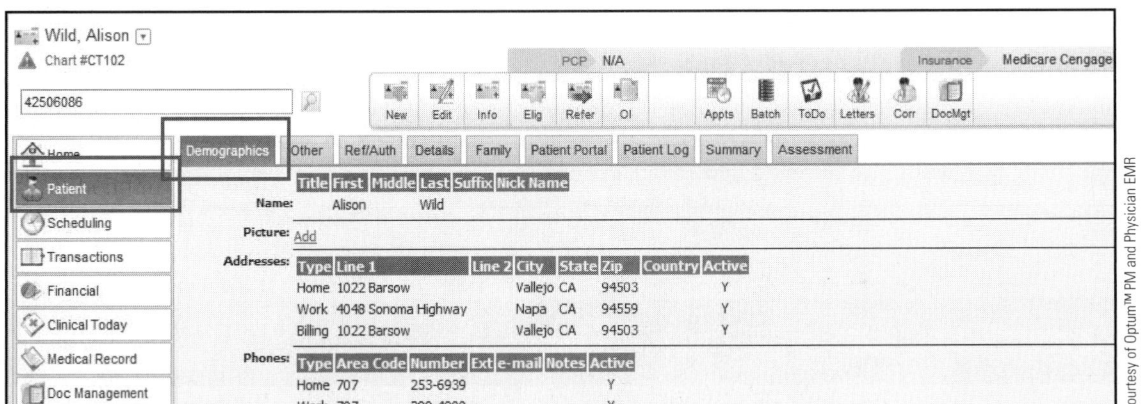

Figure 3-9 Demographics Tab

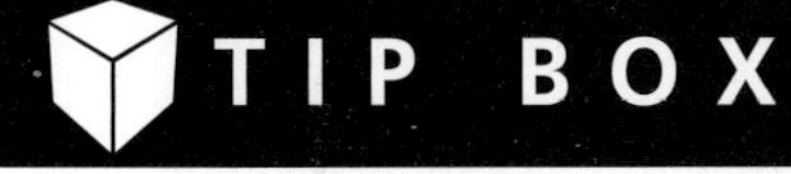

Always confirm if the *Consent, NPP,* and *HIE* were signed by the patient, and check "Yes" on the *Demographics* screen. Optum™ will automatically "date stamp" when the *Consent, NPP,* and *HIE Consent* information were entered (Figure 3-10).

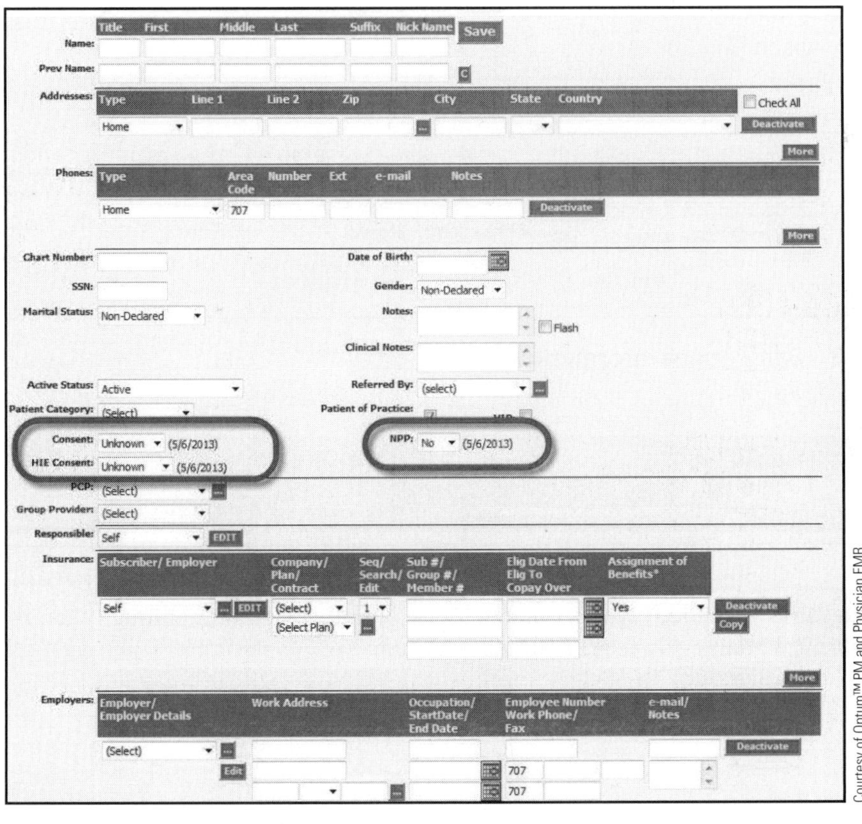

Figure 3-10 New Patient Demographic Screen with Consent Fields Highlighted

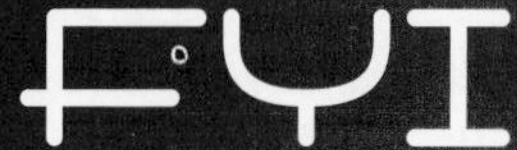

In order to complete the remainder of the demographics information, you would click *Edit* and continue the full registration process for any missing information. It is important to know that all fields should be completed, although they are not required. The pop-up will also alert you to missing information such as primary location (should be "Napa Valley Family Associates [NVFA]"), primary language, secondary language, ethnicity, race, organ donor status, and religion. To complete these fields, with the patient in context, you would click on the *Patient* module. Select the *Details* tab. Click on *Edit* in the *Display Patient Details* screen, complete the information, then hit *Save*. There are additional fields in the *Details* box, which may or may not be used by the practice.

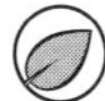 **Print the completed Demographics screen, label it "Activity 3-5," and place it in your assignment folder.**

ACTIVITY 3-6: Print the Patient Demographics Report

Medical practices may find it useful to print a patient's demographic report for a variety of reasons. Some practices will give a copy of the printed report to a patient at check-in to verify information and to make any necessary corrections/updates. Following this workflow will help identify inconsistencies between the patient information and information stored in your practice management software.

1. Pull a patient into context (Alison Wild).
2. Click the *Patient* module. Optum™ PM and Physician EMR displays the *Demographics* tab.
3. Click the *Print* icon in the upper-right corner of the *Demographics* page. Optum™ PM displays a *File Download* dialog box. (**Note:** It may take a little time to generate the report.)
4. Click *Open* to view the report (Figure 3-16). (Alternatively, you can click *Save* to save a copy of the report to your computer.)

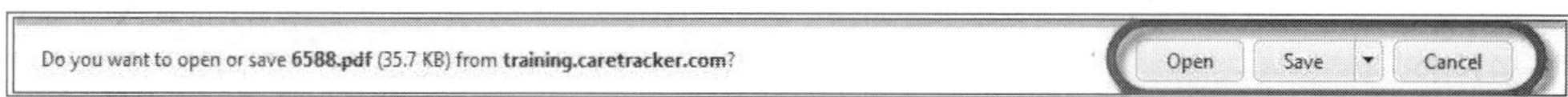

Figure 3-16 Open, Save, or Cancel Report
Courtesy of Optum™ PM and Physician EMR

5. The *Demographics* report (Figure 3-17) will open on your screen as a PDF.

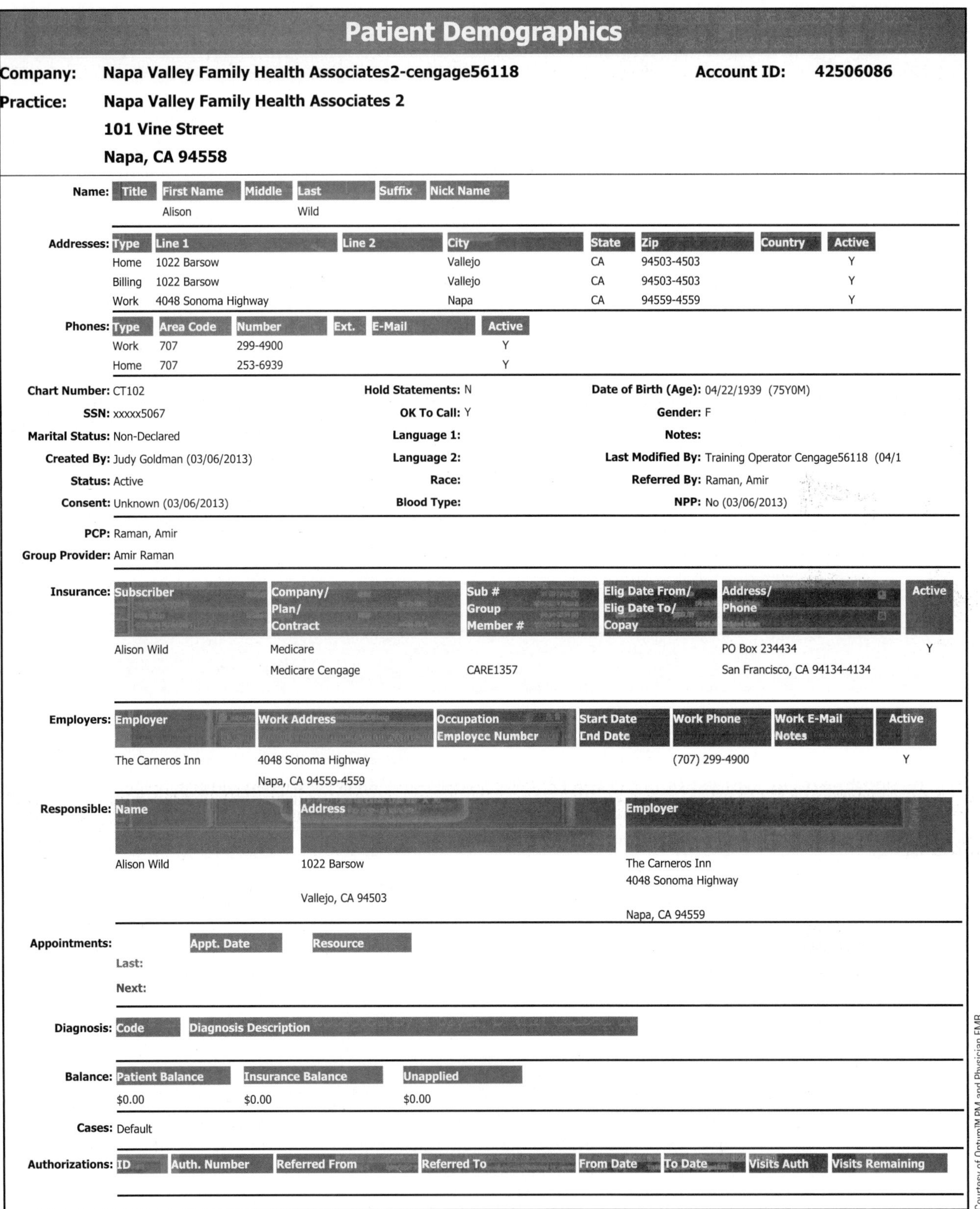

Patient Demographics

Company: Napa Valley Family Health Associates2-cengage56118 **Account ID:** 42506086

Practice: Napa Valley Family Health Associates 2
101 Vine Street
Napa, CA 94558

Name:

Title	First Name	Middle	Last	Suffix	Nick Name
	Alison		Wild		

Addresses:

Type	Line 1	Line 2	City	State	Zip	Country	Active
Home	1022 Barsow		Vallejo	CA	94503-4503		Y
Billing	1022 Barsow		Vallejo	CA	94503-4503		Y
Work	4048 Sonoma Highway		Napa	CA	94559-4559		Y

Phones:

Type	Area Code	Number	Ext.	E-Mail	Active
Work	707	299-4900			Y
Home	707	253-6939			Y

Chart Number: CT102 **Hold Statements:** N **Date of Birth (Age):** 04/22/1939 (75Y0M)
SSN: xxxxx5067 **OK To Call:** Y **Gender:** F
Marital Status: Non-Declared **Language 1:** **Notes:**
Created By: Judy Goldman (03/06/2013) **Language 2:** **Last Modified By:** Training Operator Cengage56118 (04/1
Status: Active **Race:** **Referred By:** Raman, Amir
Consent: Unknown (03/06/2013) **Blood Type:** **NPP:** No (03/06/2013)

PCP: Raman, Amir
Group Provider: Amir Raman

Insurance:

Subscriber	Company/ Plan/ Contract	Sub # Group Member #	Elig Date From/ Elig Date To/ Copay	Address/ Phone	Active
Alison Wild	Medicare Medicare Cengage	CARE1357		PO Box 234434 San Francisco, CA 94134-4134	Y

Employers:

Employer	Work Address	Occupation Employee Number	Start Date End Date	Work Phone	Work E-Mail Notes	Active
The Carneros Inn	4048 Sonoma Highway Napa, CA 94559-4559			(707) 299-4900		Y

Responsible:

Name	Address	Employer
Alison Wild	1022 Barsow Vallejo, CA 94503	The Carneros Inn 4048 Sonoma Highway Napa, CA 94559

Appointments:

	Appt. Date	Resource
Last:		
Next:		

Diagnosis:

Code	Diagnosis Description

Balance:

Patient Balance	Insurance Balance	Unapplied
$0.00	$0.00	$0.00

Cases: Default

Authorizations:

ID	Auth. Number	Referred From	Referred To	From Date	To Date	Visits Auth	Visits Remaining

Courtesy of Optum™ PM and Physician EMR

Figure 3-17 Patient Demographics Report for Alison Wild

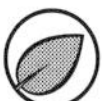

TIP BOX

The *Patient Demographics* report cannot be printed from the *Demographics* window that displays when you click on the *Edit* button in the *Name Bar*.

Print the Demographics report, label it "Activity 3-6," and place it in your assignment folder.

PROFESSIONALISM CONNECTION

Patients may become frustrated when they are asked if there have been any changes since the last office visit. Some individuals may even become aggravated when you ask to see their insurance card. This is particularly true when the patient just had a recent visit. Your choice of words and tone of voice can make the process less cumbersome. The following statement is an example of a positive directive: "Mr. Timmons, I know you were just in last week, but I just need to make certain that nothing has changed since your last visit, such as your insurance information, telephone number, etc."

ACTIVITY 3-7: View and Perform Eligibility Check—Electronic Eligibility Checks

The *Eligibility* application enables you to view a history of eligibility checks. It also enables you to electronically check eligibility with the primary insurance as well as the secondary insurance saved in *Patient Demographics*. Optum™ PM and Physician EMR automatically performs eligibility checks every evening for all patients scheduled for appointments for the next five days. Automated batch eligibility checks are performed for a patient once every 30 days regardless of the number of appointments scheduled for the patient during that month. However, it is sometimes necessary to perform individual eligibility checks periodically throughout the treatment and payment cycle or for any walk-in patients. The eligibility check helps to identify potential payer sources, reducing the number of denied claims or bad debt write-offs, and decrease staff hours required for performing manual eligibility checks.

Your student version of Optum™ PM does not have the electronic eligibility feature. To perform the simulated workflow of an eligibility check, you would click the *Elig* button on the dashboard, and then access the payer website or call the insurance company to verify eligibility when electronic access is not available (Figure 3-18).

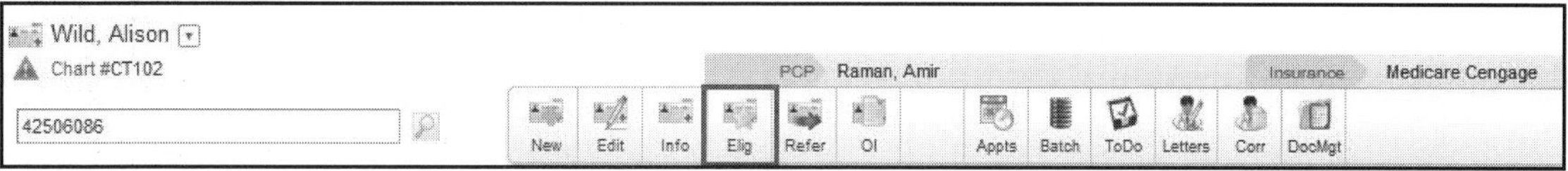

Figure 3-18 Patient Eligibility Button
Courtesy of Optum™ PM and Physician EMR

To Perform an Eligibility Check:

1. Pull patient Alison Wild into context and then click *Elig* on the *Name Bar*. Optum™ PM displays the *Eligibility History* dialog box containing a list of eligibility checks performed for the patient and additional details about the most recent eligibility check. By default, the *Insurance* list displays all active insurances. However, to view the eligibility history for inactive insurances listed under the patient demographics, select the *Show Inactive* checkbox. (**Note:** The insurance information displayed will be different than the insurance information listed in the patient's demographics. This is due to the fact that this is a simulated activity.)
2. To view details of previous eligibility checks, click on a specific line. Click *Print* to print the details if necessary.
3. Click *Elig*. Optum™ PM displays the eligibility details at the bottom of the window. The amount of information sent from an insurance company varies from plan to plan (Figure 3-19). (**Note**: Keep this activity in mind as you complete later activities. Because your student environment is not live, all patients will show as being ineligible when you run an eligibility check.)

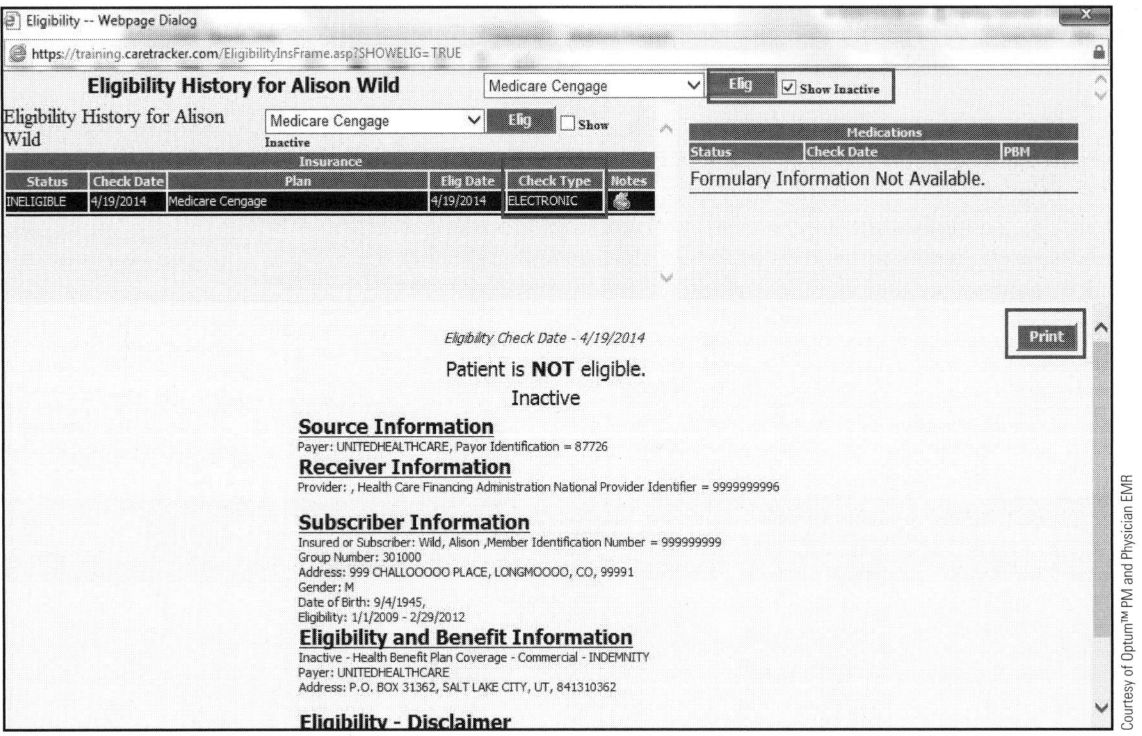

Courtesy of Optum™ PM and Physician EMR

Figure 3-19 Eligibility Check

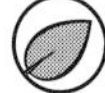 **Print the Eligibility screen, label it "Activity 3-7," and place it in your assignment folder.**

4. Click "X" in the upper right corner to close out of the *Eligibility* screen.

MINI-CASE STUDIES

Case Study 3-1

Repeat Activity 3-1 (Searching for a Patient by Name) for each of the following patients:

a. Alec Winfrey

b. Jim Mcginness

Case Study 3-2

Repeat Activity 3-5 (Edit Patient Demographics) and update *PCP* to the same as the *Group Provider* noted for each of the following patients. Assume that an NPP form has been signed and that requisite consent has been given by each patient.

a. Alec Winfrey

b. Jim Mcginness

Case Study 3-3

Repeat Activity 3-6 (Print the Patient Demographics) for each of the following patients:

a. Alec Winfrey

b. Jim Mcginness

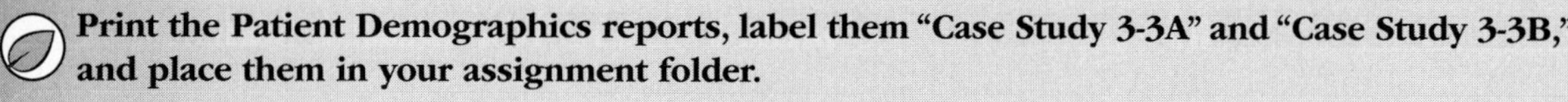

Print the Patient Demographics reports, label them "Case Study 3-3A" and "Case Study 3-3B," and place them in your assignment folder.

Resources

The Optum PM and Physician EMR Help home page represents a wealth of information for the electronic health record (https://training.caretracker.com/help/CareTracker_Help.htm).

National Healthcare Association. (n.d.). *Certified electronic health records specialist (CEHRS™)*. Retrieved from http://www.nhanow.com/health-record.aspx

U.S. Department of Health and Human Services. (n.d.). *Summary of the HIPAA privacy rules*. Retrieved from http://www.hhs.gov/ocr/privacy/hipaa/understanding/summary/

U.S. Department of Health and Human Services, National Institutes of Health. (n.d.). *What health information is protected by the privacy rule?* Retrieved from http://privacyruleandresearch.nih.gov/pr_07.asp

CHAPTER 4

Appointment Scheduling

LEARNING OBJECTIVES

1. Book appointments.
2. Check in patients.
3. Create a batch, accept payments, print patient receipts, run a journal, and post the batch.

NVFHA MANAGER CHALLENGE

Answering the phones and scheduling appointments are two of the most challenging tasks in the medical office. These tasks require an individual who is highly organized, can multitask, and has great communication skills. How you communicate with patients is critical to the practice. Not only are you gathering information concerning a patient's health, you must gather accurate information regarding the patient's insurance so that billing the visit is seamless, and revenue is collected in an expedient manner.

Imagine holding the key to your provider's home and controlling which guests have the authority to enter the home and at what times. In some respects, this is similar to what you do when scheduling appointments. Instead of holding the key to the provider's house, you hold the key to the provider's workplace. However, this is only half of the scenario; you must also be cognizant of the severity of the patient's symptoms, the time constraints that prevent the patient from taking the "next available" appointment, and that you have obtained the necessary information for billing.

Consider the desired characteristics of a scheduler as you practice scheduling patients using Optum™ PM and think of ways this task impacts billing and coding. The first step to being a good scheduler is becoming familiar with the software!

ACTIVITY 4-1: Book an Appointment

Booking appointments in Optum™ PM and Physician EMR takes place in the *Book* application of the *Scheduling* module. Both patient and non-patient appointments (e.g., meetings) are booked in this application. You must have a patient in context in the *Name Bar* to book a patient appointment. Three methods are used to book appointments (Figure 4-1):

- Scheduling directly in *Book*: This allows you to book patient and non-patient appointments by manually moving the schedule to a specific day and clicking on a specific time. You can use the *Book* filters to view the schedule for a specific time, day, location, and provider. Scheduling appointments directly from *Book* gives you the advantage of seeing appointment times that can be double-booked.

- Using *Find*: This allows you to search for the next available appointment time based on specific appointment criteria you set. When searching appointment availability, you can filter your search by provider, location, appointment type, date, day, and time.
- Using *Force*: This allows you to double-book appointments and to book an appointment during a different appointment-type time slot. Forced appointments appear outlined in blue on the schedule.

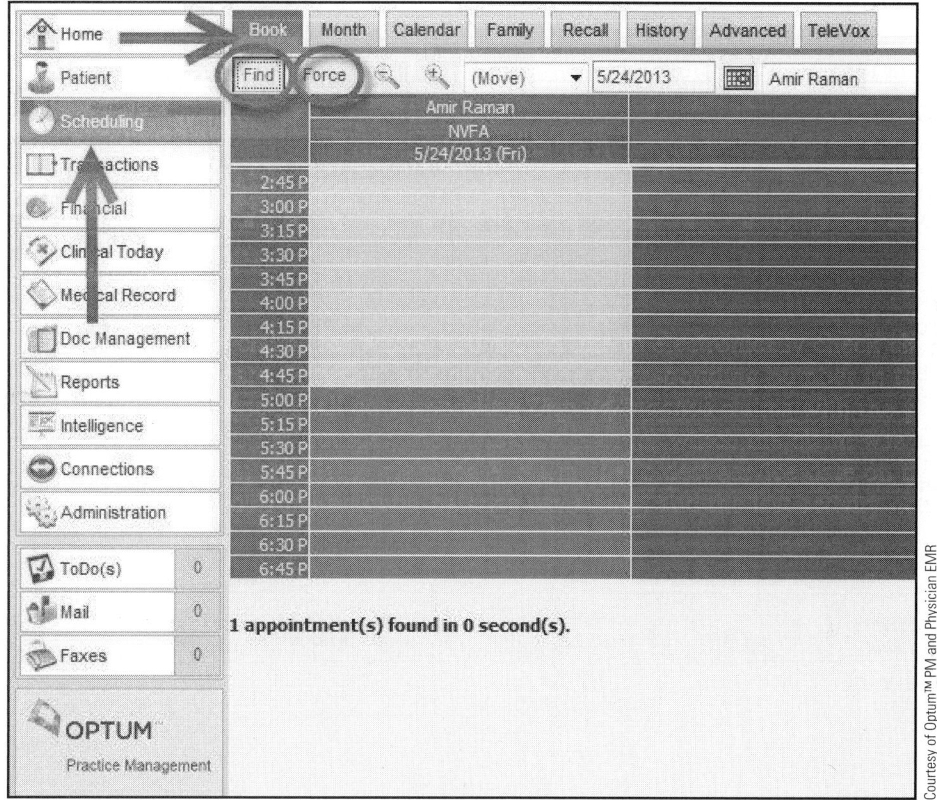

Figure 4-1 Screenshot of Book, Find, Force

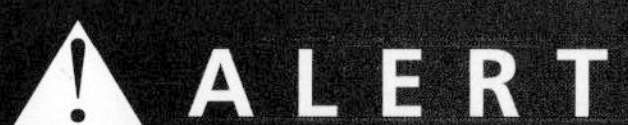

You will need to schedule appointments for Activity 4-1 on today's date. Even though these activities are simulated, you want to avoid booking too far in advance because that would affect future patient visit and billing activities.

To Book an Appointment

1. Using patient data in Table 4-1, schedule an appointment for each patient on today's date.

Table 4-1 Patient Appointments to Be Scheduled

Patient Name / ***Provider***	**Complaint**	**Type of Appointment: Record Date/Time Selected**
Alison Wild / *Dr. Raman*	Urinary symptoms	1st available/Est. Pt. Sick / Date: ________ Time: ________
Alec Winfrey / *Dr. Raman*	Productive cough; shortness of breath	1st available/Est. Pt. Sick / Date: ________ Time: ________
Jim Mcginness / *Dr. Raman*	Back pain, 6 weeks, discuss possible MRI and referral to orthopedist	1st available/Est. Pt. Sick / Date: ________ Time: ________

2. Pull the patient for whom you are booking an appointment into context on the *Name Bar*.
3. Click the *Scheduling* module. Optum™ PM and Physician EMR opens the *Book* application by default.
4. Display the desired date using one of the following options:
   a. Select an option from the *Move* list to display the schedule for specific time increments such as Next Day, Next Week, 2 Months, and so on.
   b. Manually enter a date in MM/DD/YYYY format or click the *Calendar* icon to display the schedule for a specific date.
5. Select the provider, location, and the number of days to display, and then click *Go* (Figure 4-2).

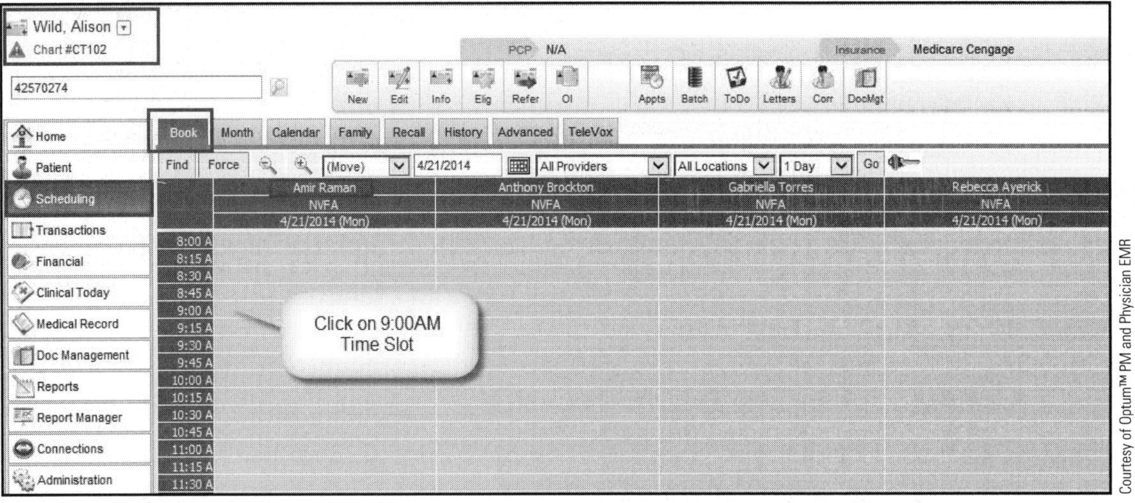

Figure 4-2 Book Appointment for Alison Wild

6. Click on the time slot for which you are booking the appointment. (If the schedule is displayed for multiple providers and locations, be sure to click the time slot in the appropriate column.) The application displays the *Book Appointment* window.

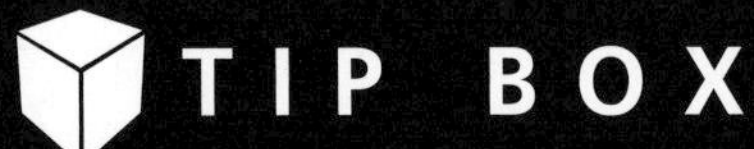

If the patient has existing appointments scheduled, the application displays the *Existing Appointments* window. Click *Book Appointment* at the bottom of the window to book a new appointment.

7. From the *Appointment Type* list, select the appointment type. When you select an appointment type, Optum™ PM and Physician EMR automatically populates the *Task* and *Duration* fields (Figure 4-3).

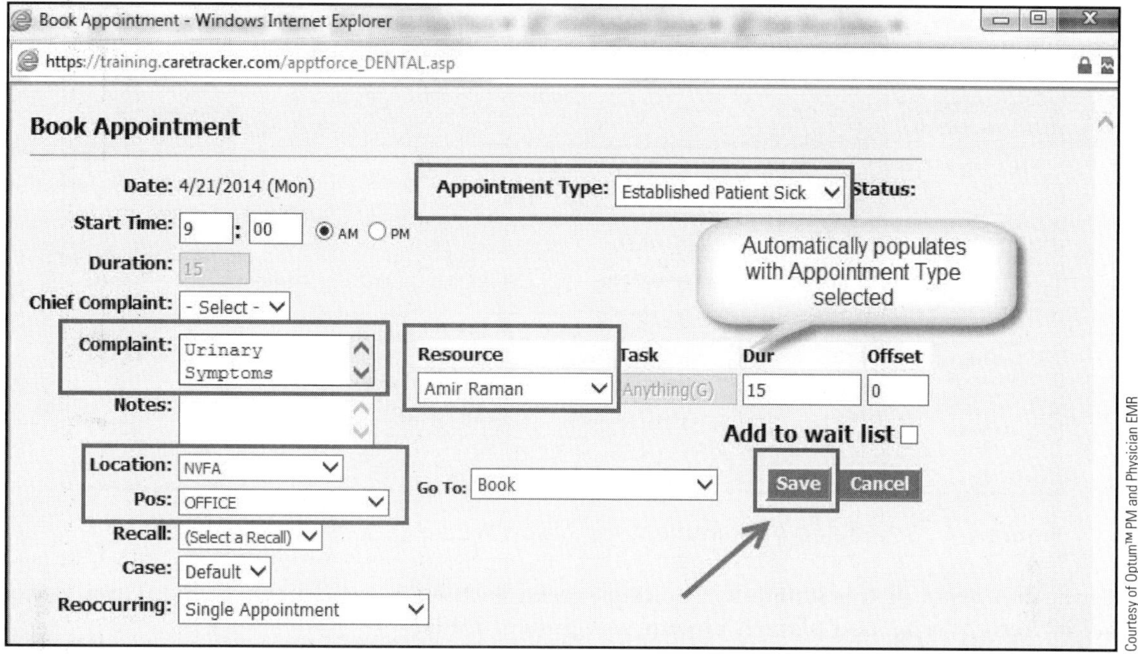

Figure 4-3 Book Appointment Window for Alison Wild

8. From the *Resource* list, select the resource (i.e., provider) needed for the appointment.

9. There are two options for entering a *Chief Complaint* (you can only use one):

   a. From the *Chief Complaint* list, select a chief complaint from the drop-down list. This list is populated with the favorite complaints selected in the *Chief Complaint Maintenance* application in the *Administration* module. (This is not available in your student version. You will use the "free text" option.)

   b. Free text the chief complaint in the *Complaint* box (see Figure 4-3). In the *Complaint* box, enter (free text) the patient's complaint as noted in Table 4-1. (The application will display the complaint in brackets [[ ]] next to the patient's name on the schedule.)

10. In the *Notes* box, enter any notes about the appointment (there are no notes associated with the patients in Table 4-1). (Notes appear in parentheses next to the patient's name on the schedule and also appear when you move your mouse over the appointment on the schedule.)

Do not use any symbols when entering appointment notes or patient complaints. Using symbols will cause an error when you try to print encounter forms.

11. From the *Location* list, select "NVFA."

12. From the *Pos* (Place of Service) list, select "OFFICE."

13. (Optional): To link the appointment to an open recall for the patient, select the recall from the *Recall* list. (Do not link an appointment in this activity.)

14. Click *Save*. The application schedules the appointment (Figure 4-4).

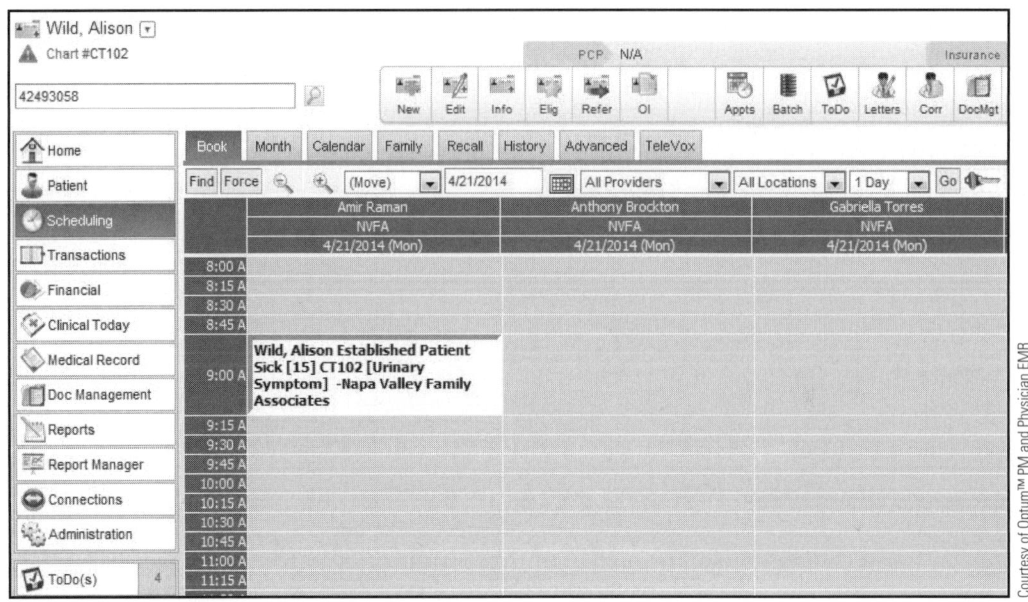

Figure 4-4 Scheduled Appointment for Alison Wild

Print a screenshot of the Schedule/Booking screen with each patient scheduled (from Table 4-1), label it "Activity 4-1," and place it in your assignment folder.

PROFESSIONALISM CONNECTION

At times it may be necessary to double-book appointments. This often occurs during flu season, or when a patient is acutely ill and needs to be seen the day of the appointment request. When this is the case, always check with the provider first. Make certain that the provider is on board with being double-booked. If you are unable to accommodate the patient, weigh all other options before discontinuing the call. Check to see if any other providers are available to see the patient, or when possible, refer the patient to an urgent care facility connected with your organization. Always demonstrate a caring attitude toward the patient, and when unable to accommodate the patient's specific preferences, offer an apology while you work to explore additional options for the patient.

ACTIVITY 4-2: Check In Patient from the Mini-Menu

For a patient encounter to be generated in the electronic medical record (EMR), the patient must be checked in when he or she arrives for an appointment. Checking in a patient changes his or her Optum™ PM and Physician EMR status to "Checked In," and verifies that the patient's billing and demographic information is complete. You can check in a patient in Optum™ PM and Physician EMR in the following places:

- In the *Book* application of the *Scheduling* module, using the mini-menu drop-down feature (Figure 4-5).
- From the *Appts* button in the *Name Bar.*
- From the *Appointment List* on the *Dashboard.*
- From the *Appointment* tab in *Clinical Today*,

To Check In Patient from Mini Menu:

1. Click the *Scheduling* module. Optum™ PM opens the *Book* application by default.
2. With or without the patient in context, move the schedule to display the appointment for the patient you want to check in (check in patient Alison Wild for her appointment scheduled in Activity 4-1). This can be done by manually entering in the date in the *Date* box, by clicking the *Calendar* icon, or by selecting a time period from the *Move* list.
3. Left-click the name of the patient you want to check in and select *Check in* from the mini-menu (see Figure 4-5). Optum™ PM changes the patient's status to "Checked In" and highlights the patient's appointment in green in both the *Book* application and the *Appointment List* in the *Front Office* section of the *Dashboard*. Additionally, Optum™ PM and Physician EMR records the check-in time and displays the patient's wait time in the *Appointment List* (Figure 4-6). Checking in a patient from the mini-menu will pull the patient into context.

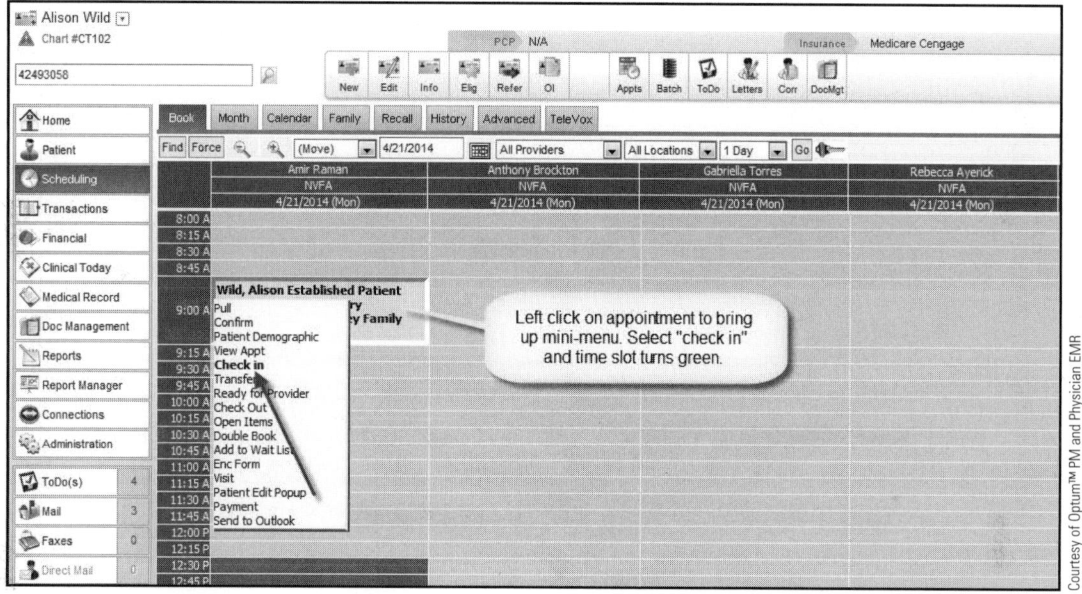

Figure 4-5 Mini-Menu Check-In

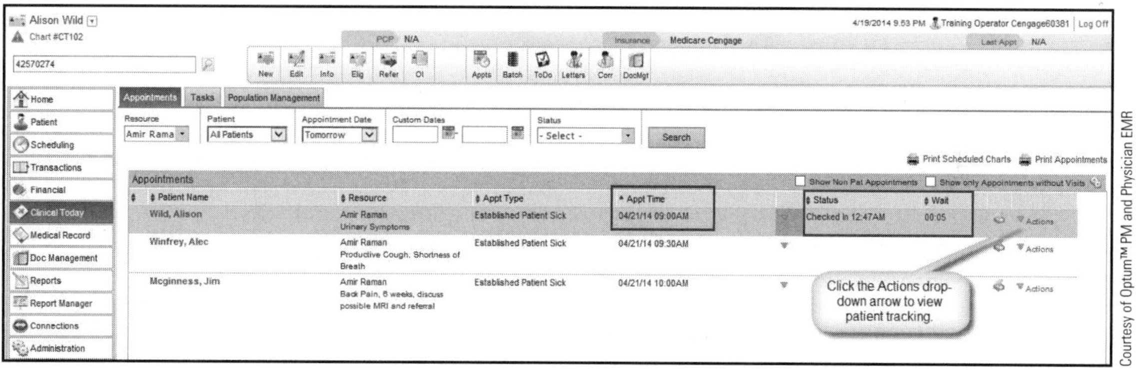

Figure 4-6 Check-In Wait Time

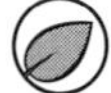

Print a screenshot of the Schedule screen with the patient checked in, label it "Activity 4-2," and place it in your assignment folder.

ACTIVITY 4-3: Setting Operator Preferences

The *Batch* application is used for setting defaults for both "Financial" and "Clinical" components. The "Financial" portion of the batch establishes defaults and assigns a name to a batch (group) of financial transactions you will be entering into Optum™ PM and Physician EMR. A new financial batch is created daily to enter financial transactions into Optum™ PM and Physician EMR, for example, charges, payments, and adjustments. This helps identify transactions linked to the batch, the date of each transaction, and the operator who entered it into the system. Setting up the financial batch helps identify a group of charges or payments and helps run reports to balance against the actual charges or payments entered.

The "Clinical" batch settings are typically set up only once and are used to set preferences and pre-populate fields common to your workflow (Figure 4-7). The "Clinical" batch settings are in the middle and lower sections of the *Operator Encounter Batch Control* dialog box. Setting the defaults here can speed up scheduling by having default *Resource* and *Location* defined.

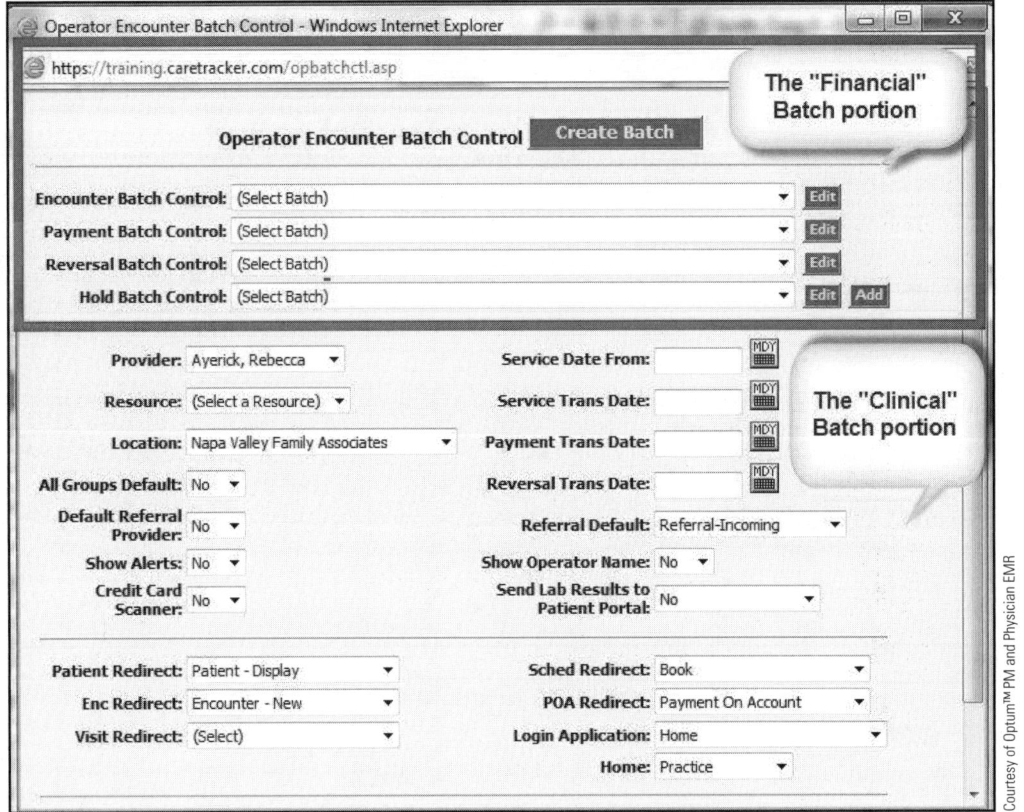

Figure 4-7 Financial and Clinical Components of a Batch

The first time you log in to Optum™ you will be prompted to create a batch. Activities related to searching for a patient or scheduling a patient do not require that a batch be created. For the activities related to financial and clinical, you will need to have a batch open. The *Batch* application enables you to set up operator preferences based on the workflow for your role. This reduces the number of clicks required to get from one application to the other, making navigation through Optum™ PM and Physician EMR easy.

To To Set Operator Preferences:

1. With no patient in context, click *Batch* on the *Name Bar*. Optum™ PM and Physician EMR displays the *Operator Encounter Batch Control* dialog box.

2. By default, Optum™ PM and Physician EMR assigns redirects, making it easy to navigate from different applications within Optum™ PM and Physician EMR. The default redirects are based on the most commonly used workflow.
3. Click *Edit* if the fields are grayed out. Otherwise, enter (or confirm if already populated) the information, following the instructions for the available redirects described in Table 4-2. These are located in the lower section of *the Operator Encounter Batch Control* dialog box (Figure 4-8).

Table 4-2 Batch Redirects

Redirects	
Field	**Description**
Patient Redirect	Launches the selected application after editing a *Demographic* record in the *Patient* module. You can also change this setting in the *Demographic* application if necessary. (Select "Patient – Display.")
Enc Redirect	Launches the selected application after saving a *Charge* in the *Transactions* module. (Select "Encounter – New.")
Visit Redirect	Launches the selected application after a visit is saved in the *Visit* application. (Select "(Select).")
Sched Redirect	Launches the selected application after an appointment is booked via the *Book* application of the *Scheduling* module. (Select "Book.")
POA (Payment on Account) Redirect	Launches the selected application after a payment is entered via the *Pmt on Acct* application of the *Transactions* module. (Select "Payment On Account.")
Login Application	Launches the selected application when you log in to Optum™ PM and Physician EMR. (Select "Home.")
Home	If the *Login Application* is set to "Home," you can select which *Home* module application to display by default; for example, the *Management, Meaningful Use, Messages,* or *News* applications. (Select "Practice.")
Click *Save*	Screen will be saved with selections made.

Courtesy of Optum™ PM and Physician EMR

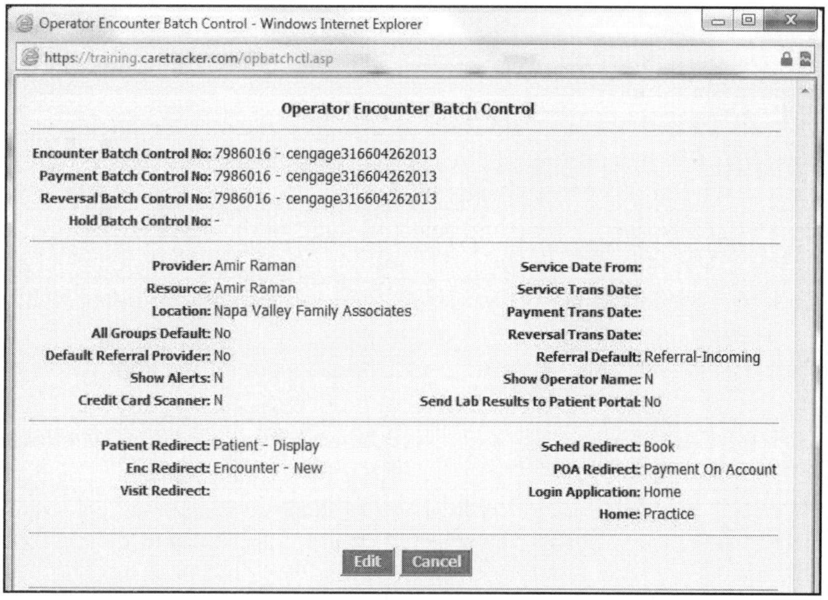

Operator Encounter Batch Control - Windows Internet Explorer
https://training.caretracker.com/opbatchctl.asp

Operator Encounter Batch Control

Encounter Batch Control No: 7986016 - cengage316604262013
Payment Batch Control No: 7986016 - cengage316604262013
Reversal Batch Control No: 7986016 - cengage316604262013
Hold Batch Control No: -

Provider: Amir Raman
Resource: Amir Raman
Location: Napa Valley Family Associates
All Groups Default: No
Default Referral Provider: No
Show Alerts: N
Credit Card Scanner: N
Service Date From:
Service Trans Date:
Payment Trans Date:
Reversal Trans Date:
Referral Default: Referral-Incoming
Show Operator Name: N
Send Lab Results to Patient Portal: No

Patient Redirect: Patient - Display
Enc Redirect: Encounter - New
Visit Redirect:
Sched Redirect: Book
POA Redirect: Payment On Account
Login Application: Home
Home: Practice

Edit Cancel

Courtesy of Optum™ PM and Physician EMR

Figure 4-8 Operator Encounter Batch Control

Print a screenshot of the Operator Encounter Batch Control screen, label it "Activity 4-3," and place it in your assignment folder.

ACTIVITY 4-4: Create a Batch

Having set up your operator preferences in the *Operator Encounter Batch Control* in Activity 4-3 and with the dialog box in display, you will now create a batch. Reference the instructions and fields in Table 4-3 as you complete your batch details.

Table 4-3 Batch Details, Field and Instructions

Batch Details	
Field	**Instructions**
Provider	From the *Provider* list, select the name of the billing provider associated with the batch. **Note:** The *Admissions* application accessed via the *Dashboard* and the *Charges* application in the *Transactions* module displays the billing provider set up in the batch.
Resource	From the *Resource* list, select the servicing provider. In most instances, the billing provider and the resource are the same. **Note:** The *Book* application in the *Scheduling* module and the *Appointment* application in the *Clinical Today* module display the resource set up in the batch.
Location	From the *Location* list, select the location associated with the batch. **Note:** The *Admissions* application accessed via the *Dashboard* and the *Book* application in the *Scheduling* module displays the location set up in the batch.
All Groups Default	By default, the *All Groups Default* list is set to "No." Change the list to "Yes" if necessary. This displays patient financial information for the current group or all groups in the practice based on the setting selected. If "Yes" is selected, you can only see the financial transactions for the groups that you have access to as an operator. This setting mostly benefits multi-group practices and also determines the default value in the *Open Items* application of the *Financial* module and *Edit* application of the *Transactions* module.
Default Referral Provider	By default, the *Default Referral Provider* list is set to "No." Change the field to "Yes" if there is no referring provider in the patient's demographics or if there is no active referral/authorization for the patient. This sets the billing provider as the referring provider.
Show Alerts	In the *Show Alerts* field, select "Yes" to enable Optum™ PM to display the *Patient Alert* window; otherwise select "No." The *Patient Alerts* window notifies users when key information is missing from a patient's demographics or when there are other issues with a patient's account.
Credit Card Scanner	The *Credit Card Scanner* field is set to *"No"* by default. Your student version of Optum™ will NOT have this feature. In a real practice setting, select *"Yes"* if your group uses a credit card scanner to process payments by credit card.
Service Date From	Click the *Calendar* MDY icon and select the start of the service dates included in the batch.
Service Trans Date	Click the *Calendar* MDY icon and select the service transaction date included in the batch.
Payment Trans Date	Click the *Calendar* icon MDY and select the payment transactions date included in the batch.
Reversal Trans Date	Click the *Calendar* icon MDY and select the reversal transactions date included in the batch.
Referral Default	By default, the *Referral Default* list is set to "Referral-Incoming." Select a referral type based on your practice specialty. The selected option will display as the default option when the *Ref/Auth* application is accessed via the *Name Bar* or *Patient* module.
Show Operator Name	Select "Yes" to display the operator's name on the Optum™ PM and Physician EMR interface. Select "No" if you do not want the operator's name displayed.
Click *Save*. The batch information is saved.	
Note: Click *Edit* to make changes if necessary.	
Click "X" on the right-hand corner to close the dialog box.	

Courtesy of Optum™ PM and Physician EMR

To Create a Batch:

1. Click *Edit*, and then click *Create Batch*. The *Batch Master* dialog box displays (Figure 4-9).

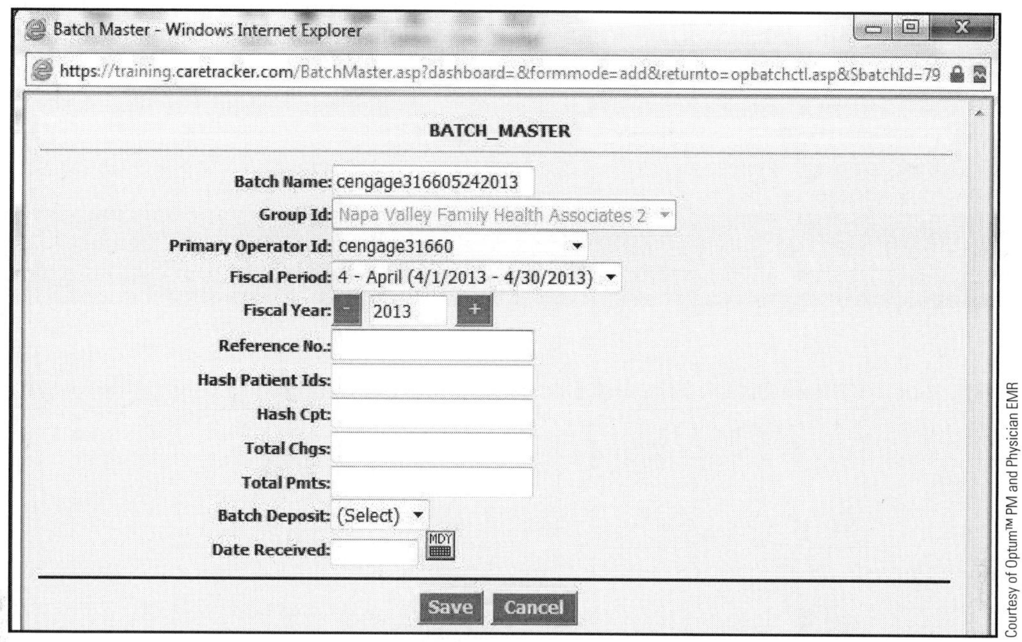

Figure 4-9 Batch Master Dialog Box

2. By default, the *Batch Name* field displays a batch identification name. The name consists of your username followed by the current date. (**Note:** You can edit the batch name if necessary to identify the types of financial transactions associated with the batch; for example," copayment5132014.") Do not use symbols when editing the name. Name this Batch "Copayment" (Figure 4-10).

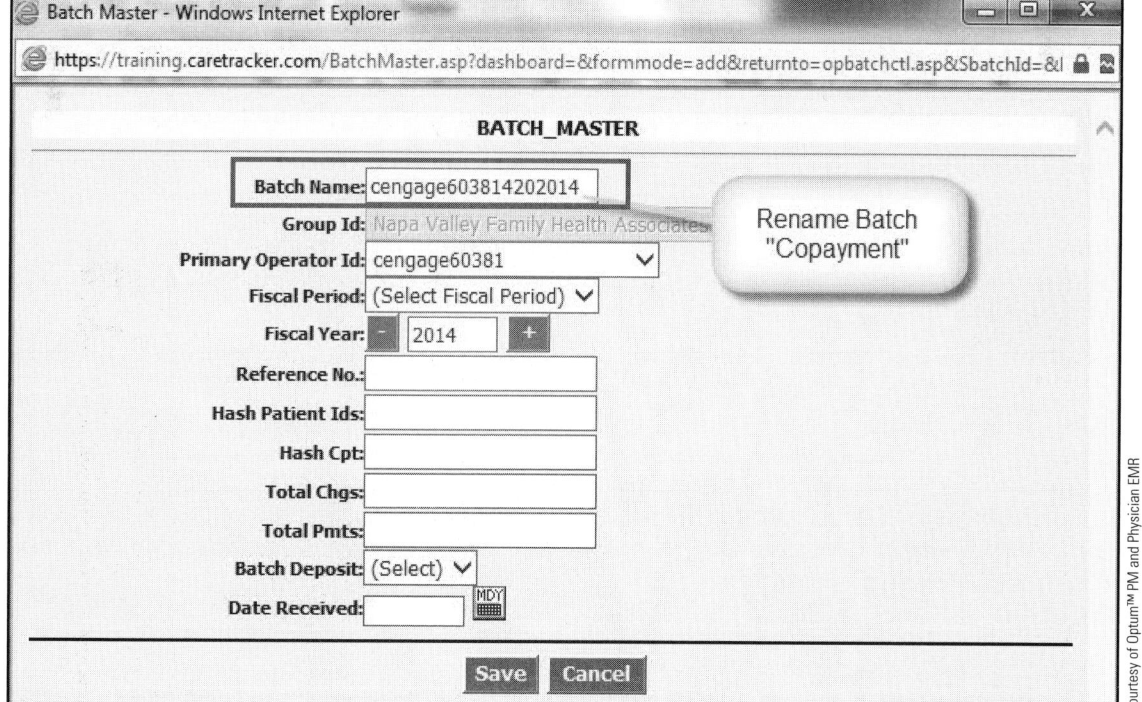

Figure 4-10 Rename Batch Copayment

3. By default, the *Group Id* displays the name of your group.
4. By default, the *Primary Operator Id* displays your username.
5. In the *Fiscal Period* list, click the period (period/year/month) in which you scheduled patients in Activity 4-1 to post related financial transactions. The list will only display fiscal periods that are currently open. If the desired *Fiscal Period* does not display or no *Fiscal Period* displays, you must open the period to continue creating your batch.

TIP BOX

To open a fiscal period, click the *Administration* module and then click the *Open/Close Period* link in the *Financial* section under *System Administration*. Select the period/year/month you want to open by selecting "OPEN" under *Status*, and then clicking *Save*.

6. By default, the *Fiscal Year* displays the current financial year set up for your company.
7. (Optional – Leave Blank) In the *Hash Patient Ids* box, enter the sum of all patient Optum™ PM and Physician EMR ID numbers pertaining to the charges associated with the batch. This is to ensure that a charge is entered for all patients associated with the batch. (**Note:** In a live practice, the biller would utilize this feature when entering charges.)
8. (Optional – Leave Blank) In the *Hash Cpt* box, enter the sum of all CPT® codes pertaining to the charges associated with the batch. This is to ensure that a charge is entered for all procedures. Example: If two patients are seen for the day, and the CPT® codes selected on the encounter form for the first patient are 71101 and 99213, and for the second patient are 71101 and 99203, calculate the *Hash CPT* by adding 71101 + 99213 + 71101 + 99203 = 340618. (**Note:** In a live practice, the biller would utilize this feature when entering charges.)
9. (Optional – Leave Blank) In the *Total Chgs* box, enter the sum of all charges that are associated with the batch. (**Note:** In a live practice, the biller would utilize this feature when entering charges.)
10. (Optional – Leave Blank) In the *Total Pmts* box, enter the sum of check(s) that are associated with the batch. (**Note:** In a live practice, the biller would utilize this feature when entering payments.)
11. (Optional – Leave Blank) In the *Batch Deposit* list, select the *Deposit ID* to link to a deposit number, if using the *Batch Deposit* application. (This feature is not active in your student version.) (**Note:** In a live practice, the biller would utilize this feature when entering payments.)
12. In the *Date Received* box, enter the date the encounter was received in MM/DD/YYYY format or click the *Calendar* MDY icon and select the date. (Leave Blank.)
13. Click *Save*. Optum™ PM and Physician EMR displays the *Operator Encounter Batch Control* dialog box with the new batch information (Figure 4-11).
14. Now, further edit your batch by updating the provider, resource, location, and so on (the middle section of the *Operator Encounter Batch Control* box). Select the *Provider* (Amir Raman), *Resource* (Amir Raman), and *Location* (Napa Valley Family Associates).
15. Click *Save*.
16. Write down your "Encounter Batch Control No." for future reference. (Should include "Copayment")
______________________________.

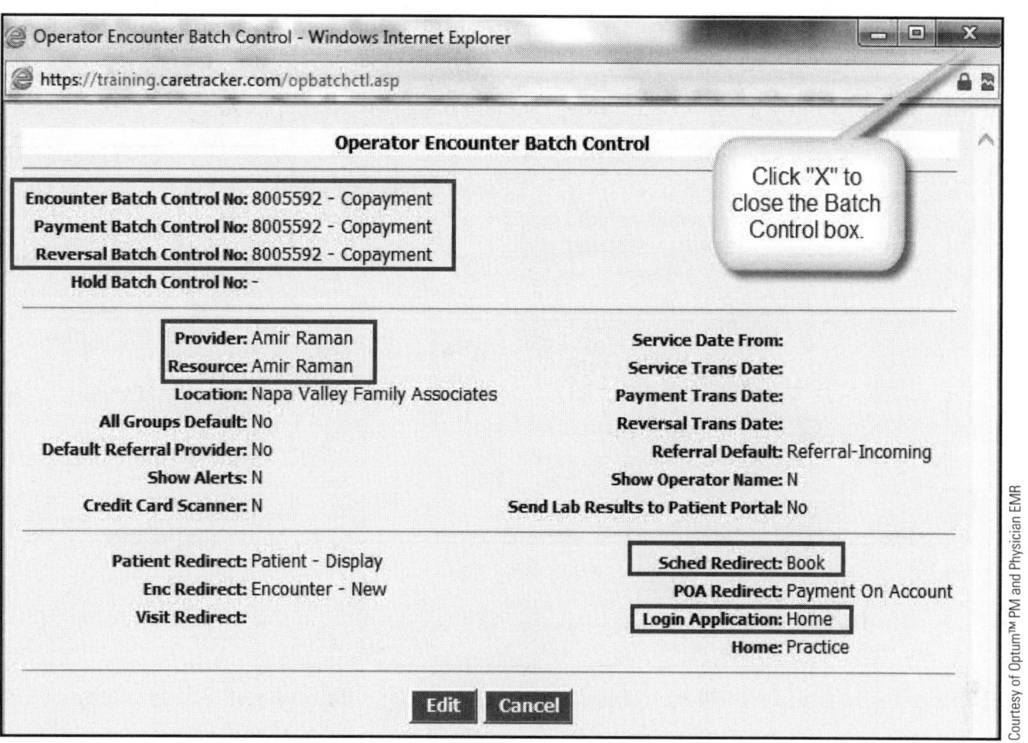

Figure 4-11 Operator Encounter Batch Control Dialog Box

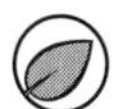

Print a screenshot of the Batch screen, label it "Activity 4-4," and place it in your assignment folder.

17. Click "X" in the top right-hand corner to close the dialog box.

ACTIVITY 4-5: Accept/Enter a Payment

The *Payments On Account (Pmt on Acc)* application is used to record patient payments. Typically you will accept a patient's copayment at the check-in process. A copayment is a predetermined (flat) fee that an individual pays for health care services in addition to what the insurance covers. For example, some health maintenance organizations (HMOs) require a $10 "copayment" for each office visit, regardless of the type or level of services provided during the visit. Copayments are not usually specified by percentages. You can access the *Payments on Account* application from the following locations within practice management:

- *Scheduling* module > *Book* tab > left-click on the patient's appointment in the schedule to display Scheduling Mini-Menu > Select *Payment* link
- *Name Bar* > *Appts* button > *Actions* menu > *Payment* link
- *Transactions* module > *Pmt on Acct* tab
- *Transactions* module > *Charge* tab

1. Pull patient Alec Winfrey into context.
2. In the *Transactions* module, click on the *Pmt on Acct* tab.
3. From the drop-down list at the top of the screen, select whether the payment is being made by the *Patient* or *Responsible Party*. (Select *Patient*.)

4. If a patient is paying a portion of his or her balance, enter the dollar amount of the payment in the *Amount* box. (Enter "$35.00.")

   (**Note:** If the patient is paying his or her entire balance, click *Pay Bal.* Optum™ PM and Physician EMR automatically pulls the patient's balance into the *Amount* box.)

5. From the *Payment Type* list, select the payment method. (Select "Payment – Patient Check.") (**Note:** If the payment type is credit card, you would select the *Process Credit Card* checkbox.)
6. If the payment method is a check, enter the check number in the *Reference #* box (Enter "2014" as the check number.) The reference number will print on the patient's receipt.
7. From the *Method* list, select how to apply the payment to the patient's account:
   a. If you are collecting a copayment for a patient who does not have an outstanding balance, select "Force Unapplied." Optum™ PM and Physician EMR creates an unapplied balance for the patient that is applied to the patient's private pay balance when his or her charges are saved. (Select "Force Unapplied" and check the *Copay?* box.)
8. In the *Trans. Date* box, enter the transaction date to which you want to link the payment. (Select the date of the financial batch you created.) This date will pre-populate if you selected the date in your batch defaults.
9. (FYI Only) If you want to override the copayment amount recorded in the patient's demographic record for a specific appointment:
   a. Select the *Copay?* checkbox. (**Note:** This field is selected by default when an appointment is linked to the payment.)
   b. In the *Appt* box, select the appointment date to which the copay applies.

TIP BOX

The *Plan Name* and *Copay Amt* fields display the insurance plan and copay amount saved in the patient's demographics, if applicable. These fields are read-only.

10. The *Go To* field defaults to the redirect option selected in the operator's batch. You can select a different option if needed (Figure 4-12). (Select "Payment on Account.")

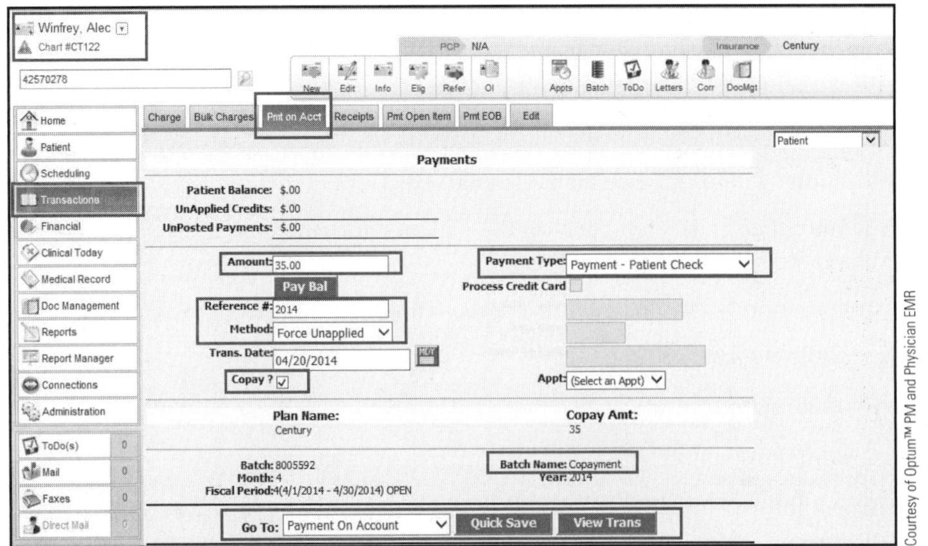

Figure 4-12 Enter Payment on Account

TIP BOX

To view a summary of the transaction prior to saving (Figure 4-13), click *View Trans.*

Figure 4-13 View Transaction

11. Click *Quick Save*. Optum™ PM and Physician EMR saves the payment information and launches the application selected in the *Go To* field (see Figure 4-12).
12. You can view the payment in the *Open Batch* field under *Billing* on the *Dashboard* (Figure 4-14).

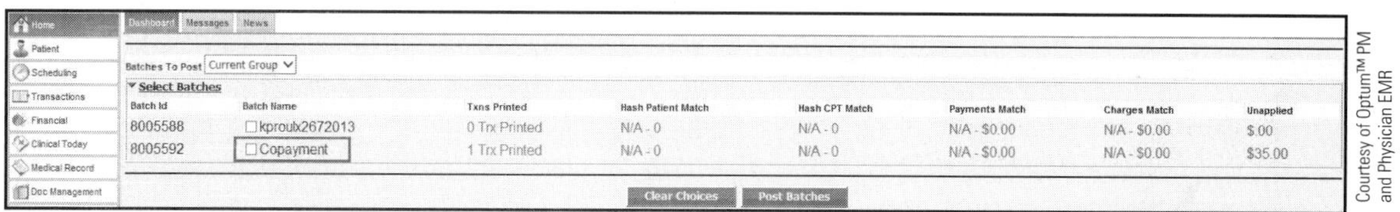

Figure 4-14 Open Batches

You will later print a receipt from the Receipts tab in the Transactions module (Activity 4-6).

PROFESSIONALISM CONNECTION

Some patients feel that medicine and money should never mix; however, a medical office is a business and must conduct itself as such. This means that collecting the copayment prior to the visit makes the most business sense. Once the appointment is completed, the services have been rendered and the patient may not be as willing to meet his or her financial obligations. When possible, the collection of payments should be performed outside of the reception area; however, when this is not possible, the collection of payments should be handled in a discreet manner. You may use a phrase such as the following: "Mrs. Barrett, what method of payment will you be using today to meet your copayment requirement?" This sentence illustrates that payment is expected, but you are willing to work with the patient by accepting a mode of payment that works best for her.

ACTIVITY 4-6: Print Patient Receipts

Having entered the payment information in Activity 4-5, now print a receipt from the *Receipts* tab in the *Transactions* module. Receipts in Optum™ PM and Physician EMR identify a patient's previous balance, the activity of charges and payments for that date of service, and the new patient balance.

1. With the patient in context (Alec Winfrey), click the *Transactions* module.
2. When the *Transactions* module opens, click on the *Receipts* tab.
3. From the drop-down list at the top of the screen, select who you would like to view the receipt from, *Patient* or *Responsible Party*. (Select *Patient*.)
4. Select the date of service for which you need to print a receipt from the *Receipts* list. (Select the date of the payment received, which should also be the same date as your batch.)
5. When a date of service is selected, the receipt displays on the screen.
6. Click on the *Print* button (Figure 4-15), or right-click on the receipt.
   a. When you right-click, a gray pop-up menu appears. Select *Print*, and the receipt will print.

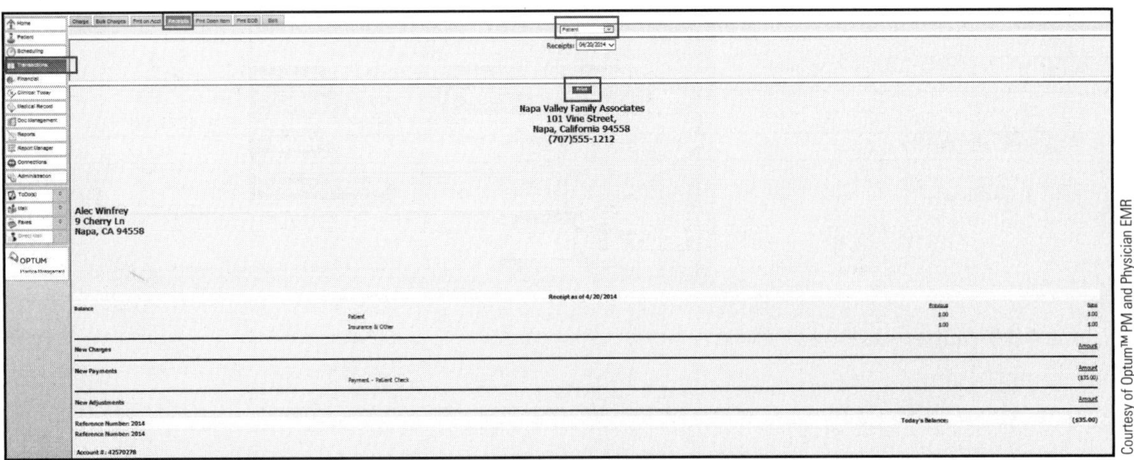

Figure 4-15 Print Patient Receipt

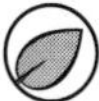 **Print the Patient Receipt, label it "Activity 4-6," and place it in your assignment folder.**

ACTIVITY 4-7: Run a Journal

Now that you have entered copayments, you will complete the process by running a journal and posting your batch as your end-of-day workflow. You must run a journal prior to posting your batch (Activity 4-8) to verify that you have entered all the financial transactions correctly in Optum™ PM and Physician EMR. Journals provide a summary of financial transactions, for example, charges, payments, and adjustments.

It is important to identify and correct any errors before a batch is posted. Once a batch has been posted, the transactions linked to it are locked in the system and must be reversed to be corrected. Posted errors can only be corrected by reversing the transaction on the patient's account, which occurs in the *Edit* application of the *Transactions* module. It is highly recommended that you run a journal to make sure that your transactions balance for the day is correct before posting your batch. Posted batches are accessible any time so you can always access an old journal from the *Historical Journals* link (Figure 4-16) under the *Financial Reports* section of the *Reports* application, which alleviates the need to save paper copies of journals.

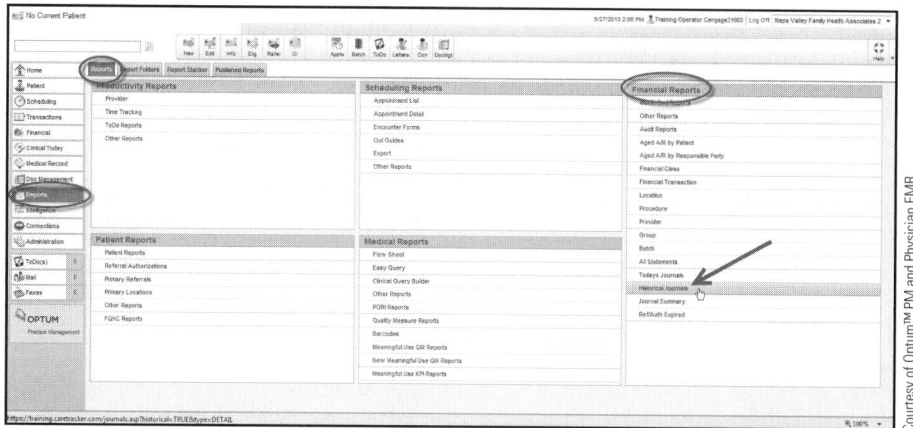

Courtesy of Optum™ PM and Physician EMR

Figure 4-16 Historical Journals Link

To Run a Journal:

1. Click the *Reports* module.
2. Click the *Todays Journals* link under the *Financial Reports* section (Figure 4-17). Optum™ displays the *Todays Journal Options* screen (see Figure 4-18). All of your group's open batches are listed in the *Todays Batches* box.

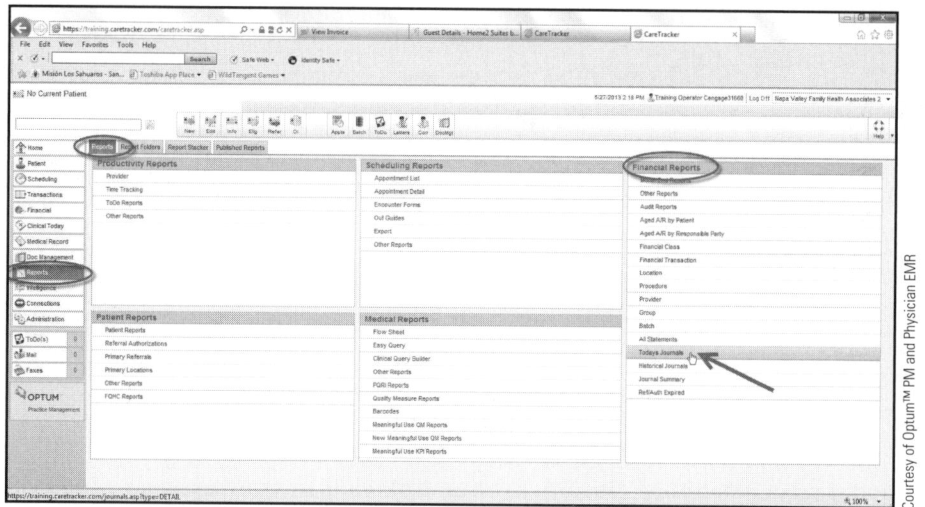

Courtesy of Optum™ PM and Physician EMR

Figure 4-17 Todays Journals Link

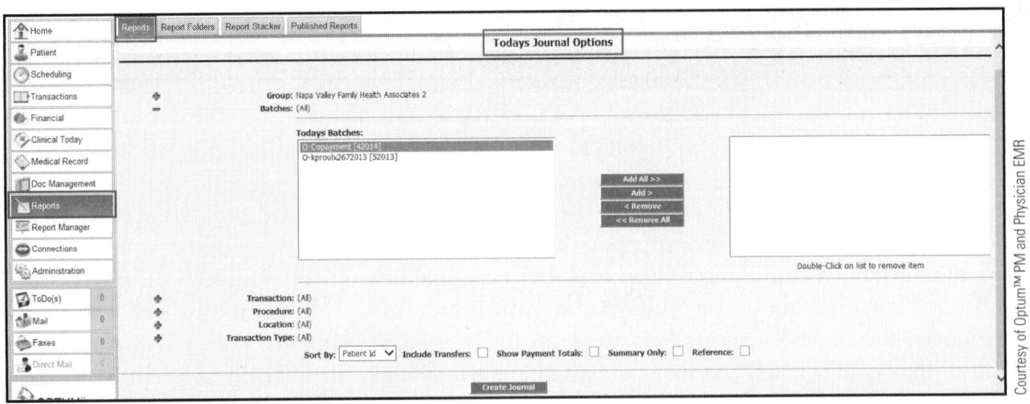

Figure 4-18 Todays Journal Options

3. Select a batch to include in the journal either by double-clicking on the batch name or by clicking on the batch and then clicking *Add* (Figure 4-19). Optum™ PM and Physician EMR adds the selected batches to the box on the right. (Add batch "Copayment.")
4. From the *Sort By* list drop-down, select "Entry Date."
5. Select the *Show Payment Totals* checkbox (Figure 4-19).

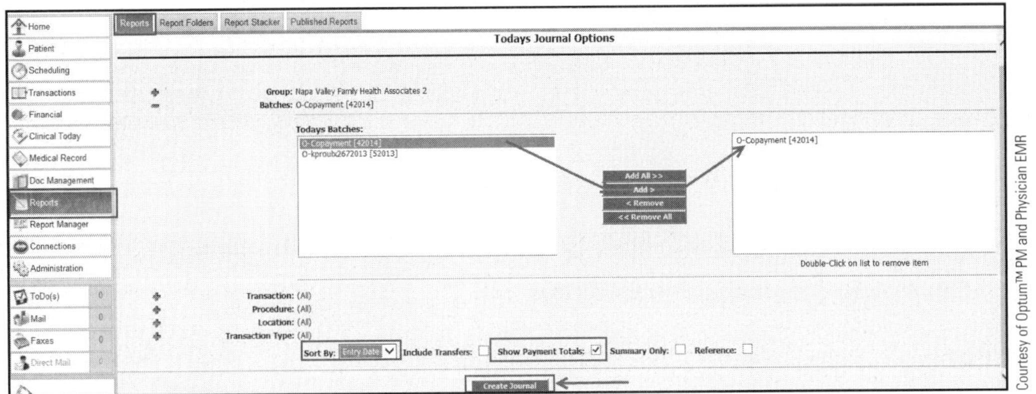

Figure 4-19 Select a Batch for the Journal

6. Click *Create Journal*. Optum™ PM generates the journal (Figure 4-20).

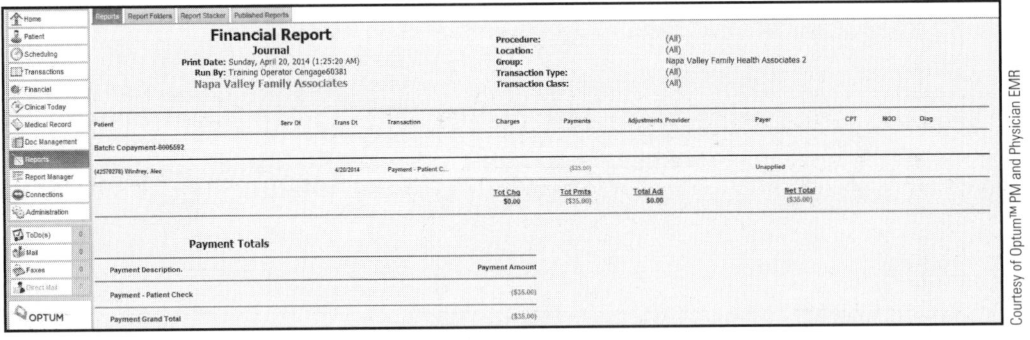

Figure 4-20 Journal

7. To print, right-click on the journal and select *Print* from the shortcut menu.

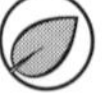 **Print the Journal screen, label it "Activity 4-7," and place it in your assignment folder.**

ACTIVITY 4-8: Post a Batch

1. Click the *Administration* module. The application opens the *Practice* tab.
2. Click the *Post* link under the *Daily Administration* > *Financial* header (Figure 4-21). Optum™ PM displays a list of all open batches for the group.

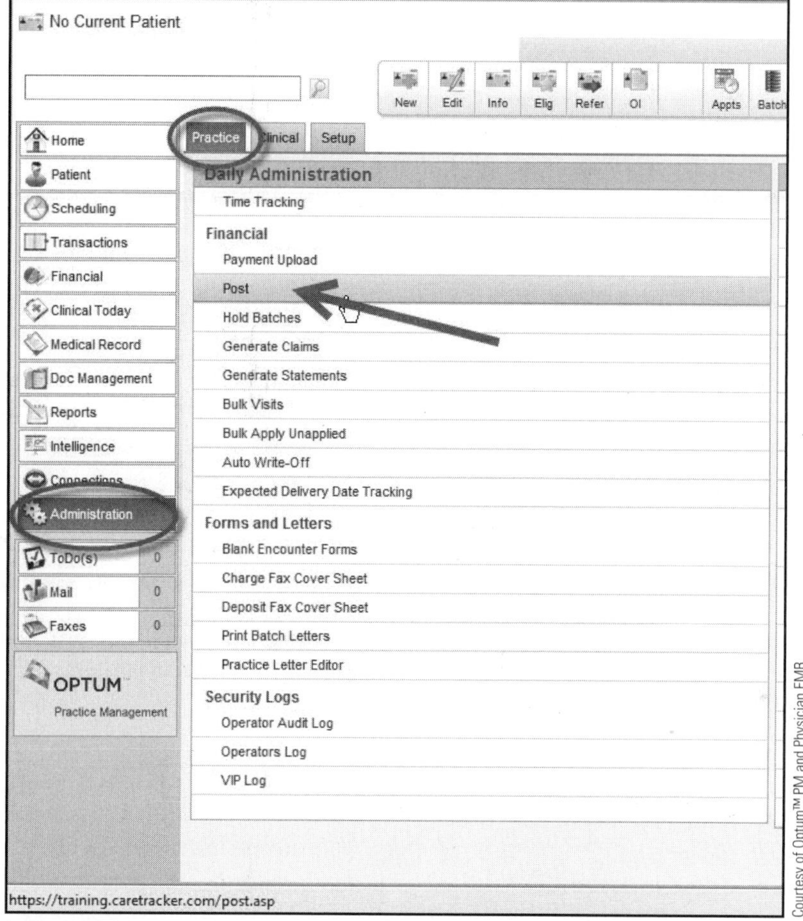

Figure 4-21 Post Link

3. Select the checkbox next to the batch you want to post. (Select batch "Copayment.")

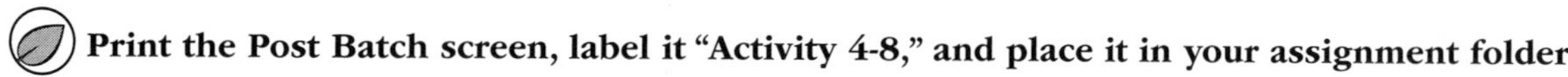
Print the Post Batch screen, label it "Activity 4-8," and place it in your assignment folder.

4. Click *Post Batches* (Figure 4-22).

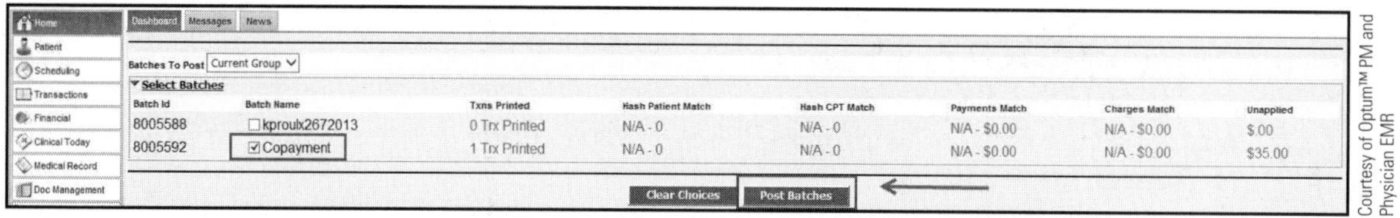

Figure 4-22 Post Batches

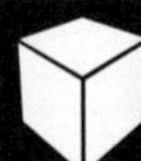

TIP BOX

- Although not required, it is recommended to only post a batch after a journal has been generated and balances verified.
- As a best practice, you should close out your batch at the end of each day; however, wait until instructed to do so in a particular activity in this text.
- All transactions must be posted before running any *Month End* report in Optum™, and *Periods* cannot be closed with open batches linked to them.
- A password may be required to post a co-worker's batch.

MINI-CASE STUDIES

Case Study 4-1

Repeat Activity 4-2 (Check In Patient from the Mini-Menu) for each of the following patients. They all had appointments scheduled earlier in the chapter:

a. Alec Winfrey

b. Jim Mcginness

Print a screenshot of the Schedule screen showing that each patient has been checked in, label it "Case Study 4-1," and place it in your assignment folder.

Case Study 4-2

Repeat Activity 4-5 (Accept/Enter a Payment) for patient Jim Mcginness, who had an appointment scheduled earlier in the chapter. Create a new batch and name it "CaseStudyCh4." Enter the copay amount that is entered in Jim's patient demographics screen ($35.00, paid by Check #5513).

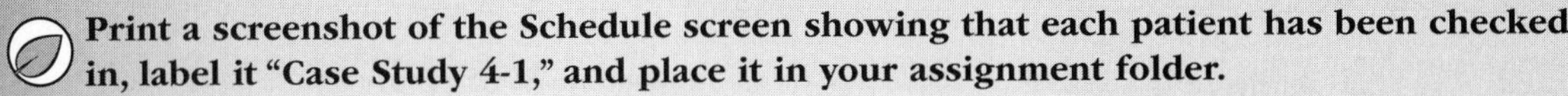

NVFHA MANAGER CHALLENGE

In a hurry, the check-in desk did not confirm Jim's demographic information or scan a copy of his current insurance card. Jim's employer changed to a new health insurance plan, BC/BS of California (ID #BCBS987) on the first day of last month. His new copay is $20.00. Keep this in mind and think about how the erroneous copayment will affect the billing function in later activities.

Case Study 4-3

Repeat Activity 4-6 (Print Patient Receipts) for patient Jim Mcginness.

Print a receipt for Jim Mcginness, label it "Case Study 4-3," and place it in your assignment folder.

(*Continues*)

MINI-CASE STUDIES (*Continued*)

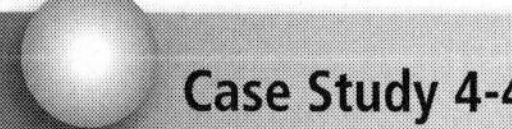

Case Study 4-4

Repeat Activity 4-7 (Run a Journal) for the "CaseStudyCh4" batch created in Case Study 4-2.

Print a screenshot of the Journal screen, label it "Case Study 4-4," and place it in your assignment folder.

Case Study 4-5

Repeat Activity 4-8 (Post a Batch) for the "CaseStudyCh4" batch created in Case Study 4-2.

Print a screenshot of the Post Batch screen, label it "Case Study 4-5," and place it in your assignment folder.

Resources

The Optum PM and Physician EMR Help homepage represents a wealth of information for the electronic health record (https://training.caretracker.com/help/CareTracker_Help.htm).

National Healthcare Association. (n.d.). *Certified Electronic Health Records Specialist (CEHRS™)*. Retrieved from http://www.nhanow.com/health-record.aspx

CHAPTER 5

Preliminary Duties in the EMR and Patient Work-Up

LEARNING OBJECTIVES

1. Review recorded training in Help regarding meaningful use and its stages, including tools within Optum™ PM and Physician EMR that assist with viewing and reading the Meaningful Use dashboard.
2. Activate the care management registries in Optum™ PM and Physician EMR.
3. List major applications of the Clinical Today module.
4. Set operator preferences in your Batch application.
5. View daily appointments in Clinical Today.
6. Perform check-in duties and track patients throughout their visits.
7. Retrieve the patient's EMR and update sections within the patient medical history panes.
8. Update the Patient Care Management application.
9. Create and print a Progress Note.

NVFHA MANAGER CHALLENGE

Although this workbook focuses primarily on billing and coding functions, it is important to have an understanding of all administrative and clinical duties a medical assistant may be tasked with. Clinical medical assistants in our practice are responsible for ascertaining that all patients are up to date on preventive testing and health maintenance goals. This means that a clinical medical assistant will be responsible for going through the patient's chart prior to the appointment and reviewing the patient's immunization status to determinine whether the patient needs testing such as a mammogram or colonoscopy, for having a plan ready, and discussing that plan with the patient during the visit (referred to as care management). Often, patients will decline testing due to scheduling constraints, but your job is to create goals that are attainable. Do you think you have what it takes to be a health care advocate? How can you, as a medical coder and biller, be a part of the team that delivers quality patient care?

Electronic Medical Records

In the first four chapters, you learned a great deal about Optum™ PM—the practice management side of the Optum™ software. This chapter introduces you to Optum™ EMR—a fully integrated, CCHIT®-certified, cloud-based EHR solution guaranteed to help providers meet meaningful use requirements. This chapter focuses on the utilization of EMRs in ambulatory care settings. For providers to obtain full reimbursement from governmental agencies such as Medicare and Medicaid, they must be in full compliance with specific guidelines set forth by those agencies.

EMRs have been in use for the past couple of decades, but their widespread adoption has skyrocketed in the past few years. This is largely due to Medicare and Medicaid financial incentives offered by the federal government for practices that meet meaningful use as well as the penalties that will take place later in the decade for not instituting EMR.

CLINICAL SPOTLIGHT

Meaningful Use

Meaningful use is the way in which electronic health record (EHR) technologies must be implemented and used for a provider to be eligible for the EHR Incentive Programs and to qualify for incentive payments. These incentives specify three components of meaningful use:

- The use of a certified EHR in a meaningful manner
- The use of certified EHR technology for electronic exchange of health information to improve quality of health care
- The use of certified EHR technology to submit clinical quality and other measures

The purpose of meaningful use is not only to institute the adoption of EMRs, but to ascertain that practices use their EHR software to its fullest. Benefits of meaningful use include complete and accurate medical records, better access to information, and patient empowerment. One of the major goals of meaningful use is to make medical records interoperable so that immediate access can be given to any provider who works with the patient. Three stages are associated with meaningful use.

Stage 1: Data Capture and Sharing Stage. This stage focuses on the following:

- Electronic capturing of health information in a coded format
- Using electronically captured health information to track key clinical conditions and communicate information for care coordination purposes
- Implementing clinical decision support tools to facilitate disease and medication management
- Reporting information for quality improvement and public health information

Stage 2: Advance Clinical Processes. This stage focuses on expanding on Stage 1 criteria to encourage the use of health information technology (HIT) for continuous quality improvement at the point of care and the exchange of health information in the most structured format possible. Criteria for Stage 2 include:

- More rigorous health information exchange (HIE)
- Increased requirements for e-prescribing and incorporating lab results
- Electronic transmission of patient care summaries across multiple settings
- More patient-controlled data

Stage 3: Improved Outcomes. This stage focuses on the following:

- Promoting improvements in quality, safety, and efficiency
- Clinical decision support for national high-priority conditions
- Patient access to self-management tools
- Improving population health

(Continues)

Clinical Spotlight *(Continued)*

Meaningful use criteria require providers to meet 14 core objectives, 5 out of 10 menu set objectives, and 6 total clinical quality measures. (In Figure 5-1A, please note that core objective C-12 was required through 2013 but will not be a requirement moving forward.) Figures 5-1A and 5-1B illustrate what is included in the core and menu set objectives.

List of Core Requirements - Final Regulation

ARRA EHR MEANINGFUL USE STAGE 1 REQUIREMENTS

CT #	CORE REQUIREMENTS (must meet all of these)
C 1	Record demographics as structured data for preferred language, race, ethnicity, date of birth, and gender (50 percent requirement).
C 2	Record and chart changes in vital signs (BP, height, weight, & display BMI); additionally, plot and display growth charts for children age 2 to 20 including BMI (50 percent requirement).
C 3	Maintain an up-to-date problem list of current and active diagnoses based on ICD-9-CM or SNOMED CT (80 percent of all unique patients admitted have at least one entry or an indication of "no problems are known" recorded as structured data).
C 4	Maintain active medication list with at least one entry or indication of "no currently prescribed medications" as structured data (80 percent requirement).
C 5	Maintain active medication allergy list with at least one entry or indication of "no known medication allergies" as structured data (80 percent requirement).
C 6	Record smoking status for patients 13 years old or older as structured data (50 percent requirement).
C 7	Provide patient with clinical summary for patients for each office visit within 3 business days (more than 50 percent for all office visits).
C 8	Provide patients with electronic copy of their health information (problems, medication, medication allergies, diagnostic test results) upon request (50 percent of patients must receive electronic copy within three days).
C 9	Generate and transmit permissible prescriptions electronically — eRx (40 percent requirement, does not apply to hospitals)
C 10	Use CPOE for medication orders directly entered by any licensed healthcare professional who can enter orders into the medical record per state, local, and professional guidelines. (30 percent for patients with at least one medication ordered through CPOE)
C 11	Implement drug-drug and drug-allergy interaction checks (functionality is enabled for these checks for the entire reporting period)
C 12	Implement capability to electronically exchange key clinical information among providers and patient authorized entities (Perform at least one test of EHR's capacity to exchange information)
C 13	Implement one clinical decision support rule relevant to specialty or high clinical priority along with and ability to track compliance for that rule.
C 14	Protect electronic health information created or maintained by the certified EHR technology through the implementation of appropriate technical capabilities (conduct or review a security risk analysis in accordance with the requirements and implement security updates as necessary)
C 15	Report ambulatory clinical quality measures to CMS or states (For 2011, provide aggregate numerator, denominator, and exclusions through attestation, 2012 submit electronically).

© Ingenix, Inc. 6 INGENIX.

Courtesy of Optum™ PM and Physician EMR

Figure 5-1A Stage 1 List of Core Requirements

The Menu Set Requirements – Final Regulation

ARRA EHR MEANINGFUL USE STAGE 1 REQUIREMENTS

CT #	MENU SET (must meet 5 of these)
M 16	Implement drug-formulary checks (generate at least one report for entire reporting period).
M 17	Incorporate clinical lab-test results into EHR as structured data (40 percent of all tests ordered with results in a positive/negative or numerical format).
M 18	Generate lists of patients by specific conditions to use for quality improvement, reduction of disparities, research, and outreach (generate at least one report with a list of patients with a specific condition)
M 19	Use certified EHR to identify patient-specific education resources and provide to patient if appropriate (10 percent requirement).
M 20	The eligible provider who receives a patient from another setting of care or provider of care or believes an encounter is relevant should perform medication reconciliation (50 percent requirement).
M 21	The eligible provider who transitions there patient to another setting of care or provider of care or refers their patient to another provider of care should provide summary care record for each transition of care and referral (50 percent requirement).
M 22	Capability to submit electronic data to immunization registries or Immunization Information Systems and actual submission in accordance with applicable law and practice (perform at least one test if the registry has the capability to receive electronically). NOTE: EP must complete one of Immunization or Syndromic Surveillance unless has an exception for both.
M 23	Capability to submit electronic syndromic surveillance data to public health agencies and actual transmission in accordance with applicable law and practice (perform at least one test unless public health agencies to not have the capacity to receive electronically) NOTE: Must complete one of Immunization or Syndromic Surveillance unless EP has an exception for both.
M24	Send appropriate reminders to patients per patient preference for preventative/follow up care during the 90 day reporting period for patients 65 and older or 5 years and younger (20 percent requirement).
M 25	Provide patients with timely electronic access to their health information, including laboratory results, problem list, medication list, and medication allergies within four business days of the information being available to the eligible provider (10 percent requirement).

INGENIX.

Courtesy of Optum™ PM and Physician EMR

Figure 5-1B Stage 1 Menu Set Requirements

ACTIVITY 5-1: Viewing the Meaningful Use Dashboard

Before we start working in the EMR side of Optum™, we need to review settings within the Practice Management (PM) side and make the appropriate adjustments to accommodate each.

The *Meaningful Use Dashboard* within Optum™ PM tracks a provider's progress toward meeting the Medicare and Medicaid EHR Incentive Program reporting requirements for the core and menu set items. The dashboard displays a progress bar next to each of the measures that has a reporting requirement. Figure 5-2A illustrates a graphing screen of the core requirements for Dr. Olivia Sherman and Figure 5-2B illustrates the graphing features of the menu set requirements for Dr. Olivia Sherman. (Dr. Sherman is not a provider in our environment.)

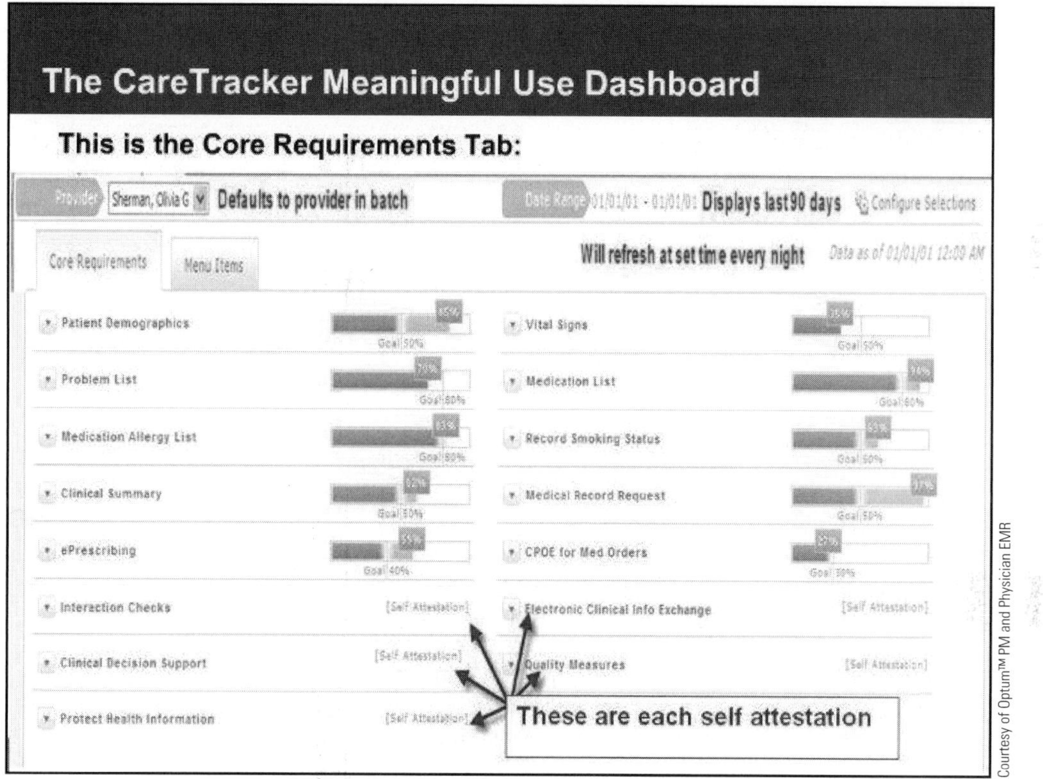

Figure 5-2A Core Requirements for Dr. Olivia Sherman

The dashboard's default date range is determined by when the provider begins the attestation period, or the date that begins the 90-day reporting period of meeting the core and menu measures listed previously. The dashboard calculates these measures over the previous 90 days. From the dashboard you can:

- Customize the requirements displayed on the dashboard for each participating provider
- View a status of a provider's progress for the last 90 days (percentages updated nightly)
- Hover over the percentage bar to review the data used to calculate the provider's percentage
- Click the *Menu Items* tab and then the drop-down arrow to download reference documents or run Key Performance Indicator (KPI) reports

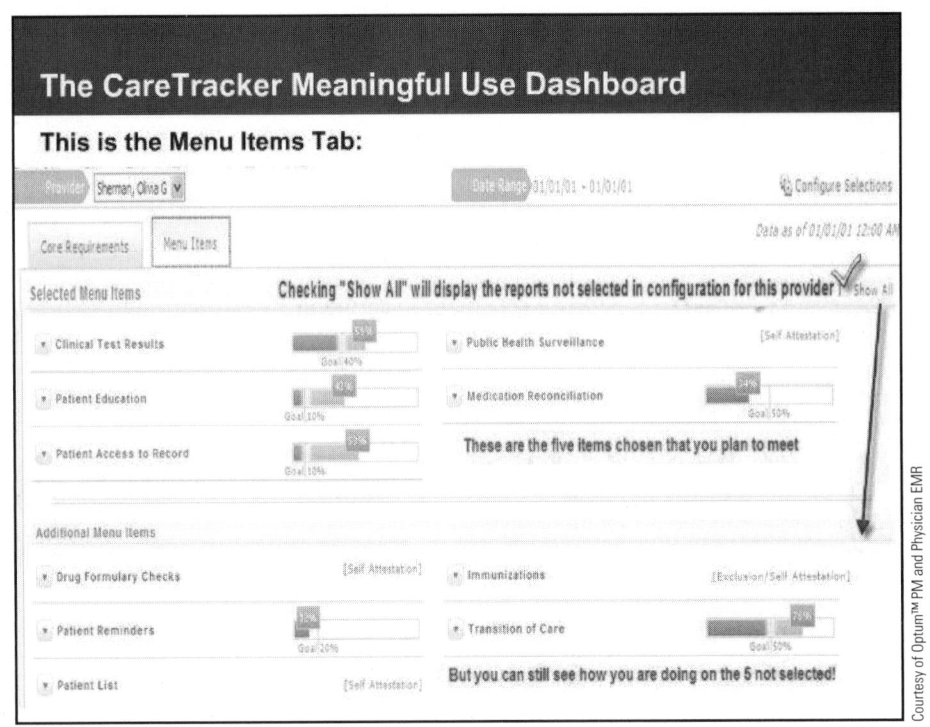

Figure 5-2B Menu Requirements for Dr. Olivia Sherman

To View the Meaningful Use Dashboard:

1. Click the *Home* module.
2. Click the *Meaningful Use* tab under the *Dashboard* tab (Figure 5-3). Optum™ PM displays the *Meaningful Use Dashboard*.

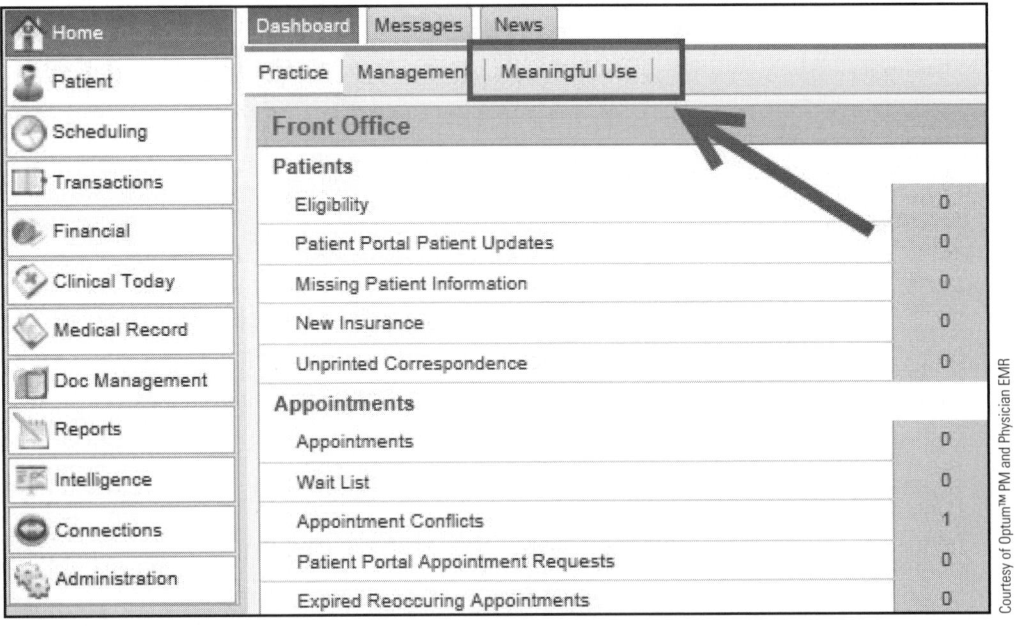

Figure 5-3 Meaningful Use Tab

3. From the *Provider* list, select the name of the provider whose data you want to view. In this case, click on "Dr. Brockton." Optum™ PM displays the provider's percentages on the *Core Requirements* tab (Figure 5-4).

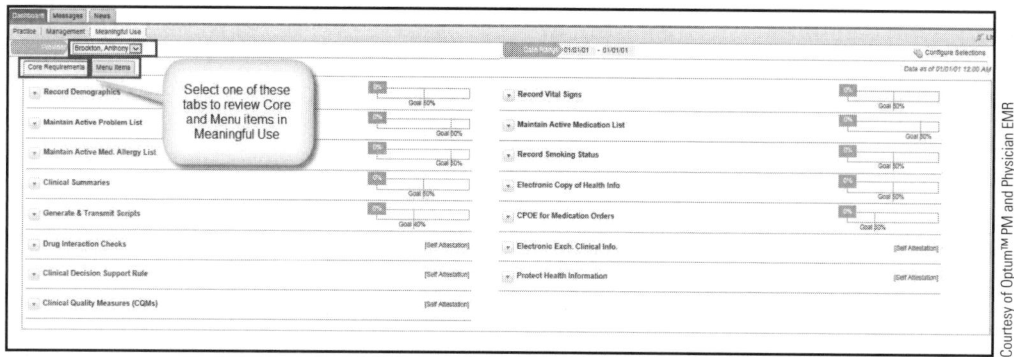

Courtesy of Optum™ PM and Physician EMR

Figure 5-4 Dr. Brockton's Core Requirements

Print a screenshot of the Core Requirements screen, label it "Activity 5-1A," and place it in your assignment folder.

4. Click the *Menu Items* tab to view the *Menu Items* requirements. On the *Menu Items* tab, select the *Show All* checkbox to view any excluded requirements.

Print a screenshot of the Menu Items screen, label it "Activity 5-1B," and place it in your assignment folder.

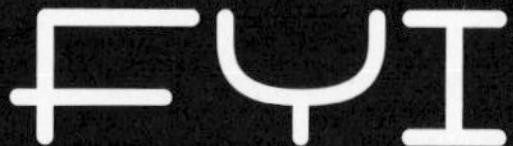

Because this is a training environment, you are only able to see the shell; no meaningful use statistics are available. Figure 5-5 illustrates what a *Core Requirements* tab looks like in a fully functional environment.

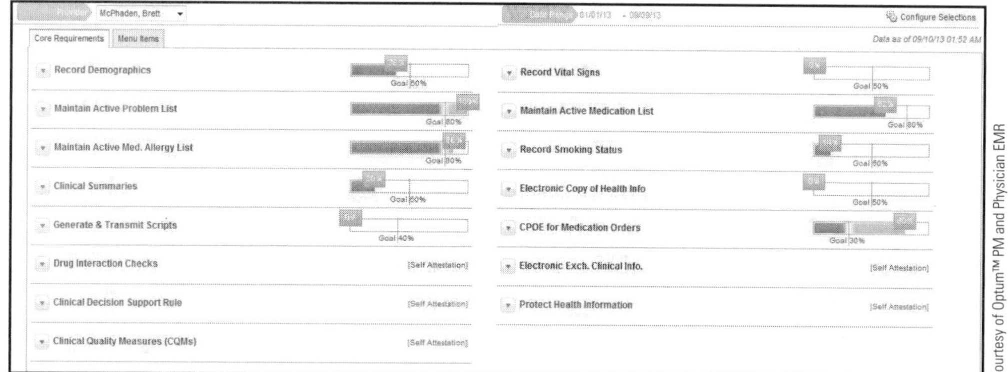

Courtesy of Optum™ PM and Physician EMR

Figure 5-5 Core Requirements in a Fully Functional Environment

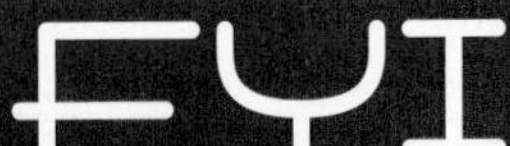

Review Recorded Meaningful Use Session 1 in Help

A number of recorded materials are available in *Help*. To view Meaningful Use Session 1, follow these instructions:

1. Log in to Optum™ and click on the *Help* icon.
2. Click on the *Training* tab.
3. Click on *Learn More,* under *Recorded Training*.
4. Scroll down and click on "Meaningful Use Session 1" *Recorded Training*. (**Note:** This is a 26:30-minute training session. To become familiar with all aspects of meaningful use, view Meaningful Use Sessions 2, 3, 4, and Meaningful Use Tools.)

PROFESSIONALISM CONNECTION

Providers will be impressed when you demonstrate knowledge of meaningful use and how and why the increased use of information technology will further improve patient safety, bring positive outcomes, and meet organizational goals.

ACTIVITY 5-2: Activating Care Management Items

The *Care Management* feature in Optum™ PM and Physician EMR allows practices to set clinical measures for health maintenance and disease management registries. The registries will assist with early identification of disease and early treatment. Keeping up to date with immunizations will help to prevent future disease and control costs associated with those diseases. This feature also assists in meeting some of the standards of meaningful use.

By default, clinical measures are turned off in Optum™ PM and Physician EMR. You need to activate the registries and measures you want to make available to the providers in your group. As you will observe, these registries will check to ascertain that the patient is up to date with preventive testing and immunizations.

After activation, the registries and measures selected are included in the *Patient Care Management* application of the *Medical Record* module and the *Care Management* application of the *Clinical Today* module. Registries are repopulated with the *Clinical Today/Population Management* tab. Once activation occurs, anytime you open the patient's chart, you can see where he or she falls within the registries and help the patient to come into compliance with testing or procedures.

1. Click on the *Administration* module, and then click the *Clinical* tab.
2. Click the *Care Management Activation* link under the *Maintenances* heading (Figure 5-6A). Optum™ PM and Physician EMR launches the *Care Management Activation* application.
3. Select the measures and registries checked in Figure 5-6B (select/click on all the boxes).

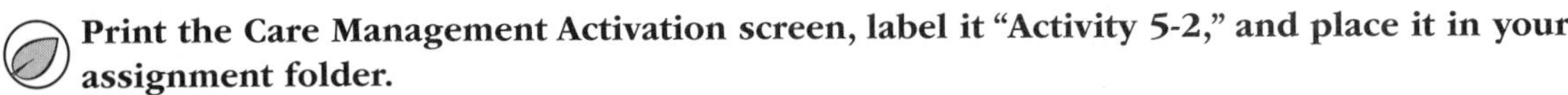

Print the Care Management Activation screen, label it "Activity 5-2," and place it in your assignment folder.

4. Click *Save* to save your settings.

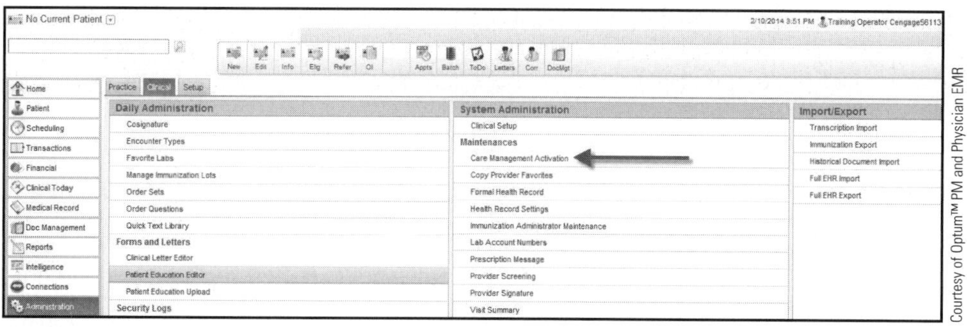

Courtesy of Optum™ PM and Physician EMR

Figure 5-6A Care Management Activation Link

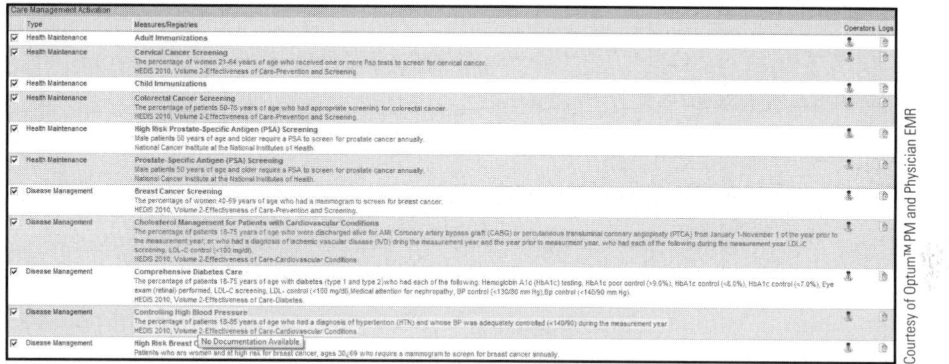

Courtesy of Optum™ PM and Physician EMR

Figure 5-6B Care Activation Measures and Registries

5. Now click on the *Clinical* tab and the *Care Management Activation* link to view the saved screen with all of the boxes checked.

PROFESSIONALISM CONNECTION

Many of the disease prevention goals set for the patient are directly connected to meaningful use and the provider's core requirement percentages. When the medical assistant is unable to get the patient to agree to these goals, it not only impacts the patient's health but the provider's meaningful use statistics. Because we are a "Pay for Performance" facility, it impacts the practice's bottom line as well. Keep this in mind as you complete activities related to *Care Management*.

NVFHA MANAGER CHALLENGE

As you proceed with this chapter, you are going to learn a great deal about working in the patient's electronic medical record (EMR). You are very fortunate to enter the medical field at a time when technology is flourishing. Electronic medical records organize the patient's information so that you know exactly where each item is stored within the patient's chart. EMRs also help medical assistants stay on task and keep up with lab reports and prescription renewals. Your challenge is to embrace the training in this chapter so that you are able to fully navigate the patient's medical record in Optum™ EMR. Consider how accurate documentation in a patient's EMR affects the billing and coding side of the practice and the revenue cycle.

ACTIVITY 5-3: Setting Operator Preferences in Your Batch Application

The *Batch* application in Optum™ PM and Physician EMR enables you to set up your operator preferences based on the workflow for your role. This reduces the number of clicks required to get from one application to the other, making navigation through Optum™ easy. As a medical assistant working in a clinical capacity, you will want your screen to open in the *Clinical Today* module each time you log in to Optum™. Selecting the appropriate setting from the *Login Application* in your *Batch* preferences will take you directly to the *Clinical Today* module after logging in.

1. To set up operator preferences, click *Batch* on the *Name Bar*. Optum™ PM and Physician EMR displays the *Operator Encounter Batch Control* dialog box.
2. Click on the *Edit* button.
3. Click on the drop-down arrow beside *Provider* and select "Dr. Raman," if he has not already been selected.
4. Click on the drop-down arrow beside *Resource* and select "Dr. Raman," if he has not already been selected.
5. Click on the drop-down arrow beside *Show Alerts* and select "Yes."
6. In the *Login Application* box, click on the drop-down arrow and select "Clinical."
7. Click on *Save*. Now every time you log into Optum™, you will be taken directly to the *Clinical Today* module.
8. Click "X" in the right-hand corner to close the dialog box.

ACTIVITY 5-4: Viewing Appointments

The *Clinical Today* module within Optum™ EMR helps to categorize and organize tasks, improving quality and efficiency throughout the day. As a result, providers and staff members are continuously in sync with one another, enhancing communications, and, ultimately, patient care.

Within Optum™ EMR the *Clinical Today* module is the area where most medical assistants working in a clinical capacity spend their time. The *Clinical Today* module works as an electronic desk. It organizes and helps manage tasks by displaying items to be worked on daily. It also automates a large number of routine tasks, thereby increasing productivity. In addition, the module helps track patient workflow efficiently by displaying information about scheduled appointments and patient movements within the clinic. The application helps track the care of one or more patients in the practice and provides instant access to a patient's medical record that includes test results, clinical information, and more.

ALERT

When you click on *Clinical Today*, the screen automatically defaults to the patients scheduled for the current date. For this activity, you will need the dates of the appointments you scheduled for patients in Chapter 4.

The *Appointments* application (Figure 5-7) consists of patient and non-patient appointments scheduled via the *Book* application in the *Scheduling* module.

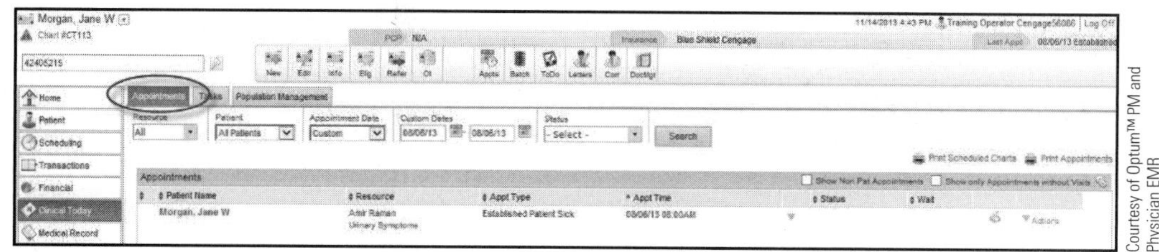

Courtesy of Optum™ PM and Physician EMR

Figure 5-7 Appointments Screen in Clinical Today

To View Appointments:

1. Click on *Clinical Today.*
2. Click on the drop-down arrow under *Resource* and select "All."
3. Click on the drop-down arrow under *Patient* and select "All Patients."
4. Click on the drop-down arrow under *Appointment Date* and select "Custom."
5. Click on the calendar beside the first box under *Custom Dates* and select the date you scheduled your patient appointments in Chapter 4. (If you scheduled your patients on different dates, select the date that you scheduled Alison Wild.)
6. Click in the second box to the right of the calendar under *Custom Dates*. The date that you inserted in the first box should automatically populate in this box.
7. In the status box, click on the drop-down arrow and select "All" (Figure 5-8).

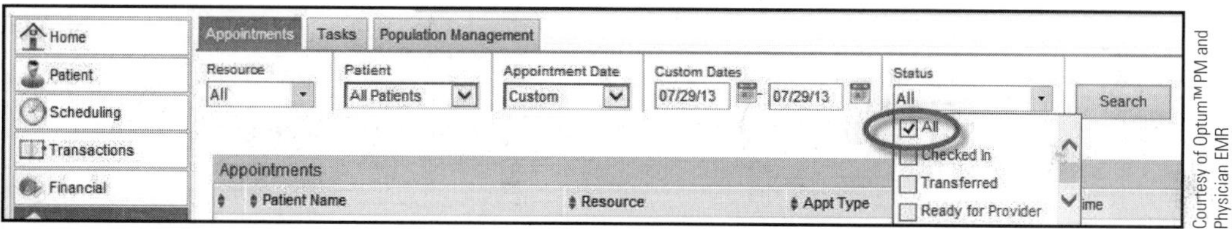

Courtesy of Optum™ PM and Physician EMR

Figure 5-8 Select All

8. Click on *Search*. The *Appointments* screen with Ms. Wild's appointment should now appear.

 **Print a screen shot of your Appointments screen from Clinical Today. Label it "Activity 5-4" and place it in your assignment folder.**

ACTIVITY 5-5: Transferring a Patient

In Chapter 4 you practiced checking in patients. Patients are typically checked in upon arrival. This cues the clinical staff that the patient is ready to be taken back to the exam room. This activity describes how to change a patient's status from "Checked In" to "Transferred." Transfer refers to the status of a patient when he or she has been taken to an exam room.

1. Click on *Clinical Today.*
2. Match the search parameters to those set in Activity 5-4. Click *Search.*

3. Alison Wild's appointment should be listed in the *Appointments* window. Her current status is green, which means that she has already been checked in. Change her status by clicking on the drop-down arrow in her *Status* column and selecting "Transfer."
4. The *Patient Location* box will pop up. Select the radio button next to "Exam Room # 1." Click *Select* (Figure 5-9).

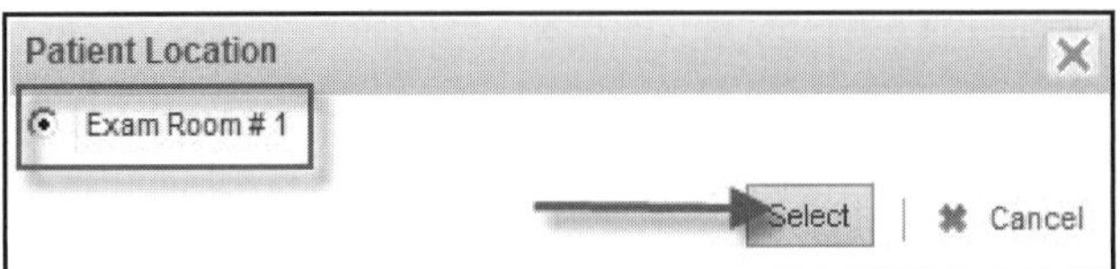

Figure 5-9 Patient Location Box

Courtesy of Optum™ PM and Physician EMR

5. Ms. Wild's entry line should now be blue, indicating that she has been transferred to the exam room. The appropriate exam room number will now appear in the *Status* column (Figure 5-10).

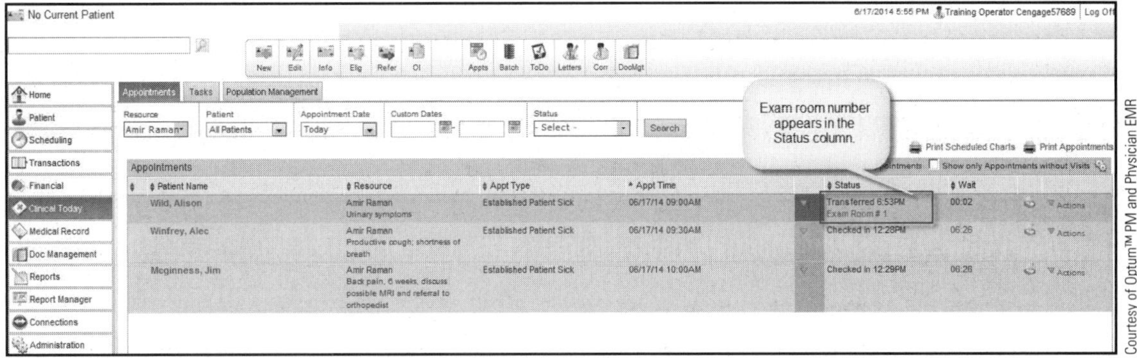

Courtesy of Optum™ PM and Physician EMR

Figure 5-10 Exam Room Status Column

PROFESSIONALISM CONNECTION

The status tab in the *Appointments* module within *Clinical Today* allows you to determine exactly where the patient is throughout the visit. It also tracks the length of time the patient spends in each area of the visit. If you happen to notice that the patient has been waiting particularly long in any area, even if it is not your assigned area, do a little investigating to establish the reason for the wait. Someone may have forgotten about the patient or may be tending to an emergency. Once you determine the reason for the wait, alert the patient and apologize for the delay. If the cirumstances causing the delay cannot be resolved within a reasonable period, offer the patient an opportunity to reschedule the appointment. The entire Napa Valley Family Health Associates staff is on the same team and need to support each other as well as the patient.

ACTIVITY 5-6: Bringing Up the Patient's Chart

Once the patient has been checked in and transferred to an exam room, you are ready to bring up his or her electronic medical record (EMR). In the case of Alison Wild, she is an established patient; however, Napa Valley Family Health Associates is in the middle of transitioning from paper records to Optum ™ PM and Physician EMR. Because Ms. Wild's chart has not yet been converted, it will need to be built from scratch. For activities related to this workbook, you will learn how to bring up the patient's chart and complete only certain functions required to continue with billing and coding activities. The clinical medical assistant will enter all of the patient's medical history, allergy information, medication list, vital signs, chief complaint, and preventive care and create flow sheets and growth charts. In addition he or she will create the progress note (acting in a provider's role) and enter all necessary information. Entering clinical data will not be included in the activities of this workbook because we are focused only on the information that is needed to complete future billing and coding activities.

1. Click on *Clinical Today*.
2. In the *Appointments* screen within *Clinical Today*, bring up the date of Alison Wild's appointment.
3. Click on Ms. Wild's name. The patient's *Chart Summary* will open in a new window (Figure 5-11).

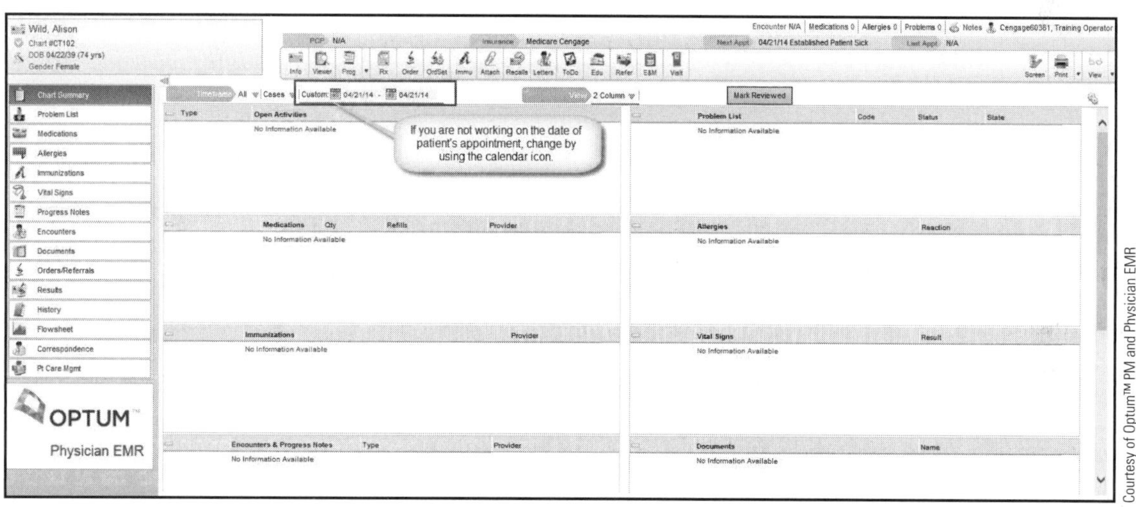

Figure 5-11 Chart Summary in New Window

ACTIVITY 5-7: Accessing Patient Care Management Items

In Activity 5-2, you activated the *Care Management* feature in Optum™, which is required prior to using the *Patient Care Management* (*Pt Care Mgmt*) application. The *Patient Care Management* application is used to update information such as the due date or interval for a test/exam and to flag a test or exam that is refused by a patient as a proactive reminder tool to improve the care management process. The patient is evaluated and moved to specific health maintenance and disease management registries based on measures that are activated within your group. Additionally, you can view a list of care management items that are complete and pending for the patient by clicking the *Pt Care Mgt* link on the *Patient Health History* pane.

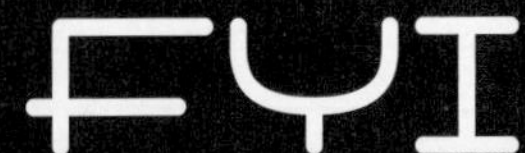

The care recommendations in the *Health Maintenance* and *Disease Management* registries are based on CDC and National Committee for Quality Assurance/Healthcare Effectiveness Data and Information Set (NCQA/HEDIS) guidelines.

Table 5-1 provides a description of each section within the *Patient Care Management* application.

Table 5-1 Sections within the Patient Care Management Application

Section	Description
Health Maintenance	This section displays all tests/exams that a patient is due for that are part of *Health Maintenance* registries.
Disease Management	This section displays all tests/exams that a patient is due for OR is required to have according to disease management measures. Click the *Expand* icon in the *Disease Management* section to view all items that are part of the disease management measure.

Courtesy of Optum™ PM and Physician EMR

The *Patient Care Management* application is used as a proactive reminder tool to improve the care management process. The application helps manage the recurring preventive care items pertinent to a patient by evaluating and moving to registries, flagging overdue items, processing order sets, and more. This helps providers to meet Meaningful Use goals.

Important: A patient is placed into a disease management measure only if the patient has an active diagnosis that triggers the ICD code rule.

To Access Patient Care Management Items:

1. If you are not in Alison Wild's medical record, access it following the steps used in Activity 5-6.
2. In the *Patient Health History* pane, click on the *Pt Care Mgmt* tab. Optum™ EMR displays the *Patient Care Management* window with all health maintenance and disease management items completed for the patient. Figure 5-12 represents what a completed *Care Management* list would look like. The list includes both pending and completed items.

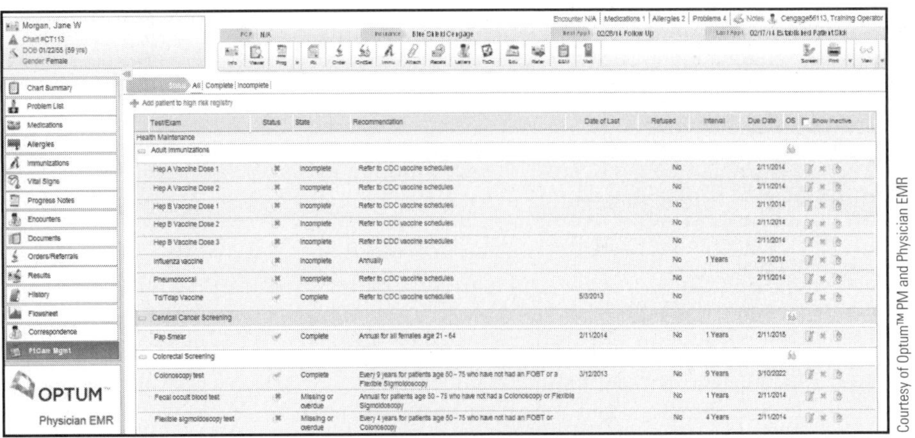

Courtesy of Optum™ PM and Physician EMR

Figure 5-12 Patient Care Management Window

3. Review the *Patient Care Management* window for Alison Wild.

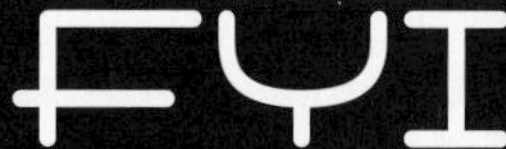

You can remove a patient care management item from the list by clicking the *Deactivate* icon. The inactive item appears dimmed and you can select the *Show Inactive* checkbox to view the item.

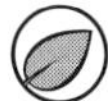 **Print a screenshot of the Patient Care Management list, label it "Activity 5-7," and place it in your assignment folder.**

CLINICAL SPOTLIGHT

Chapter 1 discussed that Napa Valley Family Health Associates is a "Pay for Performance" health care organization and that medical assistants in the practice are required to review patient Health and Disease Management registries prior to the patient's scheduled appointment. The clinical medical assistant will need to review this information and create a plan that identifies areas of concern and document steps he or she will take to bring the patient into compliance. The morning of the appointment, the plan should be shared with the provider. The provider will review the plan and make necessary adjustments. Electronic orders should be placed in the EMR prior to the appointment so that the "Catching Up" process can be performed throughout the visit. If the patient refuses any of the items listed in the plan, click on the *Edit* icon and signify that the patient refused the item. The reason for refusal should be entered in the *Notes* section of the dialog box. Sharing this information with the provider prior to patient examination gives the provider an opportunity to encourage those prevention or maintenance items that the patient refused. Consider how "Pay for Performance" relates to your position as a biller and coder.

ACTIVITY 5-8: Accessing and Updating the Progress Notes Application

Progress notes are the heart of the patient record. They serve as a chronological listing of the patient's overall health status. Data pertaining to the findings from the visit are entered into the progress note. The *Progress Notes* application displays a list of notes recorded during each patient appointment and is required for medical, legal, and billing purposes. The note includes information such as the patient's history, medications, and allergies as well as a complete record of all that occurred during the visit.

Predefined specialty and condition specific templates are available in Optum™ EMR that simplify the process of documenting a patient encounter at the point of care. Optum™ EMR provides several template types, each offering a specific layout and custom options. These options allow providers to select the template that best suits their documenting needs. Staff members can also pull in sections of a prior note and insert documents and images into templates if necessary. Standard templates can be broken down by specialty and template styles.

To Access and Update the Progress Notes Application:

1. If you are not in Alison Wild's medical record, access it following the steps used in Activity 5-6.
2. In the *Clinical Toolbar*, click the *Progress Notes* tab. If an encounter is in context, which in this case it is, Optum™ EMR displays the *Progress Notes* template window (Figure 5-13). (**Note:** If documenting a progress note that is not based on an appointment, the *Encounter* dialog box displays, enabling you to create a new encounter. If you are getting an *Encounter* dialog box, it means that you did not have an encounter in context. Repeat step 1 if necessary.)
3. By default, the *View* field displays "Template." (Skip this box at this time.)
4. In the *Template* field, click on the drop-down arrow and select "IM OV Option 4 (v4) w/A&P" (see Figure 5-13). Complete the note by navigating through each tab as directed. (**Note:** You will be instructed to enter only minimal information to complete billing and coding activities.) The provider would ordinarily work in the progress note, but because the provider is not available you will be entering the information for the provider.

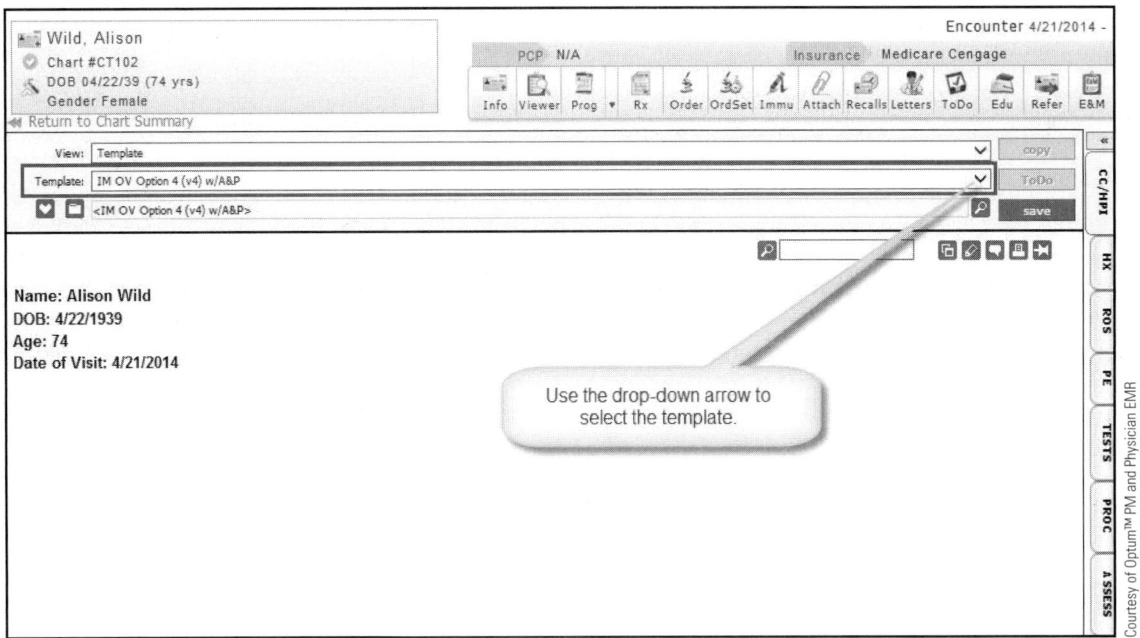

Figure 5-13 IM OV Option 4 Template

5. The *CC/HPI* tab will be showing on the right side of the screen. Place a check mark next to "Sick Visit" and "Established Patient" under *Chief Complaint*.
6. Review the note written regarding the patient's chief complaint. (**Note:** If the chief complaint was not yet entered, record "Urinary Symptoms" as the chief complaint in the *Other complaints* box.) The provider will expand a bit on the complaint by developing the History of Present Illness (HPI). Scroll down to the *HISTORY OF PRESENT ILLNESS* box and type the following:

   "Patient has a history of UTI's (1–2 infections/year). Current episode includes frequency, urgency, and burning pain upon urination (6/10). Last UTI was approximately six months ago and resolved with a ten-day treatment of Bactrim DS." Your documentation should match Figure 5-14.

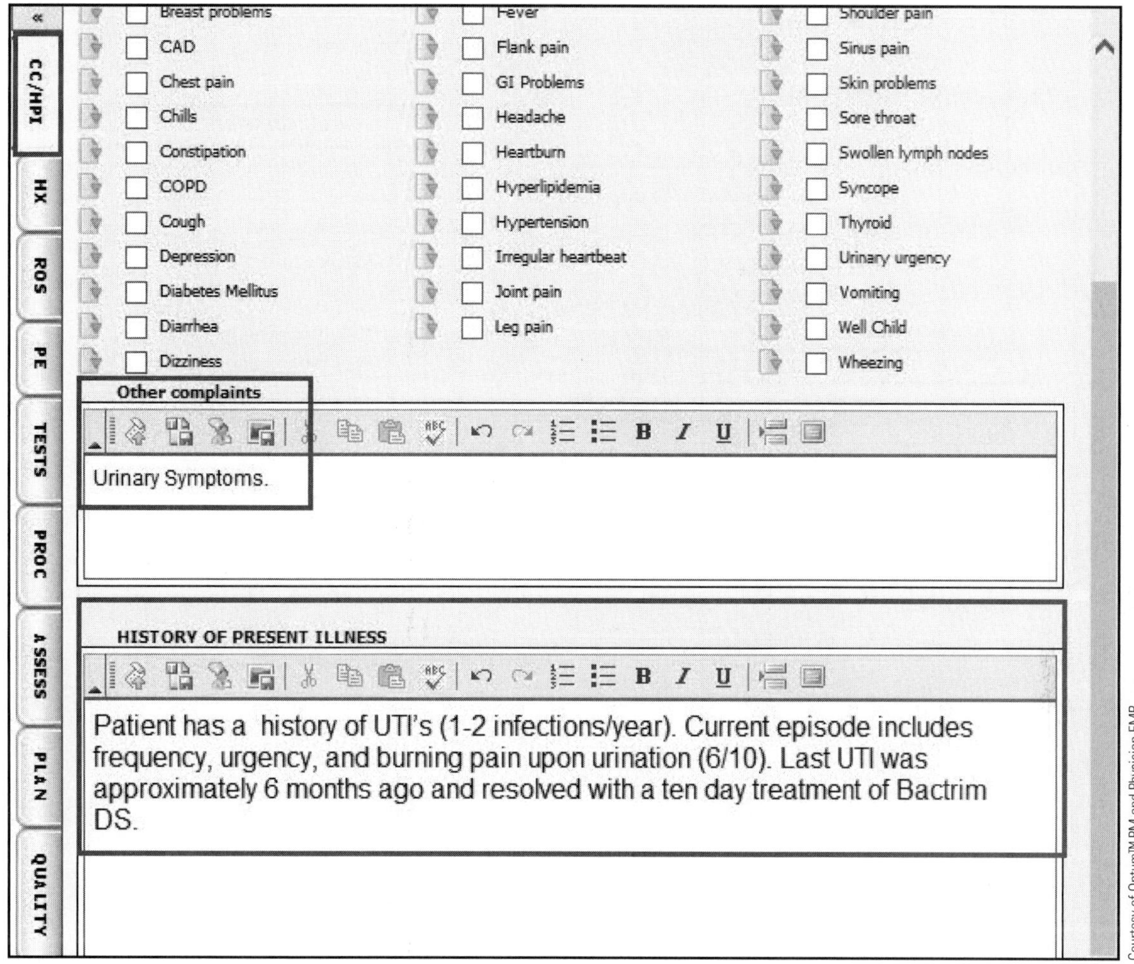

Figure 5-14 Alison Wild HPI

7. Click on *Save,* located in the yellow template box in the middle of the screen (Figure 5-15).

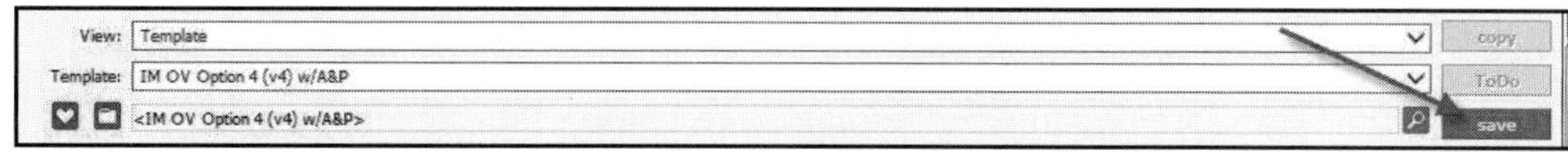

Figure 5-15 Save Button for Template Screen
Courtesy of Optum™ PM and Physician EMR

8. Skip the *HX, ROS, PE, TESTS,* and *PROC* tabs.
9. Click on the *ASSESS* tab.
10. It was discovered during the exam that the patient has hypertension. Under *Diagnoses* check the box beside *Hypertension (401.9).* The provider also diagnosed the patient with a *Urinary Tract Infection (599.0).* The final diagnosis for this visit is Dysuria (788.1). This is not an option in the list of diagnoses, so you will need to record it in the *Assessment* box (Figure 5-16).

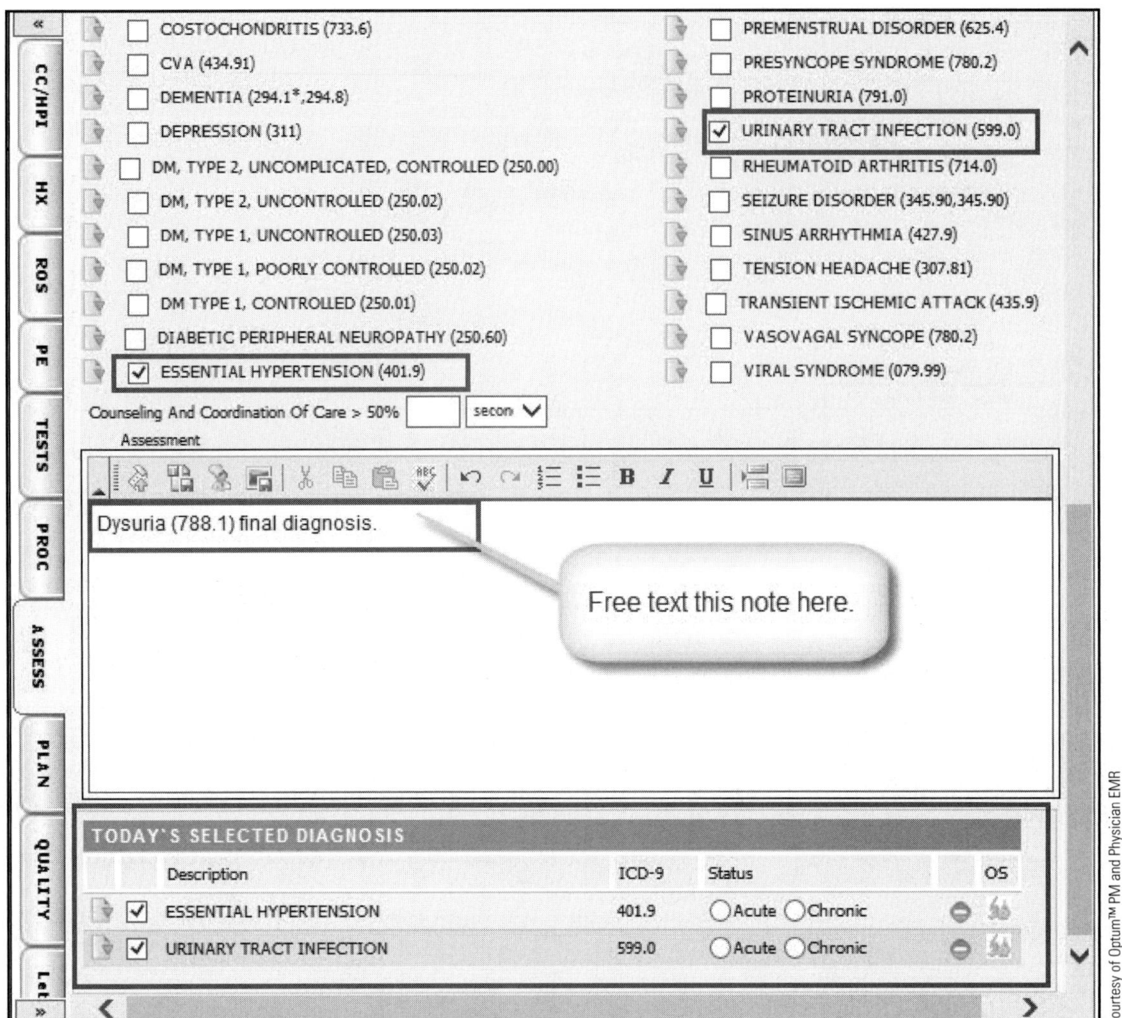

Courtesy of Optum™ PM and Physician EMR

Figure 5-16 Record ICD Code in Assessment Box

11. Click *Save* to update the progress note with the *Assessment* information.
12. Click on the *PLAN* tab to record the provider's plans. Scroll down and document the following in the *Additional Plan Details* box (Figure 5-17):

    a. Stat lab test - "Urinalysis dipstick panel by Automated test strip"

    b. Send Urine out for lab test "Urinalysis microscopic panel [#volume] in urine by automated count"

    c. Give patient educational handouts for UTI and Hypertension

    d. Bactrim DS Oral Tabs (800-160 mg), Sig 1 tab bid for 5 days, No refills

    e. Patient to return in 10 days for a Follow/Up UA and BP check

    f. Set patient up for a referral with a urologist

    PREVENTION GOALS:

    g. Patient to have her first Hepatitis B shot today

    h. Set patient up for a mammogram

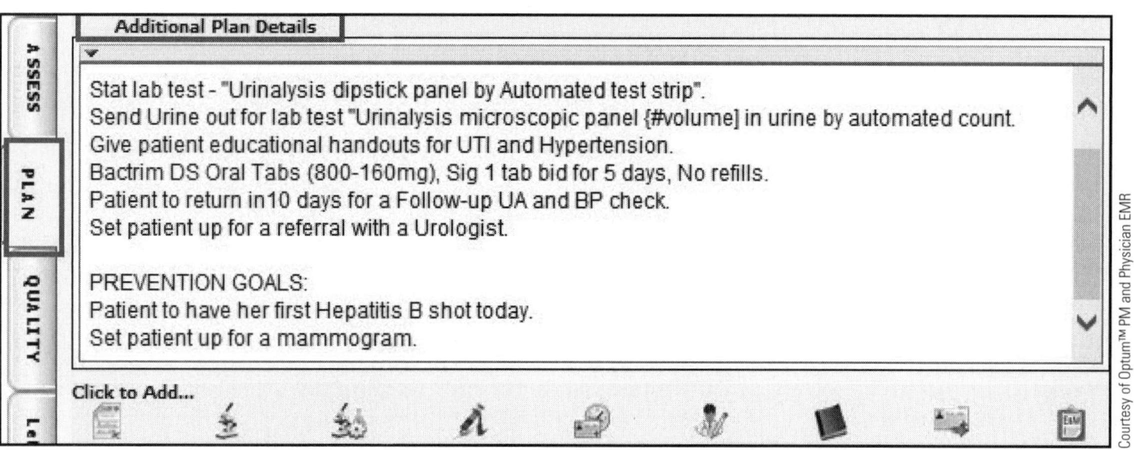

Courtesy of Optum™ PM and Physician EMR

Figure 5-17 Additional Plan Details box

NVFHA MANAGER CHALLENGE

You will refer back to the *ASSESSMENT* and *PLAN* (A&P) noted in a patient's progress note when coding and billing. Keep this in mind as you move forward with billing related tasks. You will need to be sure that all billable Evaluation and Management (E&M) and CPT® codes have been entered when saving the visit. Consider what would be the impact if all billable E&M and CPT® codes are not entered.

13. Click *Save*.

Click the green Print icon in the middle of the screen. The Clinical Note dialog box will open. Click the Print button to print a copy of the progress note. Label it "Activity 5-8" and place it in your assignment folder.

MINI-CASE STUDIES

Note: For Case Studies 5-2 and 5-3 you will need to refer to the appointment dates for Alec Winfrey and Jim Mcginness that you scheduled in Chapter 4. You will also be referencing tables with information applicable to the patients' visits.

Case Study 5-1

Repeat Activity 5-5 (Transfer Patient to Exam Room) for patients Alec Winfrey and Jim Mcginness (use "Exam Room #1").

After transferring both patients to the exam room, print a screenshot of the Appointments screen, label it "Case Study 5-1," and place it in your assignment folder.

(*Continues*)

MINI-CASE STUDIES *(Continued)*

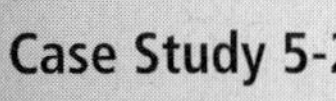

Case Study 5-2

Using the steps you learned throughout this chapter (Activities 5-6 and 5-8) and referencing information in Table 5-2, access Mr. Winfrey's medical record and create a progress note (update A&P). Mr. Winfrey is being seen today for a productive cough and shortness of breath.

Note: Select progress note template "IM OV Option 4 (v4) w/A&P."

Table 5-2 Alec Winfrey Medical Record and Progress Note

Tab	Entry
CC/HPI	*Chief Complaint*: Place a check mark in the "Sick Visit," "Established Patient," and "Cough" boxes. *Other complaints* box: Enter "Productive cough; shortness of breath" *History of Present Illness* box: Enter "Here today for cough that started 6 days ago and has gotten worse. Experiencing shortness of breath."
Skip the HX, ROS, PE, TESTS, and PROC Tabs	
ASSESS	*Diagnosis*: Pneumonia (486) *Assessment* box: Enter "Bilateral Pneumonia."
PLAN	*Additional Plan Details* box: 1. CXR 2. CBC W Auto Differential panel in Blood 3. EKG 4. Ibuprofen 800 mg oral now and instruct for every six hours while awake 5. Return visit in two days 6. Seek treatment in the ED or UC if symptoms worsen 7. Zithromax Z-Pack, one as directed

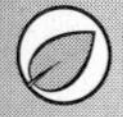
After entering all of the information provided in Table 5-2, print a progress note, label it "Case Study 5-2B," and place it in your assignment folder.

Case Study 5-3

Using the steps you learned throughout this chapter (Activities 5-6 and 5-8) and referencing the information in Table 5-3, access Mr. Mcginness's medical record and create a progress note (update A&P).

Note: Select progress note template "IM OV Option 4 (v4) w/A&P."

(Continues)

MINI-CASE STUDIES *(Continued)*

Table 5-3 Jim Mcginness Medical Record and Progress Note

Tab	Entry
CC/HPI	*Chief Complaint:* Place check marks in the "Sick Visit," "Established Patient," and "Back Pain" boxes. *Other complaints* box: Enter "Back pain, 3 weeks, discuss possible MRI and referral to Orthopedist. Patient continues to have intense lower back pain following an injury three weeks ago while lifting heavy boxes at home." *History of Present Illness* box: Enter "Patient picked up a large box at home approximately six weeks ago and immediately felt a sharp pain in his lower back. Pain started at a 5/10 and subsided to a 2/10 the following day. Pain has been steadily increasing and is now an 8/10. Patient describes pain as tight and continuous. Activity makes pain worse; sitting still in an upright position makes it feel slightly better. Patient has been taking Tylenol and using a heating pad since onset (little relief). Patient denies any numbness, tingling, or pain that radiates down either leg or previous low back pain or trauma."
Skip the Hx, ROS, PE, TESTS, and PROC Tabs	
ASSESS	*Diagnosis*: Low back pain (724.2) *Assessment*: Somatic Dysfunction-Lumbar, Pelvis
PLAN	*Additional Plan Details* box: 1. Refer for LS MRI 2. Referral to Orthopedist 3. Oxycodone-Acetaminophen 10-325 mg tabs 4. Follow-up appointment when MRI is complete

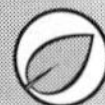

After entering all of the information provided in Table 5-3, print a progress note, label it "Case Study 5-3B," and place it in your assignment folder.

Resources

The Optum™ PM and Physician EMR Help homepage represents a wealth of information for the electronic health record (https://training.caretracker.com/help/CareTracker_Help.htm).

Department of Health and Human Services (DHHS) Centers for Medicare and Medicaid Services (CMS). (2003, June 6). *Medicare hospital manual.* Retrieved from http://www.cms.gov/Regulations-and-Guidance/Guidance/Transmittals/downloads/R804HO.pdf

U.S. Department of Health and Human Services. (2013, February 11). *Construction of LMS Parameters for the Centers for Disease Control and Prevention 2000 Growth Charts*, by Katherine M. Flegal, Ph.D., Office of the Director, National Center for Health Statistics; and Tim J. Cole, Ph.D., MRC Centre of Epidemiology for Child Health, Institute of Child Health, University College London, UK. National Health Statistics Report (No. 63). Retrieved from http://www.cdc.gov/nchs/data/nhsr/nhsr063.pdf

CHAPTER **6**

Completing the Visit

LEARNING OBJECTIVES

1. View and resolve open encounters and unsigned notes by completing and capturing the visit.
2. Access, view, sign, and print a progress note.

NVFHA MANAGER CHALLENGE

In this chapter you will learn to complete the visit and how documentation in both PM and EMR will affect your responsibilities as a biller and coder. You will refer to the A&P of the progress note to review whether all billable services have been captured.

Consider this scenario: The provider (or MA depending on workflows) selected a service code (V70.0) that is not covered by the patient's insurance (Medicare). How would you resolve this issue?

a. Confront the provider/MA who entered the code and ask why he or she used that code.

b. Confront the provider/MA and tell him or her that V70.0 is never covered by Medicare and that this is the second time this week a claim was rejected for the same code.

c. Confront the provider/MA and tell him or her that you have seen the same rejection more than once on Medicare patients. Ask the provider/MA for input as to why that might be.

d. Offer an explanation of codes that are often rejected and schedule an in-service training for all providers/staff.

e. Go to the billing supervisor first to let him or her know of the claim rejection and have him or her handle it.

f. Handle the code change yourself and do not notify the clinical MA or provider.

Discuss this scenario with your class. How billers and coders choose to handle these types of situations reflects on their knowledge and professionalism.

ACTIVITY 6-1: Access the Progress Notes Application

The *Progress Notes* application allows you to navigate the list of notes saved for the patient and click a note to view and manage from the right pane. A progress note is a document written by the clinician or provider that describes the details of a patient's encounter and is sometimes referred to as a chart note.

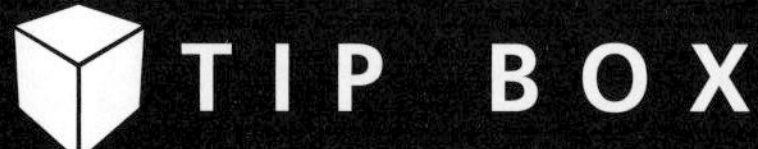

Important!! It is important to complete and sign all progress notes before any billing information is submitted to the payers.

The *Progress Notes* application displays a list of notes recorded during each patient appointment and progress note–type documents that are uploaded. Progress notes include information such as the patient's history, medications, allergies, as well as a complete record of all that happened during the visit. This information is required for medical, legal, and billing purposes. To navigate and view the progress notes listed in a patient's medical record:

- Click the *Next* and *Previous* buttons on the bottom of the *Progress Note* window to navigate through the list of notes (Figure 6-1).
- Click the *Expand/Collapse* icon in the upper-right-hand corner of your screen to maximize the view for readability.

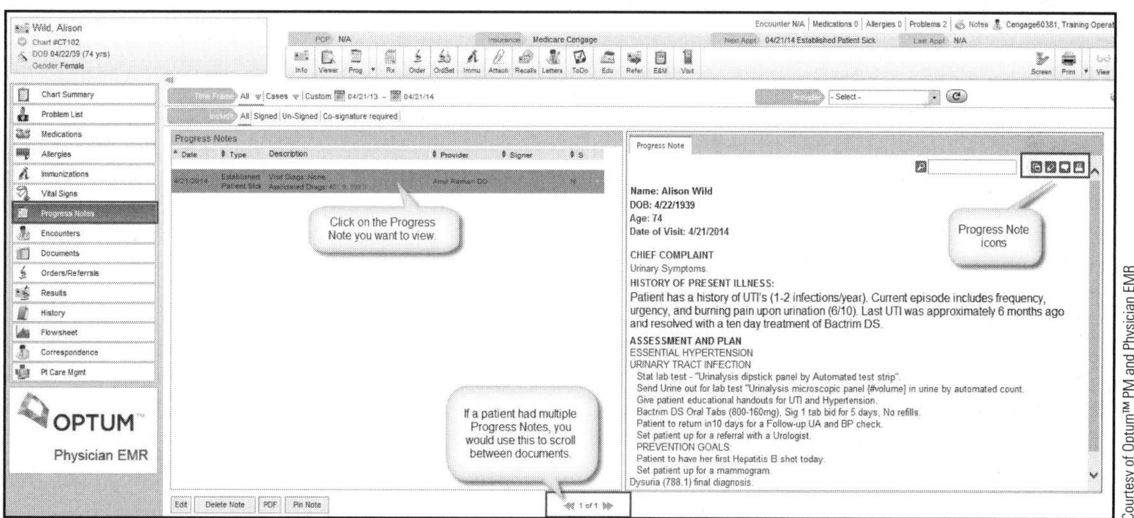

Figure 6-1 Progress Note – Next and Previous Buttons

Courtesy of Optum™ PM and Physician EMR

To Access the Progress Notes Application:

1. There are several ways to access the *Medical Record* module. Use one of the following methods:
   a. Pull the patient, Alison Wild, into context, and click the *Medical Record* module.
   b. If the patient has an appointment, click the patient's name in the *Appointments* application of the *Clinical Today* module. (Select the date of the patient's appointment that you scheduled in Chapter 4.)
2. In the *Patient Health History* pane, click *Progress Notes*.

3. The *Progress Notes* window displays with a list of signed and unsigned notes for the patient (Figure 6-2).

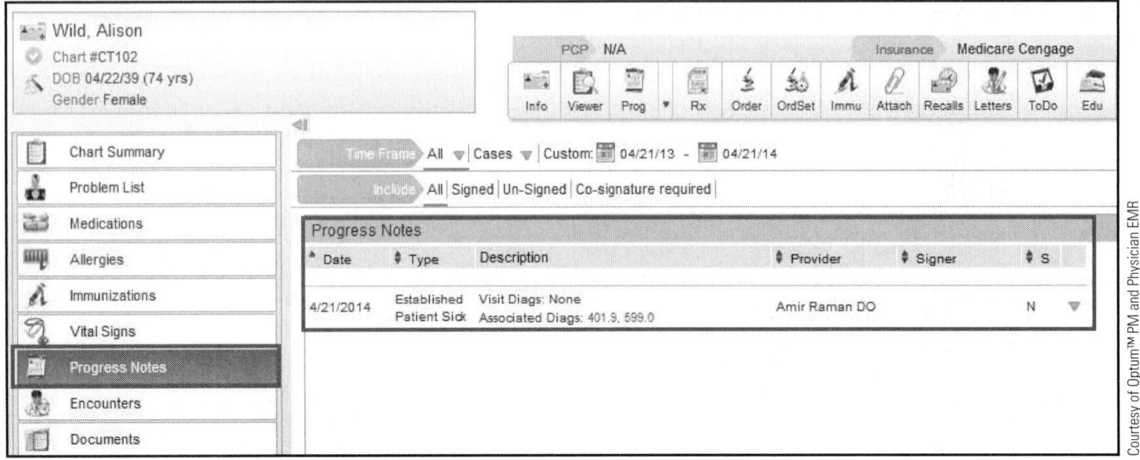

Figure 6-2 Alison Wild Progress Note

4. (FYI) The workflow would be that all tasks assigned by the provider for Alison Wild's encounter created in Chapter 5 have been completed. To confirm, scroll down to the bottom of the progress note and confirm that all orders, immunizations, referrals, and educational materials ordered in the A&P have been completed (Figure 6-3).

5. You note that the patient is to return in 10 days for a follow-up UA and blood pressure check. Make a follow-up appointment for Alison Wild with Dr. Raman for 10 days from her original encounter (Figure 6-4). (Refer to Chapter 4, Activity 4-1, if you need to review the instructions for making an appointment.)

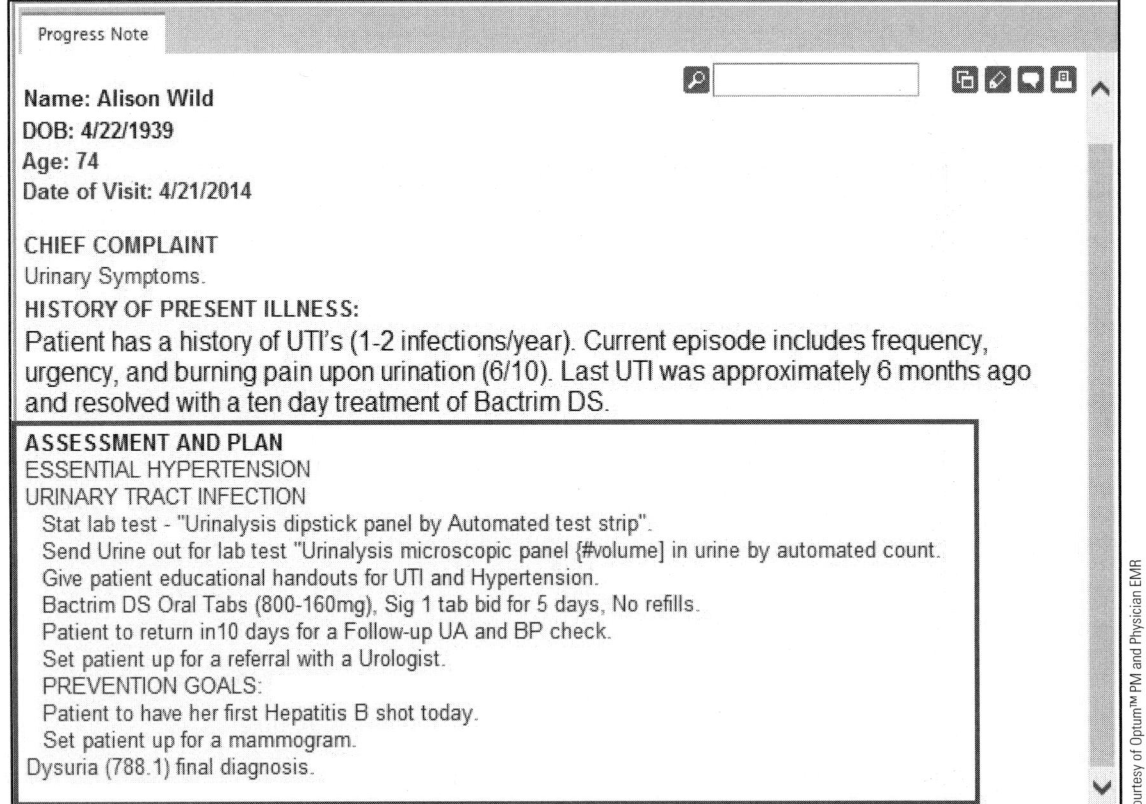

Figure 6-3 Completed A&P for Alison Wild

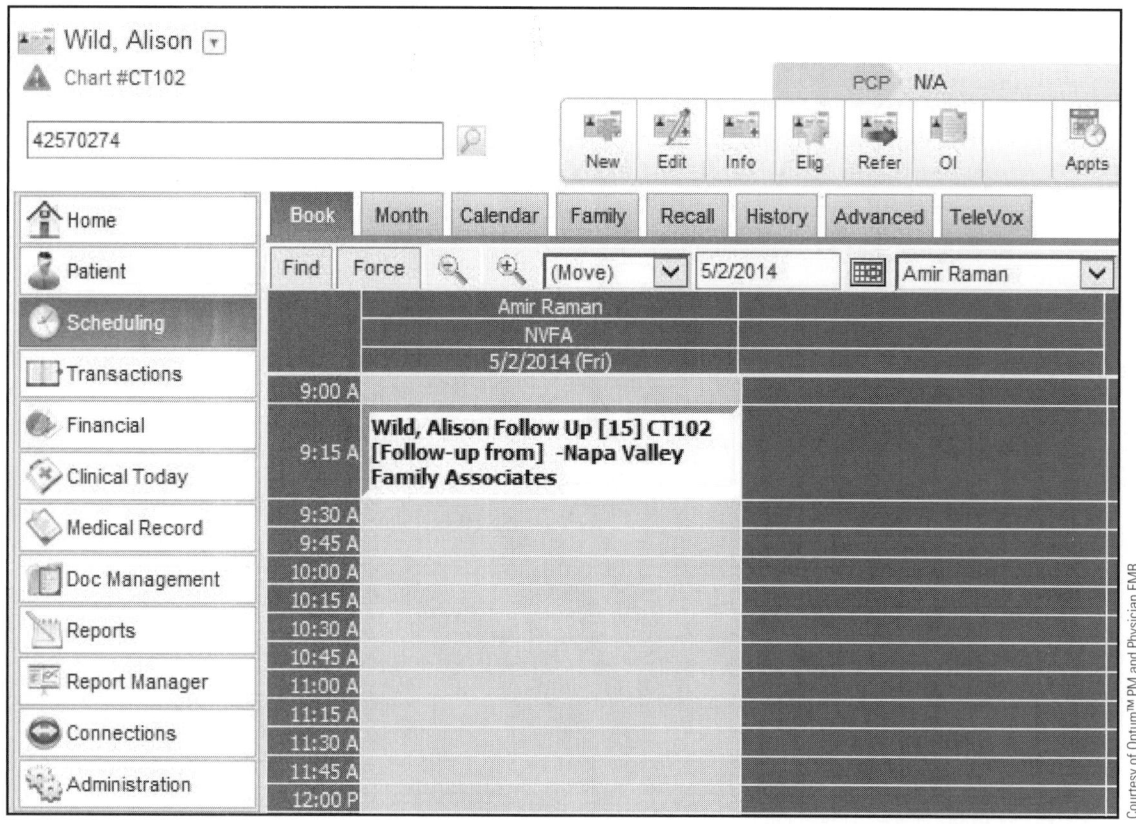

Figure 6-4 Alison Wild Follow-Up Appointment

ACTIVITY 6-2: Capture a Visit

In Chapter 5 you completed much of the patient workup to the point of completing and printing the progress note. In order for a patient visit to be billable, any open encounters must be resolved and the visit must be completed and the note signed. The provider is the person who is responsible for signing the progress note; however, to enhance your understanding of workflows in the EMR, you will be completing the visit, resolving open encounters, and electronically signing the note.

To generate claims, charges must be captured for the patient's appointment. The *Visit* application allows you to capture charges and enter procedure, NDC, and diagnosis codes for a patient's appointment. Visits can be entered into Optum™ PM and Physician EMR via several applications:

- Left-click on a patient's appointment in the *Book* application and select *Visit* from the pop-up mini-menu.
- Pull a patient into context, click the *Appts* button in the *Name Bar*, pull the appointment into context, and select *Visit* from the *Actions* menu.
- Click the *Appointments* link under the *Appointments* section of the *Dashboard* tab in the *Home* module, pull the patient appointment into context, and then select *Visit* from the *Actions* menu.
- Click the *Visits* link from the *Actions* drop-down for a patient listed in the *Appointments* application of the *Clinical Today* module.
- Click the *Visit* icon within the *Medical Record* module.

The *Visit* window contains a number of applications, but to save a visit you only need to enter the procedure and diagnosis code(s). Please note that a visit can only be edited prior to becoming a charge. For our first *Visit* activity, refer to patient Alec Winfrey's appointment that you scheduled in Chapter 4 with Dr. Raman. Access the *ASSESS* and *PLAN* tabs in the progress note (Figure 6-5) and capture the *Visit*. Mr. Winfrey is being seen today for a productive cough and shortness of breath.

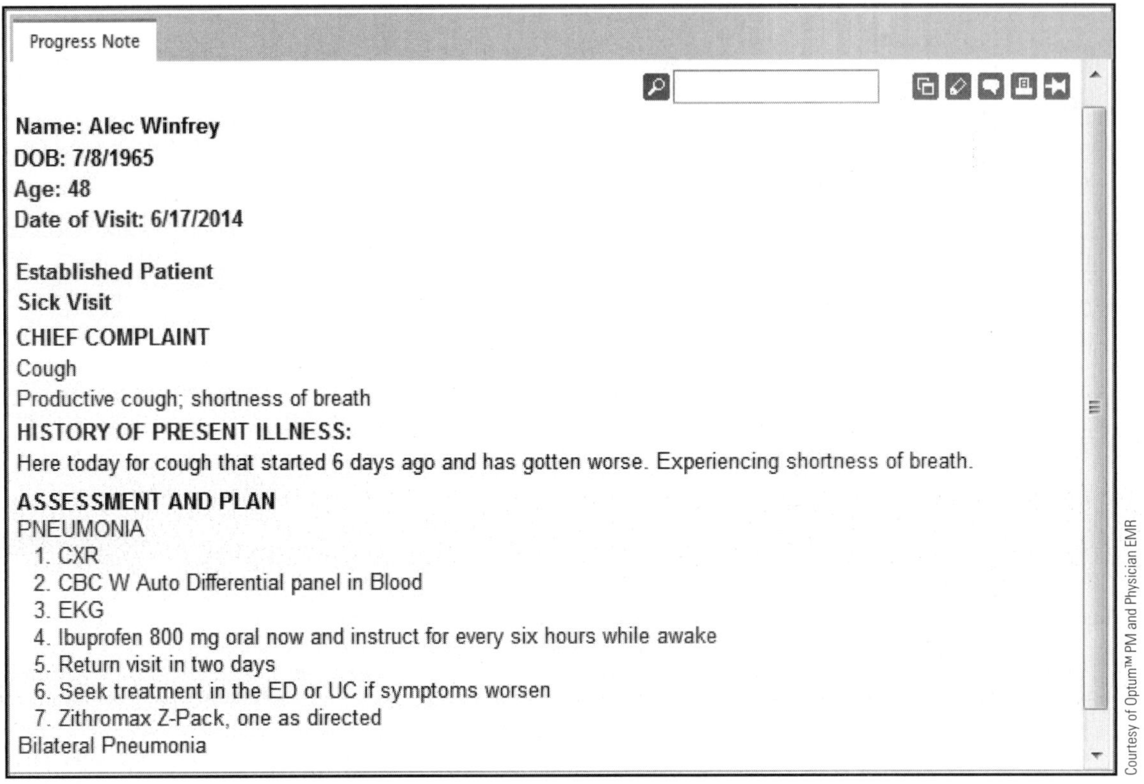

Figure 6-5 Alec Winfrey A&P

To Capture a Visit:

1. Click the *Scheduling* module. Optum™ PM and Physician EMR opens the *Book* application by default.
2. Move the schedule to display the date of service for which you want to confirm an appointment. This can be done by manually entering the date in the *Date* box, by clicking the *Calendar* icon, or by selecting a time period from the *Move* list. (Use the date from Activity 4-1 in the date box.) You may need to set the *Provider* drop-down to "All Providers" for the full schedule and all providers to display. Click *Go*.
3. Left-click the appointment for which you want to enter visit information and select *Visit* from the mini-menu drop-down. (Select Alec Winfrey's appointment.) The application displays the *Visit* window (Figure 6-6). When you first bring up the *Visit* window, it automatically displays the procedures section (*Procedures* tab located at the top left of the window).
4. The *Procedures* screen contains a list of procedure codes that mirror the CPT® codes on the encounter form. Verify that the checkboxes next to each code associated with the patient's appointment are selected: codes 99213, 71020, 36415, and 85025. (**Note:** If no *Visit* had yet been entered for the patient, the encounter form would display with no checkboxes next to procedures or diagnoses. If you see the code you want to select for the *Visit*, you can select the checkbox next to the code. Alternatively, you could enter either a code or a key term in the *Procedure Search* box to locate the desired code.)

Source: Current Procedural Terminology © 2013 American Medical Association.

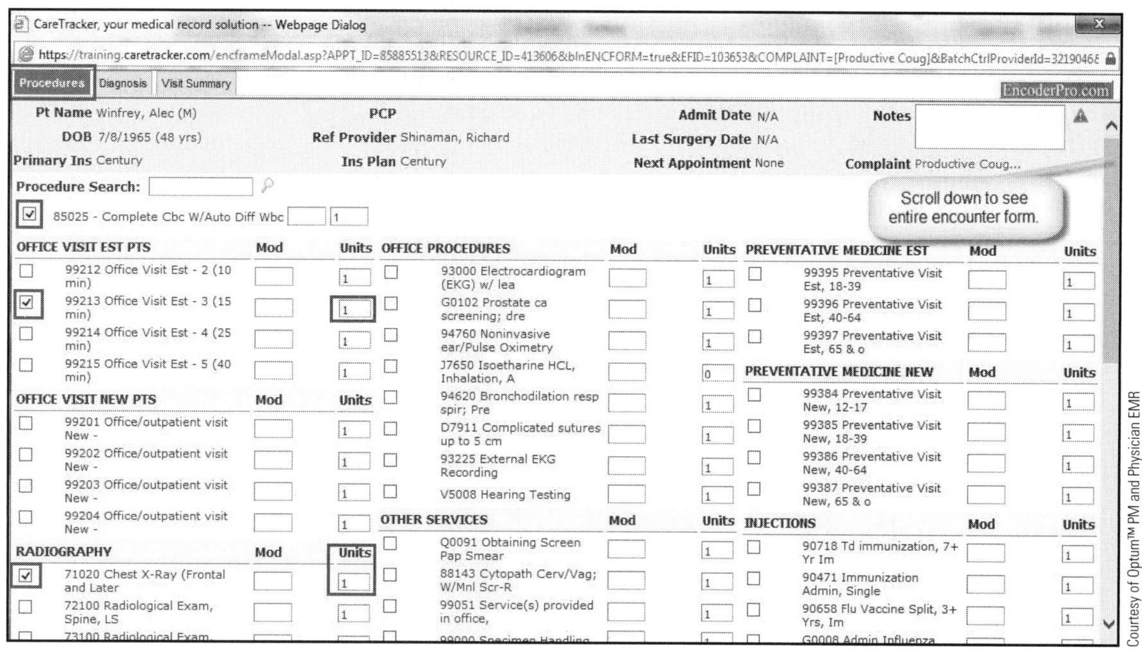

Courtesy of Optum™ PM and Physician EMR

Figure 6-6 Alec Winfrey Visit Window

NVFHA MANAGER CHALLENGE

As biller and coder, you must select and enter all service/procedure and diagnosis codes. If the codes are not already pre-populated in the A&P, do you know where to find them? **Hint:** For each of the codes you were instructed to select, there is a narrative in the A&P. For example:

- 99213 = Established patient, sick visit (15 minutes)
- 71020 = Bilateral Chest X-Ray
- 36415 = Venipuncture
- 85025 = Laboratory: CBC W Auto Differential panel in Blood

If you had not checked the verbiage in the patient's A&P of the progress note, you may have missed all the codes related to services. Consider this as you move through activities related to billing and coding.

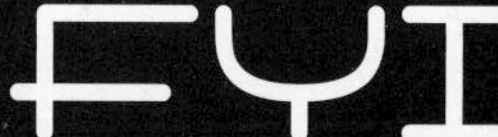

If you need to search for a CPT® code:

- Enter a partial code, a complete code, or a keyword in the *Search* field, and then click the *Search* icon. The application opens the *Procedure Search* window.
- *(Optional)* To search for an NDC Code, select *NDC Code* from the *Search Type* list and then click *Search*.
- Click on the desired procedure to select it. The codes selected from the search are added to the patient's *Visit* window and there is no limit to the number of codes you can select.

(Continues)

FYI (*Continued*)

- **Note:** If a code is not listed on the NVFHA encounter form, you will receive a pop-up warning that the code was not found. This does not mean it is an invalid code, only that it is not one of the codes included on the existing encounter form. You will still be able to add the code manually, although you may be prompted to enter the associated fee as well. If no fee is associated with the charge, you will make a note in the *Visit Summary/Billing Notes* section.

5. Enter any modifiers in the *Mod* field next to each selected procedure code, if applicable. (No modifier is required.)
6. If needed, enter the number of units in the *Units* field for each selected procedure code. (Number of units is "1" per CPT® code for this activity [as noted in Figure 6-6].)
7. Now click the *Diagnosis* tab in the *Visit* window. The application displays the *Diagnosis* application.
8. The *Diagnosis* screen displays a list of codes that mirror the ICD-9 codes on the encounter form. Select the checkbox next to each code associated with the patient's appointment. Because the type of pneumonia (organism) is not known at this stage, you will select ICD-9 code "486," as in Figure 6-7. Place a check mark next to "486" if it pre-populates. If not, scroll down the encounter form to locate it. Alternatively, you could search for the diagnosis by name or code as instructed in the FYI box.

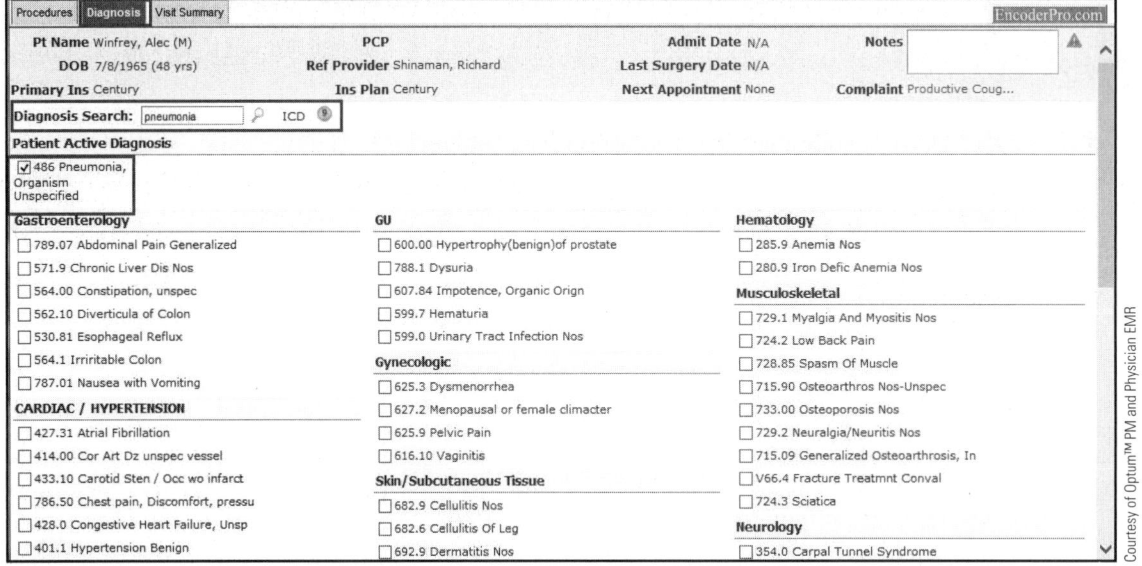

Courtesy of Optum™ PM and Physician EMR

Figure 6-7 Alec Winfrey Diagnosis Codes

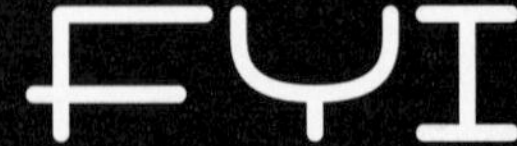

If you need to search for a diagnosis code:

- Enter a partial code, a complete code, or a keyword in the *Diagnosis Search* field, and then click *Search*. The application opens the *Diagnosis Search* window.
- Click on the desired ICD-9/ICD-10 code to select it. The codes selected from the search are added to the patient's *Visit* window.

9. Click the *Visit Summary* tab in the top left corner of the *Visit* window. Optum™ PM displays a summary of the visit information.
10. To check out the patient directly from the *Visit* application, select the *Check out Patient?* checkbox (Figure 6-8) at the bottom of the *Visit Summary* screen.
11. Review the screen (see Figure 6-8) and verify the accuracy of the information including the *Location, Place of Service (POS), Referring Provider, Insurance, Billing,* and *Servicing Provider*. (**Note:** You will reference this screen when entering a remittance (EOB) when payment is received. The amounts listed in the *Fee, Copay,* and *Extended Amount* columns should match the patient's EOB.)

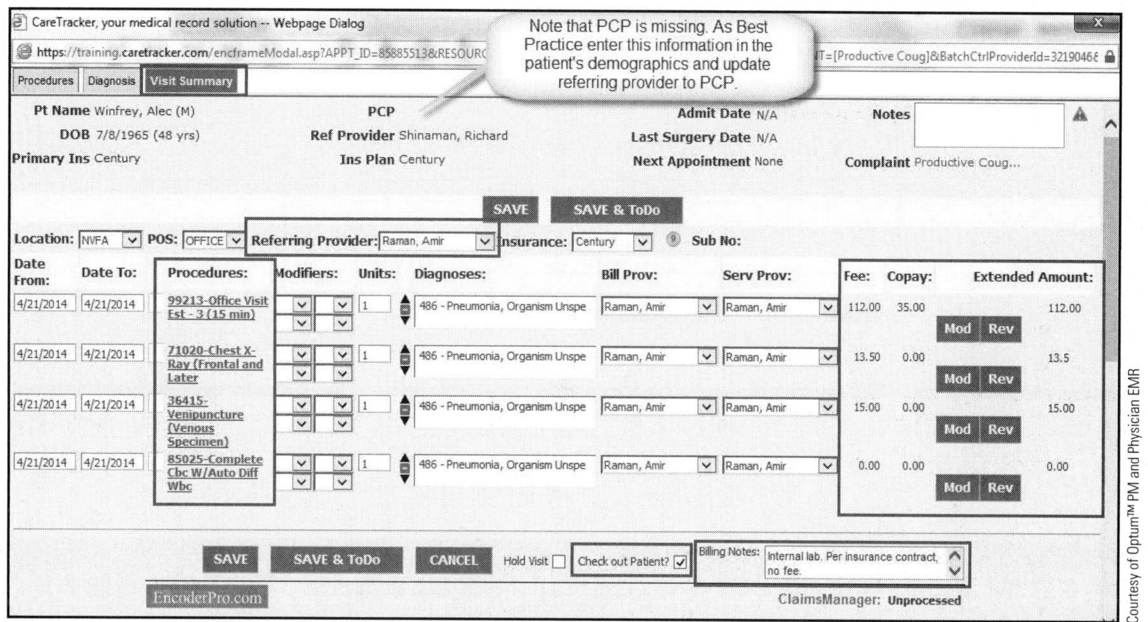

Figure 6-8 Alec Winfrey Visit Summary Window

12. (If applicable) To link the visit to a case, you would select a case from the *Case* list. (No *Case* number is associated with this visit.)
13. Select an authorization number from the *Authorization* list, if applicable (not applicable in this activity).
14. In the *Billing Notes* section, enter "Internal lab. Per insurance contract, no fee."
15. From the *Billing Type* list, select "Professional" at the bottom of the *Visit* screen (Figure 6-9).

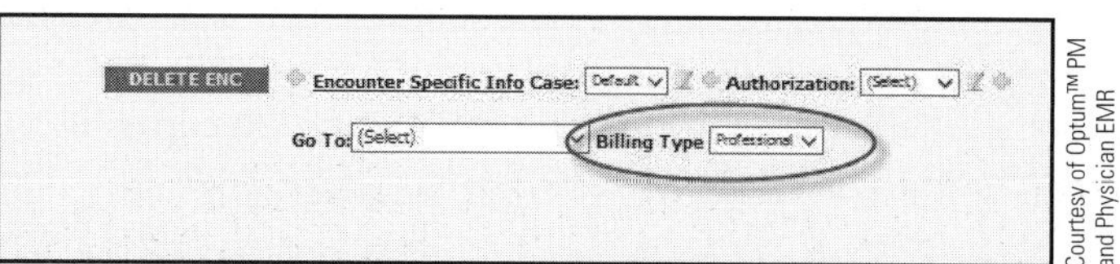

Figure 6-9 Billing Type - Professional

16. *(Optional)* Click *EncoderPro.com* to obtain coding information from *EncoderPro*. This information can be used as a guide to correct the visit information.
17. If Real Time Adjudication (RTA) is available for the payer, click *RTA* to receive preliminary payment information. RTA refers to the immediate and complete adjudication of a health care claim upon receipt by the payer from a provider. Adjudication is the final determination of the issues involving settlement of an insurance claim, also known as a claim settlement. (**Note:** RTA is not available in your student version of Optum™.)

Print a screenshot of the Visit Summary screen. Label it "Activity 6-2" and place it in your assignment folder.

18. Click *Save* at the top or bottom of the screen. When the visit is saved, the coding information is sent to *ClaimsManager* for screening. In addition, Optum™ PM and Physician EMR automatically checks out the patient on the schedule and a check mark appears next to the patient's name, confirming that the visit has been captured. Your *ClaimsManager* feature is not active in your student version of Optum™. Once you hit *Save*, you will receive a pop-up message (Figure 6-10) stating "An error occurred connecting to Claims manager. Transaction saved." Click *OK* on the pop-up. (**Note:** You must wait for this pop-up message before moving on or the transaction will not be saved.)

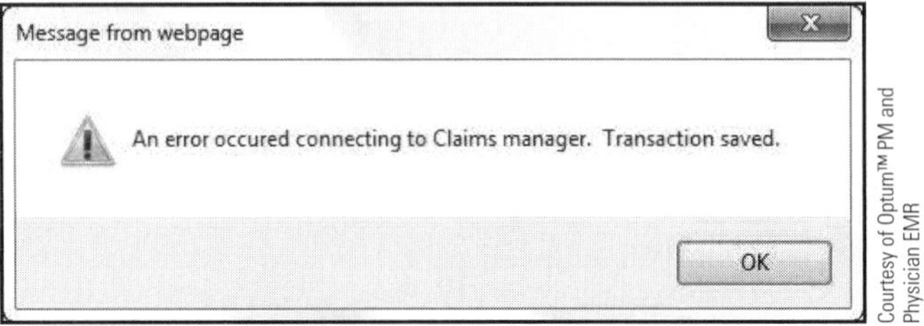

Courtesy of Optum™ PM and Physician EMR

Figure 6-10 ClaimsManager Error Message

PROFESSIONALISM CONNECTION

Using Real Time Adjudication (RTA) is becoming more commonplace as medical practices strive to remain financially viable. This is especially true for specialty practices that provide services in addition to office visits (e.g., orthopedic outpatient procedures). RTA is a relatively new concept and practices and staff may struggle to incorporate it into their billing practices. RTA does not make much, if any, change to the way an HMO insurance is handled. HMOs typically have a copay amount for office visits, hospital visits, and so on that does not vary, and patients have always paid their copay upon check-in.

RTA especially affects the workflow and common practice for Medicare and PPO insurance. Medicare and most PPOs typically have an 80/20 split. This means that once the claim is submitted, it is adjusted by Medicare or the PPO insurance company to the contracted rate for the service(s) billed. After applying the contracted rate, the insurance pays 80% (after any initial annual deductible or out-of-pocket patient requirements, if any, have been satisfied), and then the patient is responsible for the remaining 20%. Although some PPOs also have a copay requirement or a different insurance/patient split (e.g., $20 copay and 70/30 split), patients with Medicare and PPO insurance have been accustomed to waiting for the EOB from their insurance company to advise them of the contracted amount, what was paid by insurance, and what balance (e.g., 20%) the patient owes. The patient then receives a bill from the provider/practice. As practices incorporate RTA into their workflows, they will need to be sensitive to patient concerns when asking for patients to pay their "share" at the time of the visit.

Applying RTA practices to larger amounts, such as specialty outpatient services, may be even more challenging. Imagine a patient who needed an emergency outpatient orthopedic procedure and instead of getting a call from the provider's office the next day to see how he or she was doing, the call instead was to advise the patient how much his or her share of the bill was going to be. Consider how you, as a biller and coder, would incorporate this new policy of advising patients of any estimated balance due to the practice. Discuss with the class the concept of using RTA and various dialogs to use with patients.

ACTIVITY 6-3: Resolve an Open Encounter

In Optum™ PM and Physician EMR, you have the option to save a visit directly as a charge. This eliminates the additional steps of either navigating to the *Charge* screen to save the charge from the previously created visit or from having to save *Bulk Charges* via the *Missing Encounters* link on the *Dashboard*.

An encounter is an interaction with a patient on a specific date and time. Encounter types include visits, phone calls, referrals, results of a test, and more. The *Open Encounters* application displays a list of appointment-based "visit" type of encounters that do not have a corresponding clinical note and also identifies patients who have a clinical note for a specific date of service but no encounter billed for that same date. Additionally, the *Open Encounters* application displays customized encounters that require billing or a signed note. The *Open Encounters* application is accessible from the following locations:

- *Home* module > *Dashboard* tab > *Open Encounters* link (*Clinical* section) (Figure 6-11)

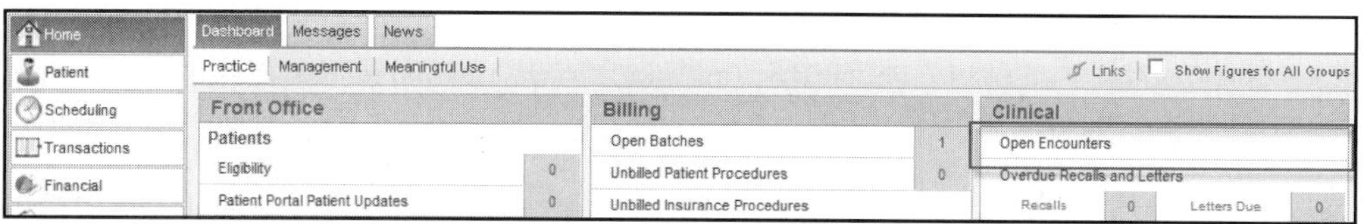

Figure 6-11 Open Encounters Link on Dashboard Tab

Courtesy of Optum™ PM and Physician EMR

- *Clinical Today* module > *Tasks* tab > *Open Encounters* (from the *Tasks* menu on the right side of the window) (Figure 6-12)

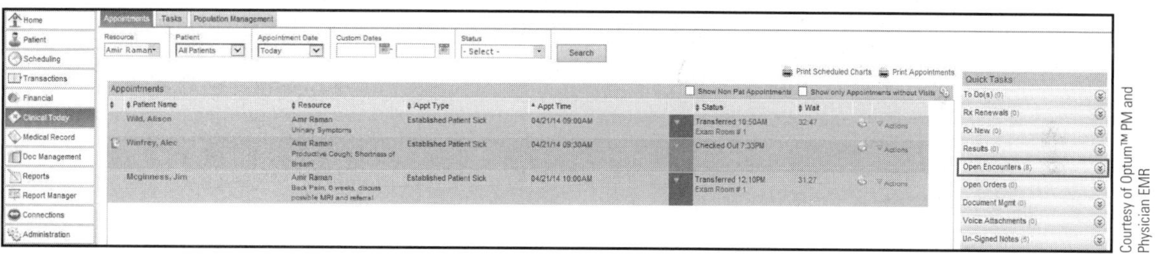

Figure 6-12 Open Encounters from the Clinical Today Module

Courtesy of Optum™ PM and Physician EMR

- An alternative method is to click the *Clinical Today* module and *Tasks* tab and view open encounter tasks in the *All Tasks* window. You can sort on the *Tasks* column to easily identify open encounter tasks.

The *Open Encounters* application helps resolve appointment-based "visit" type of encounters by entering the visit information, reviewing, transcribing (if the note contains an untranscribed file), signing the note, and then billing. Patient Alison Wild is being seen today for urinary symptoms.

To Resolve an Open Encounter:

1. Access the *Open Encounters* application from the *Home* module > *Dashboard* tab > *Open Encounters* link (*Clinical* section). If the encounter you are looking for does not display, use the drop-down feature next to *Provider*, select "All", and then click the *Change Resource* icon.

2. Find the encounter you want to resolve (Figure 6-13). (Locate the encounter you created for Alison Wild.)

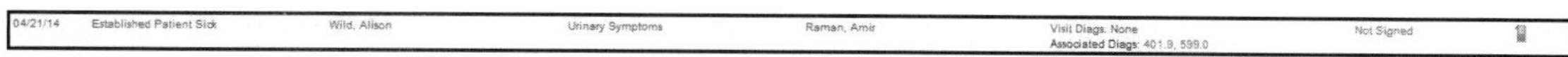

Figure 6-13 Alison Wild Open Encounter

Courtesy of Optum™ PM and Physician EMR

ADMINISTRATIVE SPOTLIGHT

An open encounter with an unsigned note, untranscribed file, is billable if visit information is captured; however, it is recommended to enter, transcribe, and sign the note, and then complete the billing.

3. Under the *Note* column, click the *Not Signed* link. The *Progress Note* application displays, enabling you to complete and sign the note. (**Note:** You are acting as a clinical MA or provider at this point.)
4. Confirm (resolve) that all items in the A&P for the encounter have been completed. Do not sign the note.
5. As best practice, perform an eligibility check on the patient before saving the visit.
6. Click on the *Visit* icon in the *Clinical Toolbar*. The *Visit* application will display. You would normally enter the codes as noted by the provider (V70.0 and 90746) (Figure 6-14), but you determine upon reviewing the patient's A&P and results of eligibility check that you need to do further research. You determine that V70.0 is an incorrect code for Medicare patients and should be coded 99213 for an established patient, sick visit. In addition, you noted on the A&P that the patient had a urinalysis; therefore, you would need to add a CPT® code for specimen handling (99000). Although the Hep B vaccine CPT® code was entered (90746), there is also a CPT® code for a fee for the injection (90471). Therefore, you will resolve the open encounter by selecting the following codes:
   - CPT® codes: 99213; 90746; 99000; and 90471

     Source: Current Procedural Terminology © 2013 American Medical Association.
   - ICD-9 codes: 599.0, 788.1, and 401.9

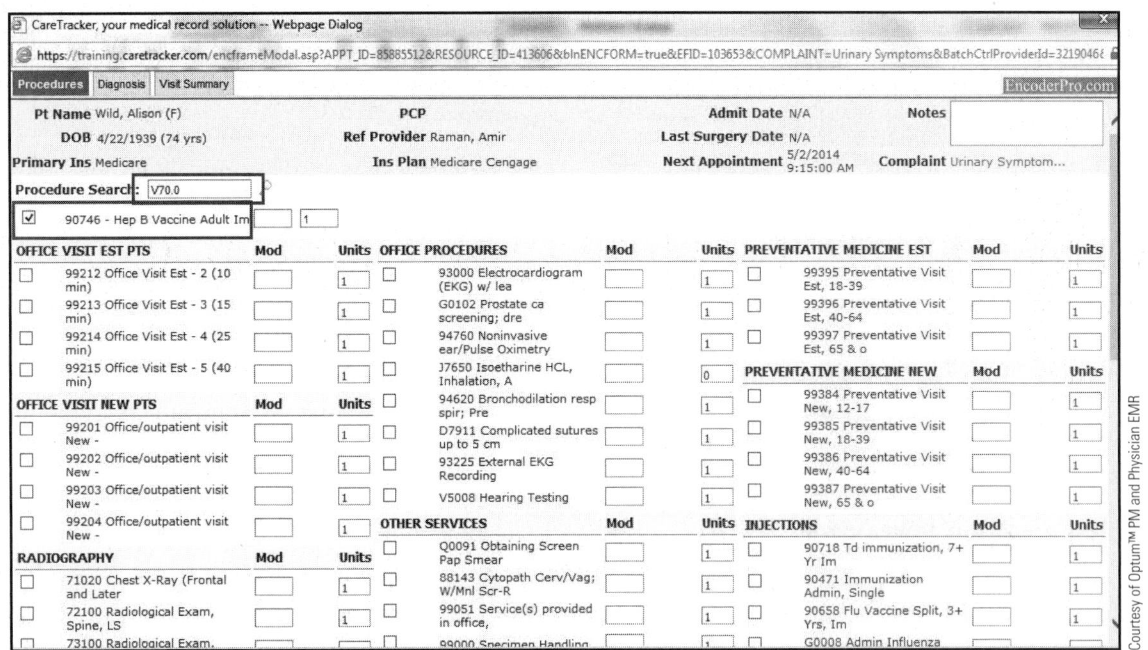

Courtesy of Optum™ PM and Physician EMR

Figure 6-14 Alison Wild Procedure Screen

7. After entering the procedure and diagnosis codes, click the *Visit Summary* tab. On the *Visit Summary* screen (Figure 6-15) click *Save*. When the visit information is saved, the icon in the *Visit* column changes to "Visit Complete." (**Note:** Refresh the *Open Encounters* screen to see the updated *Visit* column entry.)

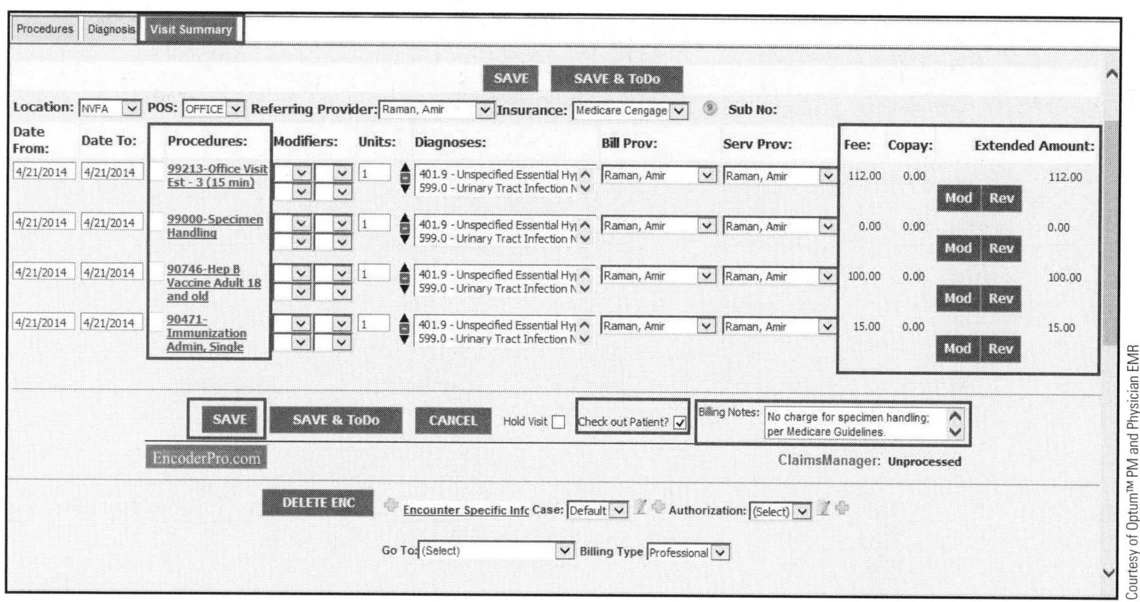

Courtesy of Optum™ PM and Physician EMR

Figure 6-15 Alison Wild Visit Summary Screen

Print a screenshot of the updated Open Encounters window, label it "Activity 6-3," and place it in your assignment folder.

8. You will sign the note in Activity 6-4. After both the note and billing processes are complete, the encounter is deleted from the *Open Encounters* application and is saved under the *Encounter* section of the patient's medical record for reference. Optum™ PM and Physician EMR updates the status of the *Note* and *Visit* columns to "Complete," and "Visit Complete."

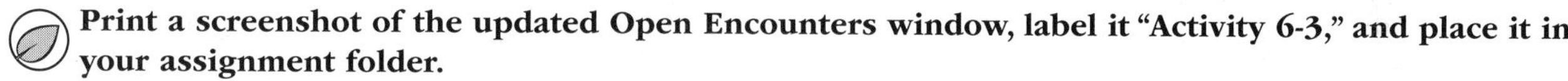

ACTIVITY 6-4: Sign and Print a Progress Note

The *Unsigned Notes* application displays a list of progress notes that are not signed or that require a co-signature by the provider set in the batch. A co-signature is required when a progress note is documented by a non-physician provider such as a physician assistant (PA) or a nurse practitioner (NP). Once again, acting as a clinical MA or provider, access the *Unsigned Notes* application (Figure 6-16) from one of the following locations:

- *Clinical Today* module > *Tasks* tab > *Unsigned Notes* (from the *Tasks* menu on the right side of the window) or click an unsigned notes task in the *All Tasks* window. You can sort on the *Tasks* column to easily identify unsigned note tasks.
- An alternative method is to click the *Clinical Today* module, and then click *Unsigned Notes* from the *Quick Tasks* menu (on the right side of the window).

The *Unsigned Notes* application lists notes that the treating and supervising provider must review and sign. You can sign the note directly from the following locations:

- *Unsigned Notes* application
- *Progress Notes* application

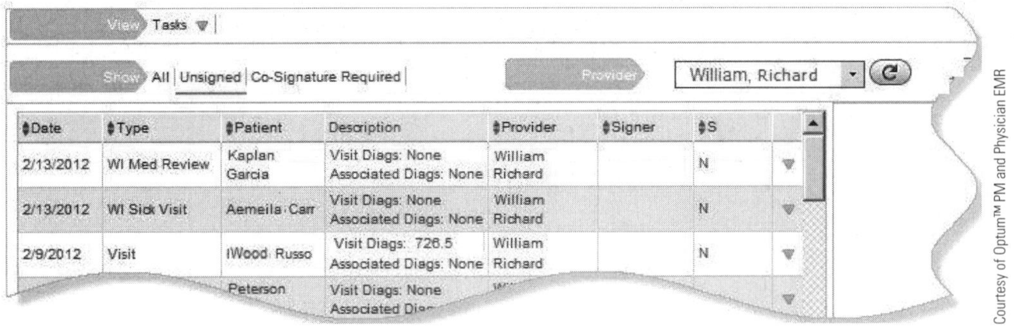

Figure 6-16 Unsigned Notes Application

It is important to know that once a progress note is signed, you can no longer make changes to it, and any open items/orders that were not completed prior to signing the note will not display within the A&P. Having confirmed that all tasks outlined in the A&P are completed, sign the note.

To Sign a Note:

1. Access the *Unsigned Notes* application by clicking on the *Clinical Today* module > *Tasks* tab > *Unsigned Notes* (from the *Tasks* menu on the right side of the window) or clicking an unsigned note under *Task* in the *All Tasks* window. You can sort on the *Task* column to easily identify unsigned note tasks.
2. Click the note to sign. The note launches on the right side of the pane. (Click the note for Alison Wild's encounter.)
3. Review the note on the right pane and click the *Sign* icon. A message prompt appears to confirm the action (Figure 6-17). Click *OK*. (**Note:** Alternatively, you could point to the *Arrow* icon in the *Action* menu and click *Edit Note* to open the note in a new window, review, make changes, and sign or co-sign the note.) Once the progress note is signed, it will disappear from the *Unsigned Notes* application.

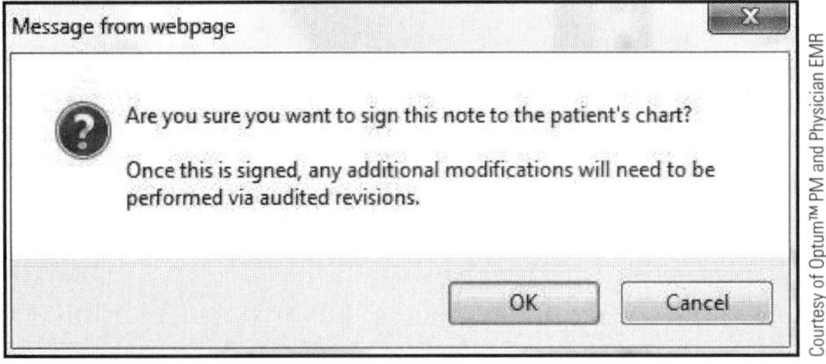

Figure 6-17 Sign Note Pop-Up Window

4. With patient Alison Wild in context, click on the *Medical Record* module.
5. Click on *Progress Notes* from the *Patient Health History* pane, and select the progress note you created for Alison Wild. The note launches on the right side of the pane.
6. Click the *Print* icon on the progress note (Figure 6-18). A *Clinical Note* dialog box will display where you can select *Print* or *PDF*.

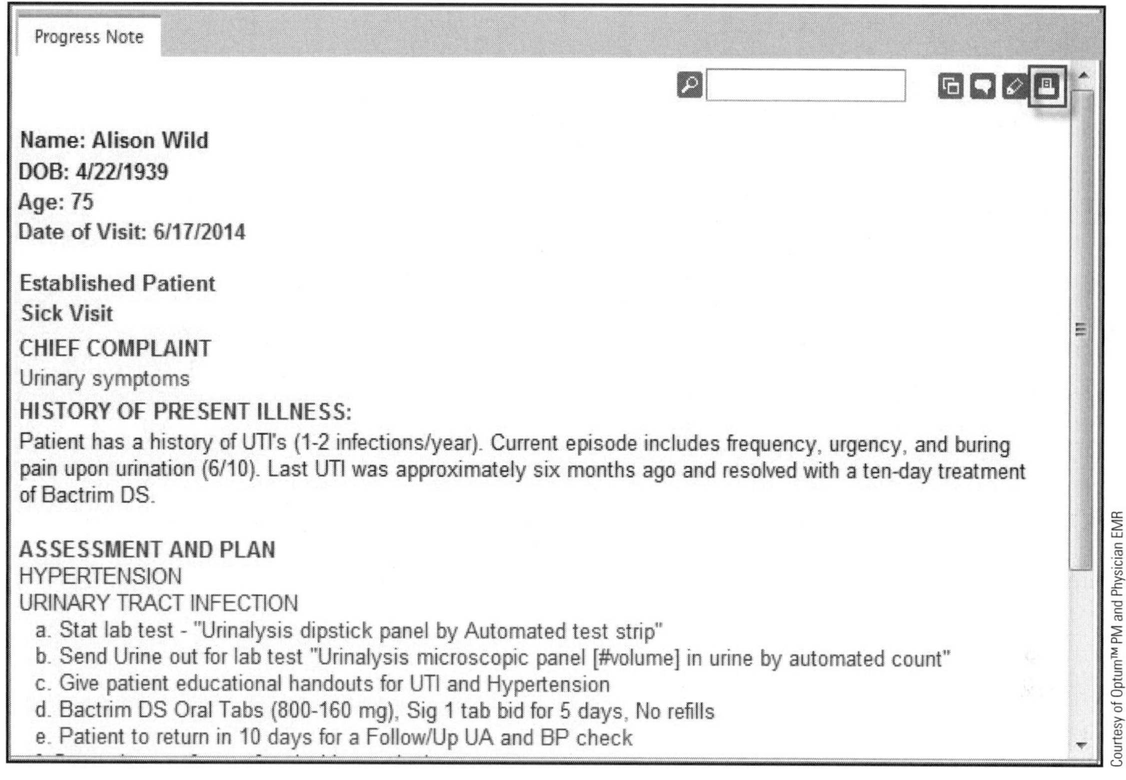

Courtesy of Optum™ PM and Physician EMR

Figure 6-18 Progress Note with Print Icon

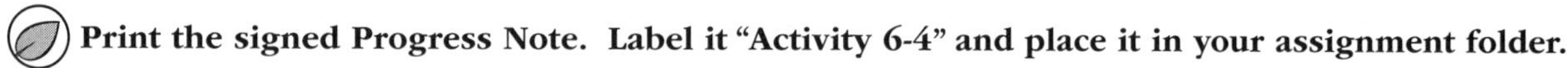
Print the signed Progress Note. Label it "Activity 6-4" and place it in your assignment folder.

7. Now access the *Open Encounters* application again from the *Home* module > *Dashboard* tab > *Open Encounters* link (*Clinical* section). Using the drop-down feature next to *Provider*, select "All", and then click the *Change Resource* icon to refresh the screen. You will note that Alison Wild's encounter is no longer listed in the *Open Encounters* link.

MINI-CASE STUDIES

If the demographic pop-up alerts you to missing information when you pull the patient into context, it is best practice to update as necessary. Update patients' PCP, subscriber numbers, and confirm (Y) to Consent, HIE, and NPP as needed.

Case Study 6-1

NVFHA MANAGER CHALLENGE

Do you recall from Chapter 4 that when Mr. Mcginness was checked in for his visit his insurance information was not updated and that no copy of his current insurance card was scanned? Consider this as you proceed with billing and coding activities and think about what effect this may have on the revenue cycle. (**Hint:** Refer back to Chapter 4 and update Jim's demographic with new insurance information before proceeding to capture his visit.) You will also note that Jim paid his former copay amount upon check-in ($35.00) and that his new insurance has only a $20.00 copay. Keep this in mind during later activities when addressing an overpayment.

a. Referring to Activity 6-2 (Capture a Visit), and using the information that follows, capture the visit for patient Jim Mcginness. Refer to the encounter you created for Mr. Mcginness in Chapter 5. Mr. Mcginness is being seen today for back pain.

- *CPT® Code*: 99203

  Source: Current Procedural Terminology © 2013 American Medical Association.

- *ICD-9 Codes*: 724.2; 739.3; 739.5

Print a screenshot of the completed visit and label it "Case Study 6-1A."

b. Once the visit has been captured, repeat Activity 6-4 and sign and print the progress note for Jim Mcginness.

Print the signed progress note and label it "Case Study 6-1B." Place both documents in your assignment folder.

Case Study 6-2

Repeat Activity 6-4 and sign and print the progress note for Alec Winfrey.

Print the signed progress note, label it "Case Study 6-2," and place it in your assignment folder.

Resources

The Optum™ PM and Physician EMR Help homepage represents a wealth of information for the electronic health record (https://training.caretracker.com/help/CareTracker_Help.htm).

Centers for Medicare and Medicaid Services (CMS). *Glossary*. Accessed from the CMS website at http://www.medicare.gov/glossary/f.html

General information: Nurse practitioner practice. (2011, April 13). Retrieved from http://www.rn.ca.gov/pdfs/regulations/npr-b-23.pdf

Health Information and Management Systems Society. (2008, August). *Real time adjudication of healthcare claims* (HIMSS Financial Systems Transactions Toolkit Task Force White Paper). Retrieved from http://himss.files.cms-plus.com/HIMSSorg/content/files/Line%2027%20-%20Real%20Time%20Adjudication%20of%20Healthcare%20Claims.pdf

CHAPTER 7

Billing

LEARNING OBJECTIVES

1. Create a batch for financial transactions.
2. Manually enter a charge.
3. Edit an unposted charge.
4. Generate electronic and paper claims.
5. Demonstrate knowledge of and perform activities related to electronic remittance including: manually posting payments and adjustments, reconciling insurance payments to the patient's account and EOB, paper claims, billing statements, and batch deposits.

NVFHA MANAGER CHALLENGE

My challenge to you is to become familiar with the many different types of insurance plans and the effects on the practice when there is an issue regarding non-covered services. In order for the medical practice to be profitable, fees will be collected from patients for services rendered. The fees and copay can be collected at the time of the visit, or you can bill the patient after a claim has been submitted to the insurance company. It is NVFHA policy that copays must be collected from the patient at the office for each encounter. Only bill the copay in a circumstance where the patient does not have any form of payment available at the time of service. Upon receipt of payment (EOB) from the insurance company and after any adjustment to the contracted rate is applied, the balance due will be billed to the patient.

Although it may be a delicate issue, you will be responsible for communicating the fees for services to patients. This discussion should take place prior to the patient's appointment with the physician to avoid an awkward situation. With the ever-changing insurance environment and mandates from the Affordable Care Act, you must verify the patient's insurance plan, deductibles, out-of-pocket amounts, and that NVFHA is in fact contracted with the patient's insurance company. If the patient's insurance is not contracted with NVFHA, the patient will be responsible for the entire fee. In some cases, patients will be forced to change providers to one that is contracted with their insurance; otherwise the costs would be unaffordable to the patient. Changing physicians is very stressful to many patients. Often they have developed relationships that span many years or decades. Therefore, it is important that you have an understanding of the various types of insurance (HMO, PPO,

(*Continues*)

NVFHA Manager Challenge *(Continued)*

Medicare, Medicaid, commercial carriers, and private pay) and how to communicate effectively with patients in an articulate and compassionate manner. Even within the many types of insurance, copays and deductibles can vary widely. Some health plans have large deductibles and large copays. Other plans may require no copay at the time of visit, but the patient will pay a percentage of the contracted rate for the service.

When you register a new patient and collect patient demographics over the phone, you will gather insurance information as well. This will help determine what type of fee or payment will be required of the patient, and confirm that our practice is contracted with the patient's insurance carrier. The office policy must be clearly stated to the patients on the telephone, by written communication (on forms patients must complete and sign), and by way of posted notices in the waiting room. Patients should be gently reminded in a very professional manner that payment will be expected at the time of service. Our automated answering system also conveys fee and payment options available.

The activities performed in this chapter mimic those duties a biller and coder perform and are crucial to the financial health of the practice. You must always review the A&Ps from the patient visits for which you are generating claims to see if all codes were billed (i.e., special handling, EKG, injections, vaccinations, etc.) and that the proper CPT® code for the visit has been captured and is a covered code with the patient's insurance. As always, you must be sure that the diagnosis (ICD) code(s) support the CPT® code(s) entered. Although you as a medical assistant cannot make changes to a progress note, you must query the provider if there are concerns about the code(s). (**Note:** For these student simulated activities, you are able to make changes and edits as needed yourself so that you become familiar with the process.)

ACTIVITY 7-1: Create a Batch for Billing and Charges

The batch is the essential component required before entering and posting any financial transaction such as charges, payments, adjustments, and refunds. Having set your operator preferences in Chapter 4 (Activity 4-3), create a *Batch* as instructed to begin your activities in this chapter.

1. Prior to creating a batch, you will need to open the fiscal period for which you will be entering activities. Go to the *Administration* module > *Practice* tab > *System Administration, Financial* headers > *Open/Close Period* link (Figure 7-1).

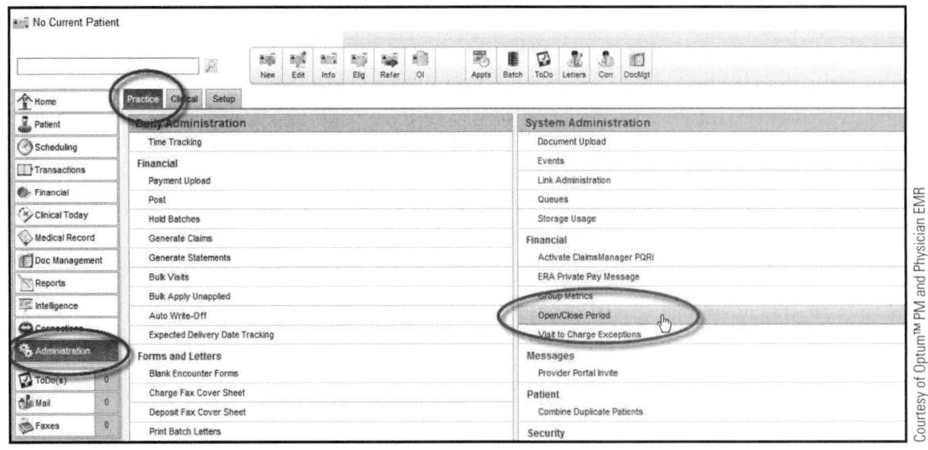

Courtesy of Optum™ PM and Physician EMR

Figure 7-1 Open/Close Period Link

2. Open the period for the activities you are posting (use the current period you are working in), and click *Save* (Figure 7-2).

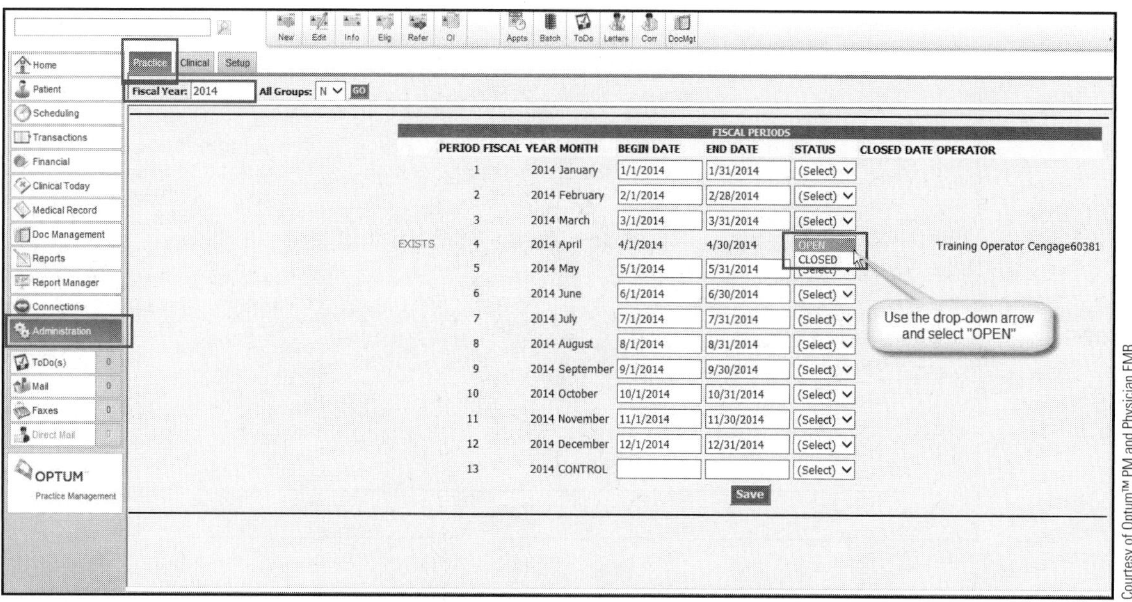

Courtesy of Optum™ PM and Physician EMR

Figure 7-2 Open Fiscal Period for Current Month/Year

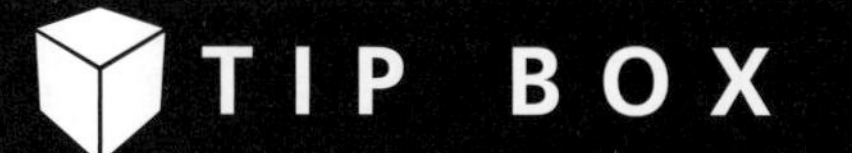

Because you may have been working in various activities in more than one period, always work in the "current" period (e.g., if you begin an activity in September, complete all the related activities in that period. If you start a new activity unrelated to a previous period [e.g., in December], you would then use the new period [December]). Although you will be instructed to complete activities and post batches, *never* close a period. In Chapter 9, Applied Learning for the Paperless Medical Office case studies, you will conclude with closing period(s) once all activities have been completed.

3. Click the *Batch* icon on the *Name Bar* and the *Operator Encounter Batch Control* dialog box will display (Figure 7-3).

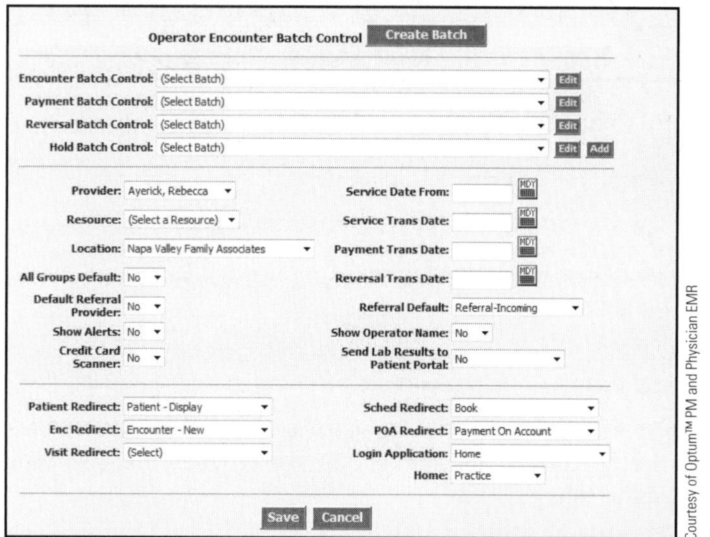

Courtesy of Optum™ PM and Physician EMR

Figure 7-3 Operator Encounter Batch Control Dialog Box

4. Click *Edit* and then click *Create Batch*. The *Batch Master* dialog box displays (Figure 7-4).

BATCH_MASTER

Batch Name: cengage56110122014
Group Id: Napa Valley Family Health Associates 2
Primary Operator Id: cengage56110
Fiscal Period: (Select Fiscal Period)
Fiscal Year: - 2014 +
Reference No.:
Hash Patient Ids:
Hash Cpt:
Total Chgs:
Total Pmts:
Batch Deposit: (Select)
Date Received: MDY
Save Cancel

Courtesy of Optum™ PM and Physician EMR

Figure 7-4 Batch Master Dialog Box

5. By default, the *Batch Name* box displays a batch identification name. The name consists of your user name followed by the current date. However, you can edit the batch name if necessary to identify the types of financial transactions associated with the batch. Name the batch "Ch7Charges" (Figure 7-5). Do not use symbols when editing the name.

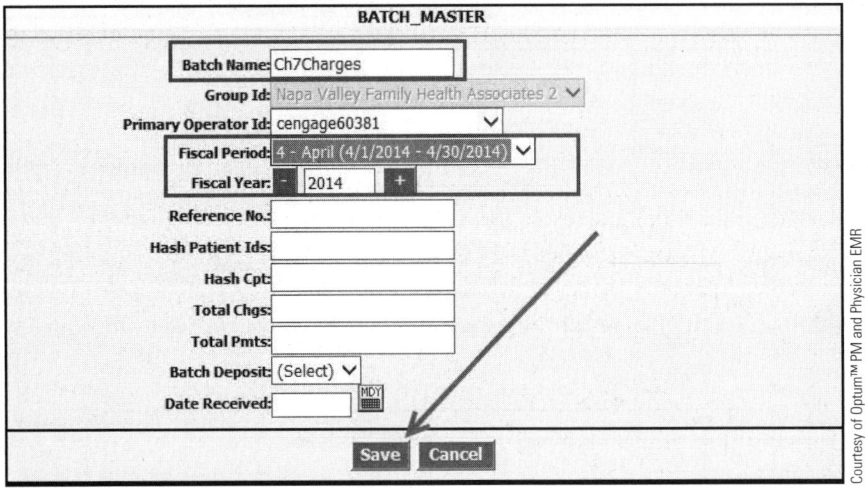
BATCH_MASTER

Batch Name: Ch7Charges
Group Id: Napa Valley Family Health Associates 2
Primary Operator Id: cengage60381
Fiscal Period: 4 - April (4/1/2014 - 4/30/2014)
Fiscal Year: - 2014 +
Reference No.:
Hash Patient Ids:
Hash Cpt:
Total Chgs:
Total Pmts:
Batch Deposit: (Select)
Date Received: MDY
Save Cancel

Courtesy of Optum™ PM and Physician EMR

Figure 7-5 Change Batch Name

6. By default, the *Group Id* displays the name of your group.
7. By default, the *Primary Operator Id* displays your user name. This cannot be changed.
8. By default, the *Fiscal Year* displays the current financial year setup for your company. Select "20XX" (the current year you are working in).
9. In the *Fiscal Period* list, click the period to post financial transactions. The list only displays fiscal periods that are currently open. Select the current month you are working in as the *Fiscal Period*.
10. In the *Date Received* box, enter the date the encounter was created in MM/DD/YYYY format or click the *Calendar* MDY icon and select the date. Select the date of Alison Wild's first appointment (the date you scheduled her appointment in Chapter 4).
11. Click *Save*. If you have more than one period open, a pop-up warning (see Figure 7-6) will appear asking you to confirm the fiscal period. Click *OK*.

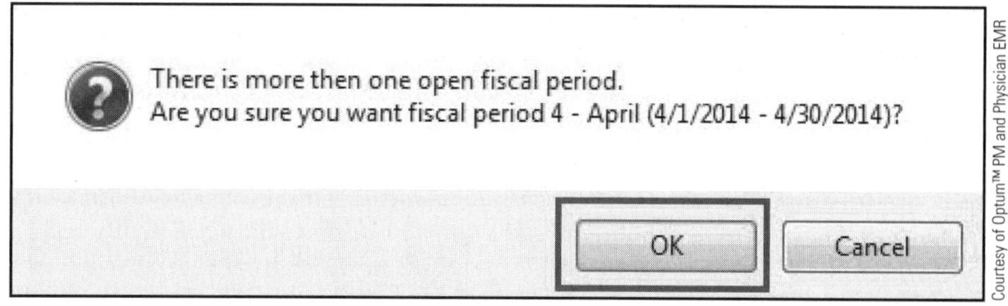

Figure 7-6 Fiscal Period Pop-Up Warning

12. Optum™ PM and Physician EMR displays the *Operator Encounter Batch Control* dialog box with the new batch information (Figure 7-7).

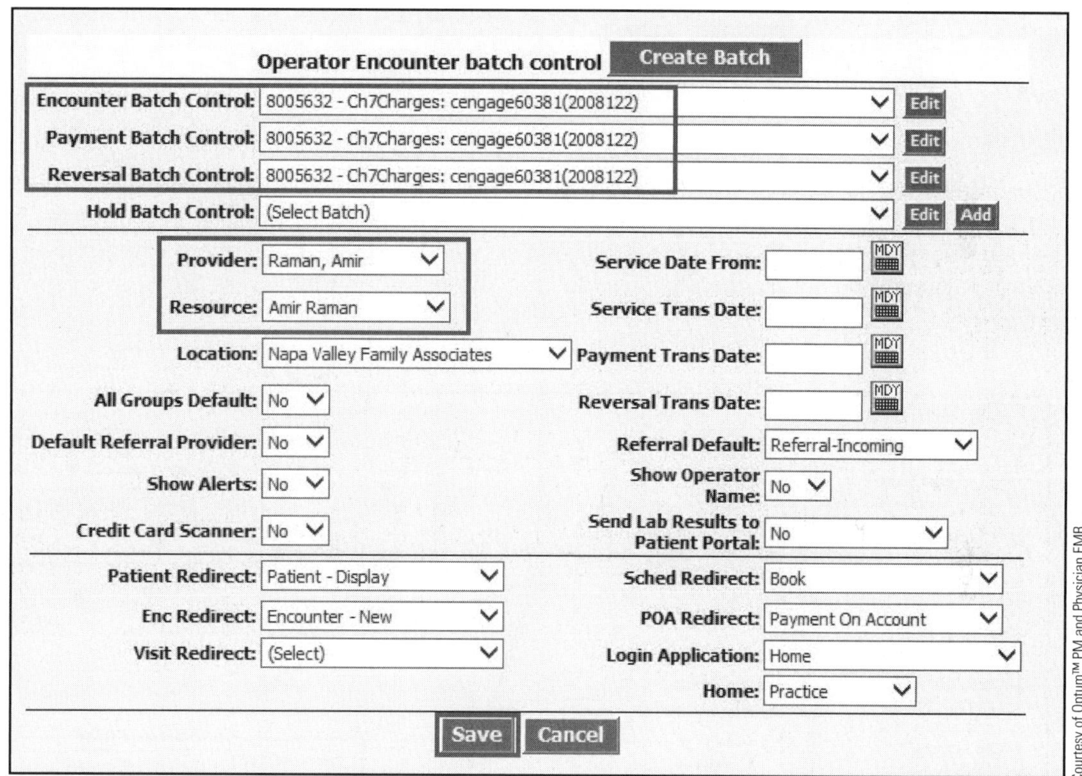

Figure 7-7 Ch7Charges Batch Information

13. You can further *Edit* your batch by using the drop-down arrow next to each field and updating the provider, resource, location, and so on, if needed. Confirm that the *Provider* and *Resource* noted in the batch match with patient Alison Wild (select "Amir Raman").

14. Click *Save*.

15. Write down your "Encounter Batch Control No." for future reference (should include "Ch7Charges"). ______________________.

Print a screenshot of the Operator Encounter Batch Control screen, label it "Activity 7-1," and place it in your assignment folder.

16. Click "X" in the upper-right corner to close the dialog box.

ACTIVITY 7-2: Posting a Patient Payment

Optum™ PM and Physician EMR provides a secure environment to ensure that the billing process goes smoothly and the quality of the information sent to insurance carriers is clean. The normal flow for a claim in Optum™ PM and Physician EMR starts with a patient appointment, followed by checking in the patient where patient information is confirmed and updated and any copay is collected. At the end of the patient visit, the services are recorded and reviewed before the claims are sent out.

Although Ms. Wild does not have a copay with her Medicare insurance, she knows that she will have an amount due after Medicare pays its portion. She does not like to owe money on her account, so at checkout, she would like to make a payment toward any balance that may be due.

1. If not already done, open the fiscal year/period in which you are entering a charge from the *Administration* module > *Practice* tab > *Open/Close Period* link (see Figure 7-2).
2. Pull patient Alison Wild into context.
3. Open the *Transactions* module. The *Charge* application displays by default.
4. Click on the *Pmt on Acct* tab.
5. In Chapter 4 you learned how to enter and print payment receipts for patients. Following the instructions in Activity 4-5, enter a payment on account for patient Alison Wild. Ms. Wild has provided a check for $50 toward any eventual balance due. Enter check number "4434" and the appointment date to be applied to the patient's payment (the appointment you created for Alison Wild in Chapter 4). Your screen should look like Figure 7-8.

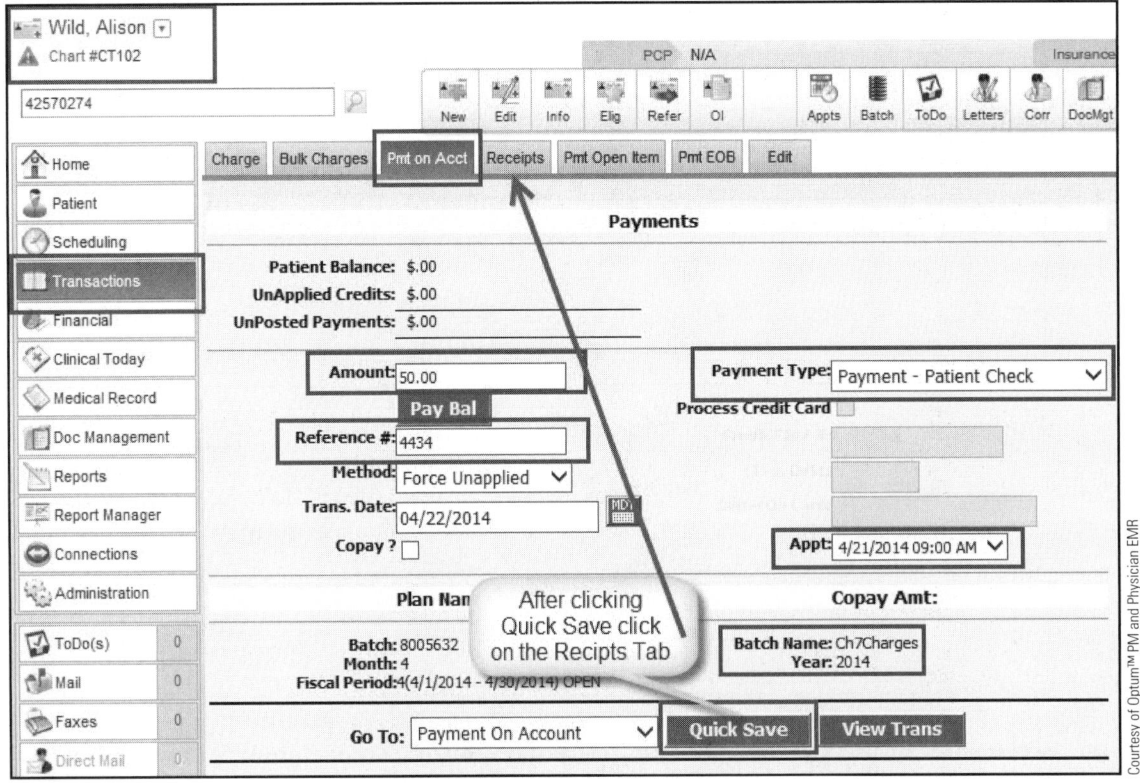

Figure 7-8 Alison Wild Payment on Account

6. Click *Quick Save*.

7. Click on the *Receipts* tab and print a receipt for Alison Wild (as in Activity 4-6).

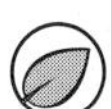

Print the receipt, label it "Activity 7-2," and place it in your assignment folder.

8. You will not post the batch at this time because you will complete additional activities before running a journal and posting a batch.

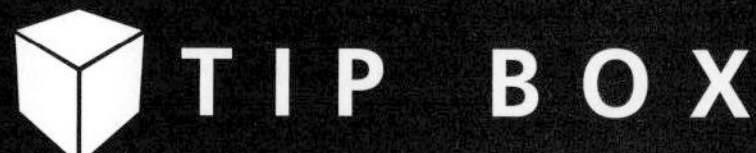

If you were through with billing activities and wanted to post the batch, you would click on the *Home* module > *Practice* tab > *Billing* section > *Open Batches* link (Figure 7-9). You would then click the checkbox next to the batch you want to post (Figure 7-10) and select *Post Batches*.

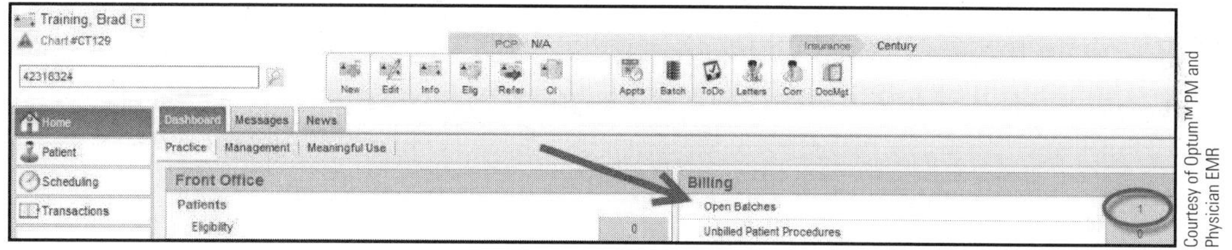

Courtesy of Optum™ PM and Physician EMR

Figure 7-9 Open Batches Link

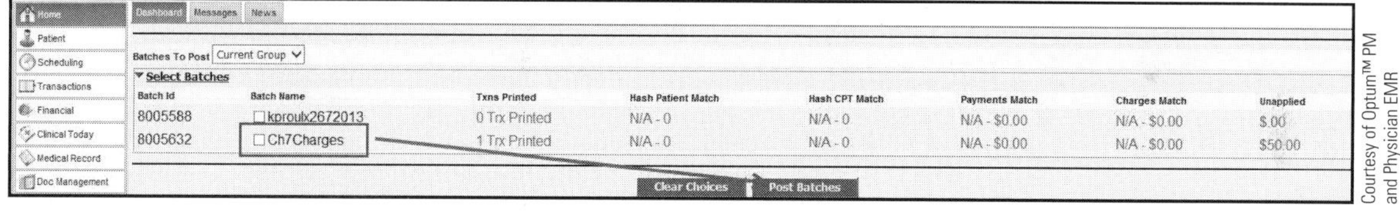

Courtesy of Optum™ PM and Physician EMR

Figure 7-10 Post Copay Batch

ACTIVITY 7-3: Manually Enter a Charge for a Patient

You will be manually entering a charge (not appointment related) in the same period as your previous activities. Follow the steps in Activity 7-1 to create a new batch using today's current month and year. (**Note:** If the fiscal period is not already open, you will need to open it before creating the batch.) Name the new batch "SmithSNF." Set the batch defaults to reflect the current period, *Provider* and *Resource* for patient (Dr. Raman), change the *Location* to "Napa Valley Skilled Nursing Facility," and so on.

1. After the current fiscal period is open and you have the new batch created, pull patient Darryl Smith into context.
2. Open the *Transactions* module. The *Charge* application displays by default, displaying the charge screen.
3. Manually enter a "SKILLED NURSING FACILITY" charge using the following charge related information:
   a. Using the *Location* drop-down, select "NVSNF." Using the [Tab] key will automatically populate the *POS* with "SKILLED NURSING FACILITY."

b. Enter *Ref Provider* "Dr. Raman."

c. If a service date was not selected when you created your batch, it must be entered in the *Date* and *Date To* fields. The date must be within the open period in your current batch. A date can either be entered manually in MM/DD/YYYY format or can be selected from the *Calendar* MDY function. In the *Date* and *Date To* fields, enter today's date (see Figure 7-11).

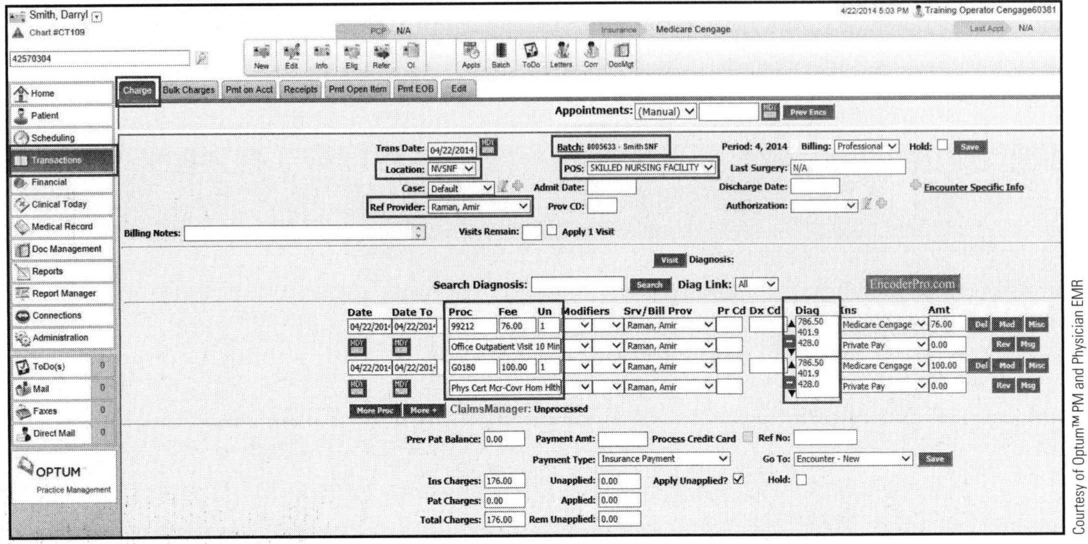

Courtesy of Optum™ PM and Physician EMR

Figure 7-11 SNF Charge

4. *Visit Diagnosis* (Figure 7-12) will be grayed out in the student environment in the center of the screen.

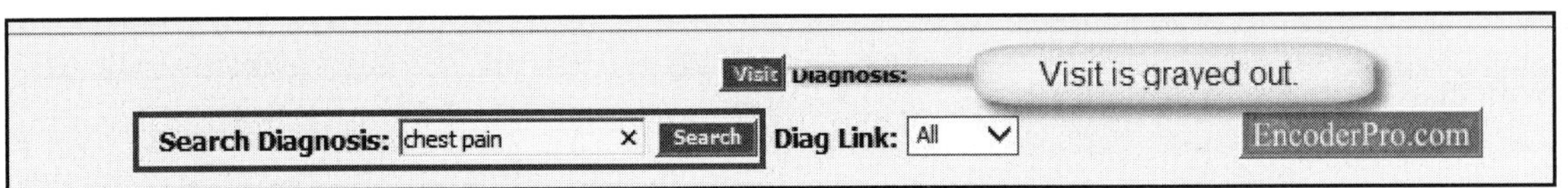

Figure 7-12 Visit Diagnosis

Courtesy of Optum™ PM and Physician EMR

5. If there have been previous ICD codes entered for this patient, you can place a check mark by the desired code to select it. If the code is not listed, type "chest pain" in the *Search Diagnosis* field and then click *Search* (it may take a few moments to populate). Click on code "786.59 (Chest pain, other)". Optum™ PM will pull in the diagnosis "786.59" to the *Diag* field (Figure 7-13).

Courtesy of Optum™ PM and Physician EMR

Figure 7-13 Search Diagnosis

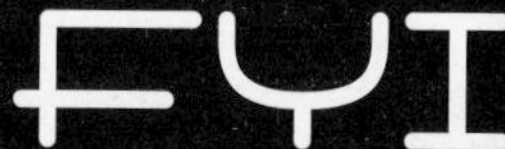

If you need to search for a diagnosis code, enter a partial code or a keyword (enter "Chest Pain") in the *Search Diagnosis* box, and then click *Search*. The application opens the *Code Search* window (Figure 7-14). Click on the desired ICD-9 or ICD-10 code to select it. The application pulls the selected code into the *Diag* box.

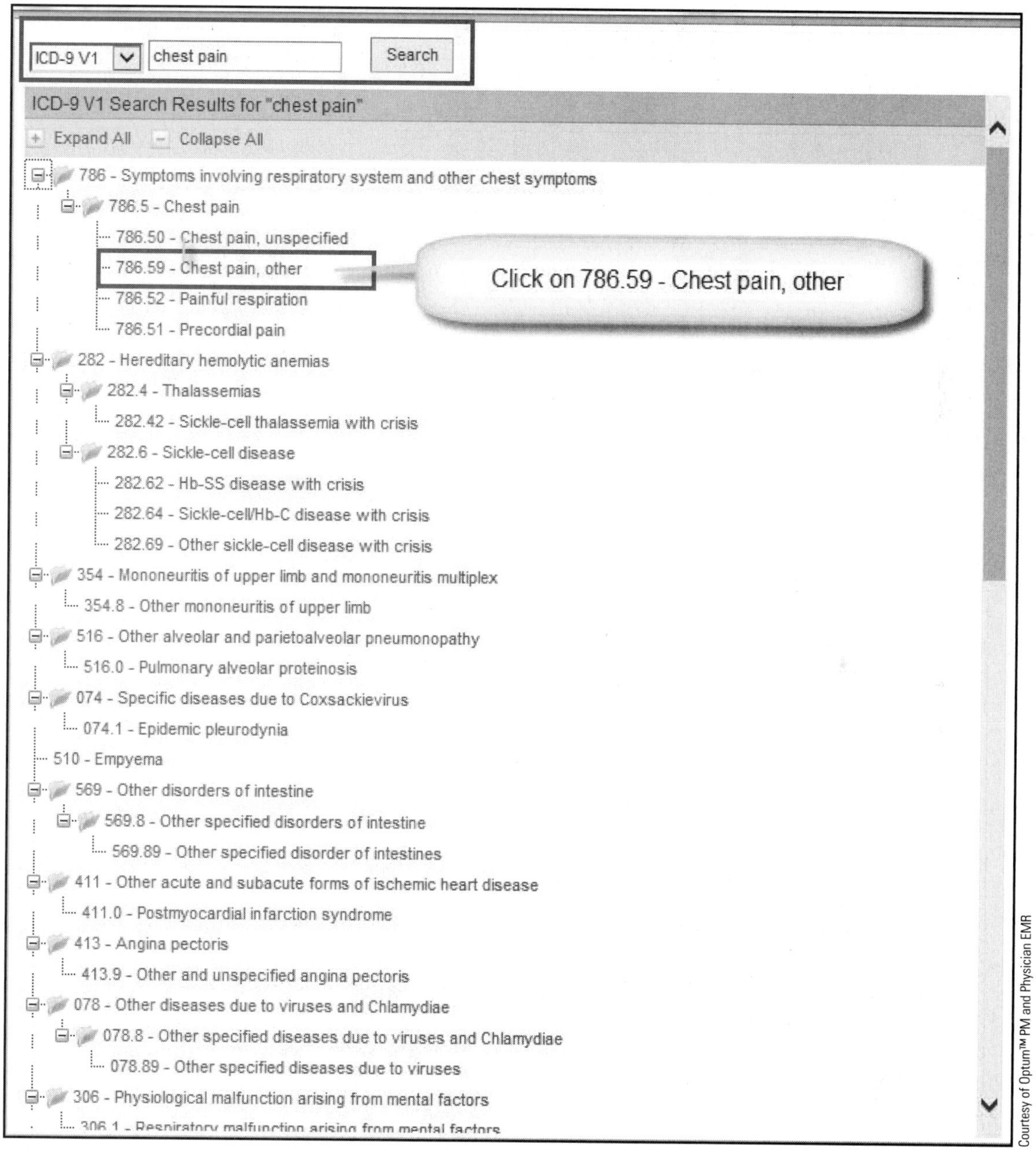

Courtesy of Optum™ PM and Physician EMR

Figure 7-14 Code Search Window

6. Repeat step 5 to add additional diagnosis codes to the *Diag* box if needed. Add ICD-9 codes: 401.9 and 428.0 (as in Figure 7-11).
7. Click on *EncoderPro.com* to review the codes selected and determine if they are appropriate for the visit/charge. Operators can also access *EncoderPro* from both the procedure and diagnosis pages in the *Visit* application.

TIP BOX

ICD-9 codes are internationally recognizable 3- to 5-digit code sets, representing medical conditions or signs and symptoms. ICD-9 is to be replaced by the ICD-10 code set on October 1, 2015. To accommodate the change to ICD-10, Optum™ now has a *View Mappings* link (Figure 7-15) that will enable you to find the ICD-10 code as needed. The *Visit Diagnosis, Visit Summary,* and *Claim Edit* screens now display a code set (9) icon next to the insurance field that indicates if the insurance company or plan is configured to receive ICD-9 or ICD-10 diagnosis codes (Figure 7-16). A diagnosis code in the *Diag* box can be removed by double-clicking on the code. The order of multiple codes can also be changed in the *Diag* box by highlighting the code to move up or down and then clicking on the corresponding up or down black arrow next to the *Diag* box.

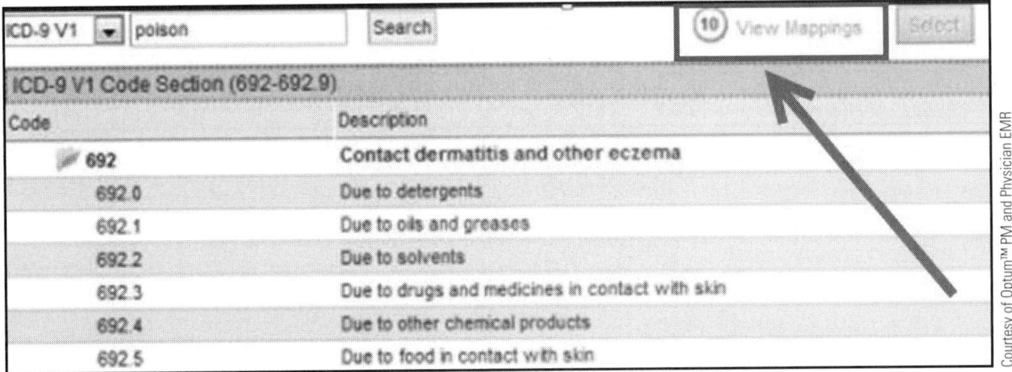

Figure 7-15 View Mappings

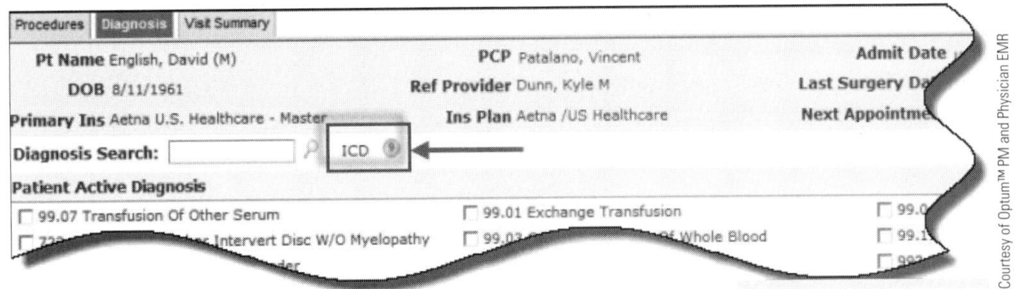

Figure 7-16 Diagnosis Code Set

Mapping Screen

The ICD mapping screen is accessed by clicking the *View Mappings* link at the top of the search results. This screen acts as a basic mapping tool, allowing the operator to see which ICD-10 codes map to the current ICD-9 codes (see Figure 7-17) and vice versa. Basic mapping is available for:

- ICD-9-CM Vol. 1 to ICD-10-CM
- ICD-10-CM to ICD-9-CM Vol. 1

The mapping screen contains several columns with information about the relationship between the ICD-9 and ICD-10 codes.

(*Continues*)

Tip Box (*Continued*)

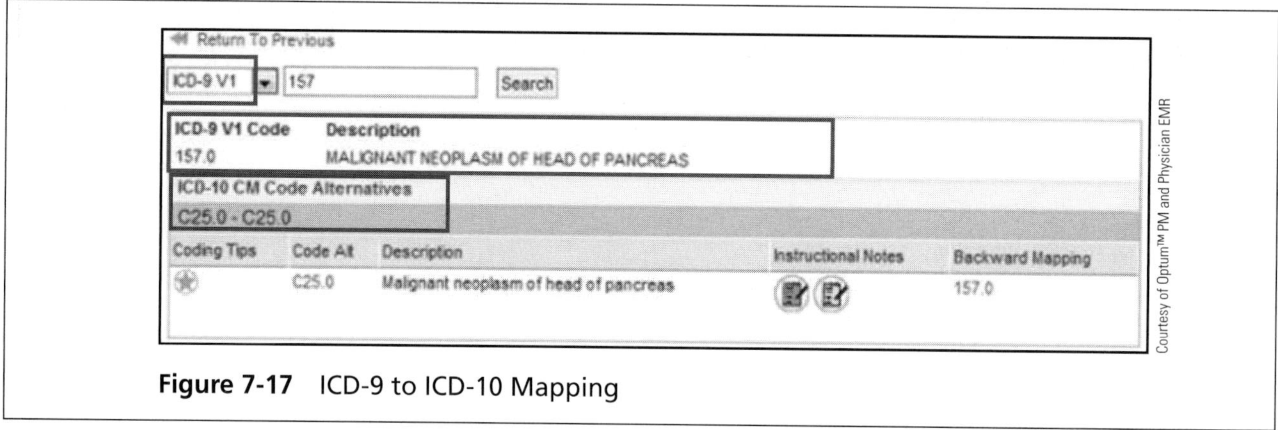

Figure 7-17 ICD-9 to ICD-10 Mapping

8. When a procedure code is entered in the *Proc* field, hit the [Tab] key and the procedure description, fee, and the amount to be charged to the patient's insurance and to the patient will be populated, and the *Modifiers* field will become the active field. Using the procedure code the provider submitted, enter the code "99212" in the *Proc* field, hit the [Tab] key, and a $76 *Fee* will automatically populate from the fee schedule.
9. Click on the *More Proc* button, which brings up another billing line. Enter CPT® code "G0180" in the *Proc* field. Hit the [Tab] key and the *Procedure Search* pop-up box will appear (Figure 7-18). Click on the code or description and the procedure will be pulled into the charge box.

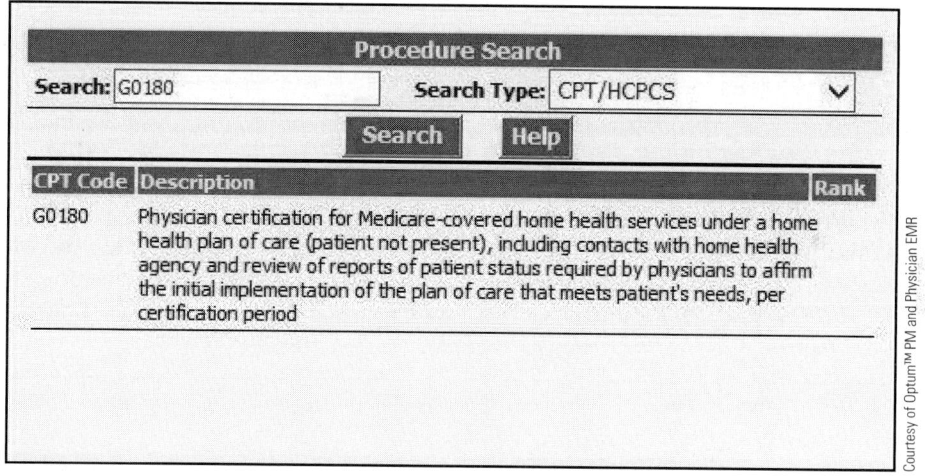

Figure 7-18 G0180 Procedure Search Window

10. Enter "$100" in the *Fee* field because this CPT® code is not on the NVFHA fee schedule.
11. Enter the provider's name (Dr. Raman) in the *Srv/Bill Prov* field from the drop-down list, if not already selected (Figure 7-19).

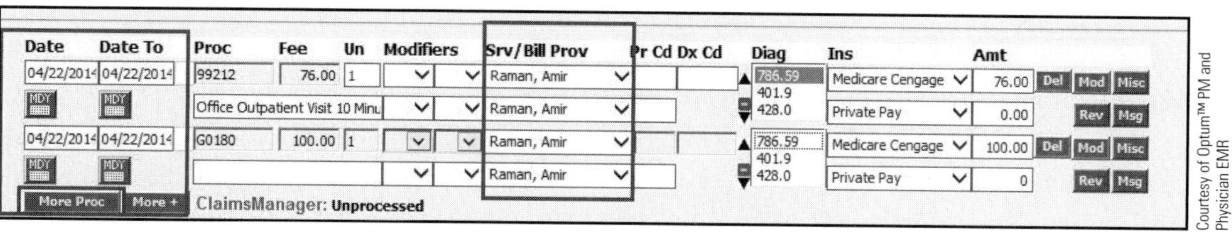

Figure 7-19 SNF Charge

Print the Charge Screen, label it "Activity 7-3," and place it in your assignment folder.

12. Click *Save*. You will receive an error message (Figure 7-20) because your student version is not connected to *ClaimsManager*. However, the transaction will be saved, and the patient is taken out of context. (**Note:** It may take a few moments for this task to save. Wait until you receive the error message "Transaction Saved" before moving on.)

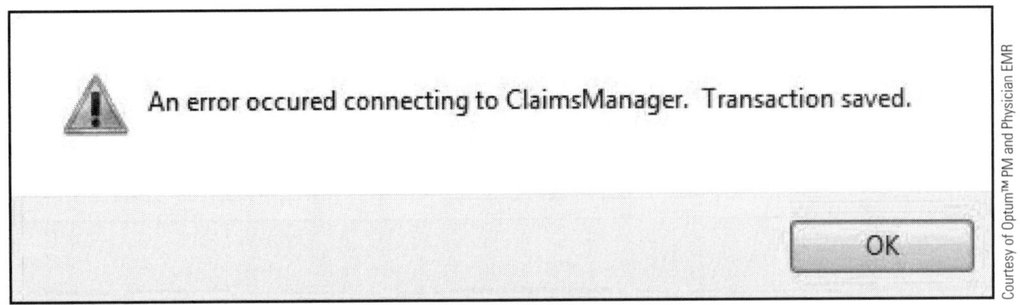

Figure 7-20 Error Message on Save When Entering a Charge

13. Click *OK* and the patient is removed from context and "Encounter Added" displays on your screen.
14. Your manually entered charge is now saved.

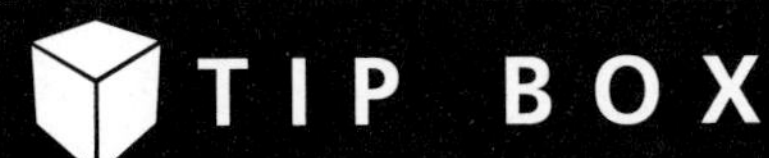

When a patient has both Medicare and a commercial insurance, always use the HCPCS code when billing injectables, DME, and others. If the HCPCS code is linked via a crosswalk code set to the CPT® code, the application will automatically pull the corresponding CPT® code onto the claim when the claim goes to the commercial insurance. Crosswalk (sometimes referred to as a "link") refers to a relationship between a medical procedure (CPT®/HCPCS code) and a diagnosis (ICD code). Not all HCPCS codes are linked via a crosswalk code set to CPT® codes.

ACTIVITY 7-4: Reversing a Charge

Although it is not required to edit charges, there will be times when you will find it necessary to edit an unposted charge (e.g., a biller is reviewing a charge and sees that the incorrect CPT® code was assigned to the claim). Using the charge entered in Activity 7-3, reverse the unposted charge.

1. Pull patient Darryl Smith into context.
2. Click the *Transactions* module. Optum™ PM and Physician EMR opens the *Charge* application.
3. Click on the *Edit* tab. When *Edit* is clicked all of the procedures entered in the patient's account along with each financial transaction linked to it will display (see Figure 7-21) beginning with the most recent date of service. Locate the procedure that needs to be entirely reversed on the patient's account (**Note:** You may need to scroll down the screen to locate the charge in question.) As biller, you have noticed that CPT® code 99212 is incorrect for SNF-related charges and you want to delete the charge so the billing is accurate, because G0180 is the accurate code for this service. You query the provider regarding codes, and he asks you to also bill CPT® code 99214.

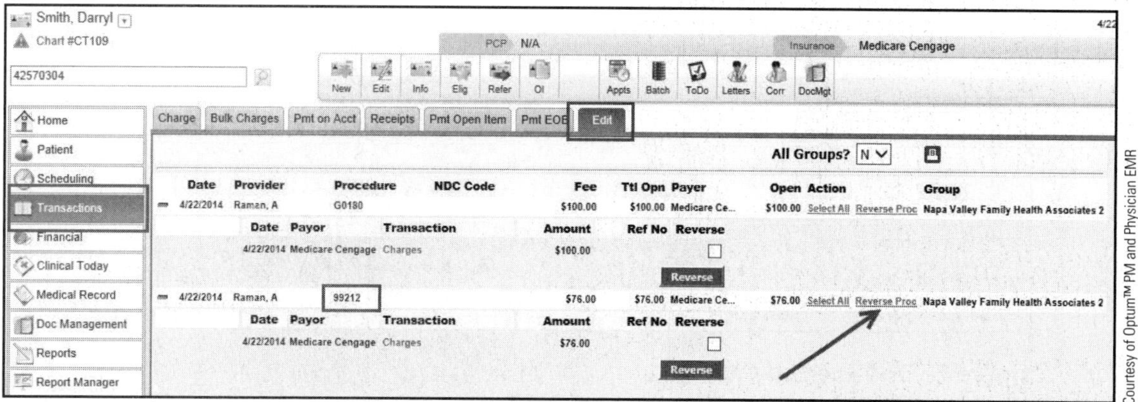

Courtesy of Optum™ PM and Physician EMR

Figure 7-21 Edit Unposted Charge for Darryl Smith

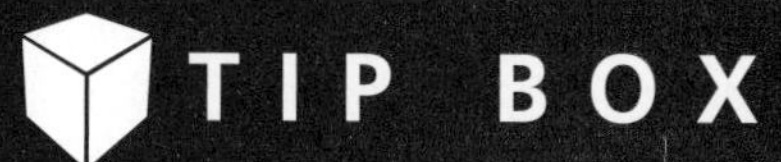

You can edit any active field, including *Location, Pos, Case, Referring Provider, Date, Modifiers, Servicing Provider, Billing Provider,* and *Diag*.

4. On the procedure line that needs to be entirely reversed, you can click on either the *Select All* link or the *Reverse Proc* link. Select the *Reverse Proc* link on the 99212 charge (see Figure 7-21).

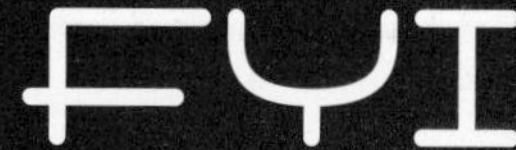

If you click on the *Reverse* button, all of the selected transactions are reversed.

5. You will receive a pop-up warning message (Figure 7-22) asking "Are you sure you want to reverse the selected Financial Transactions?" Click *OK*. The transaction will be reversed (Figure 7-23). (**Note:** If you receive the error message "The Reversal Date must be within Period Start and End Dates: xx/xx/20xx and: xx/xx/20xx" it may be due to a "compatibility" issue with your browser. Click on the compatibility icon in your web browser so that functionality is restored.)

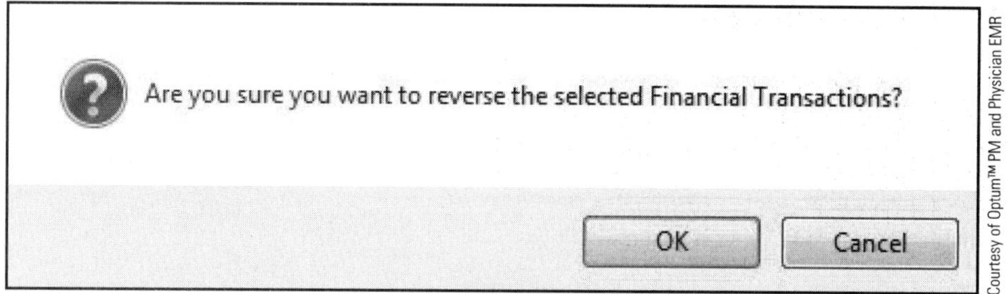

Courtesy of Optum™ PM and Physician EMR

Figure 7-22 Reverse Financial Transaction Warning

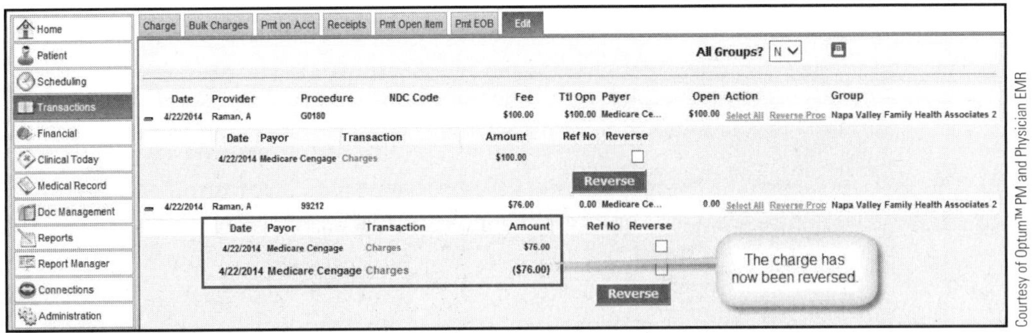

Figure 7-23 Reversed Charge

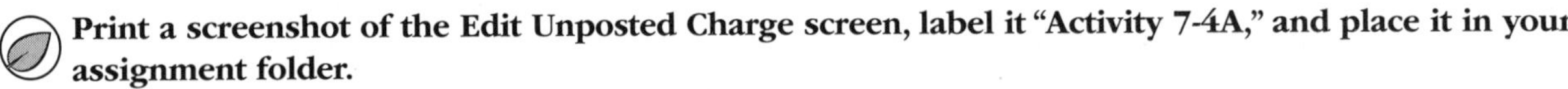

Print a screenshot of the Edit Unposted Charge screen, label it "Activity 7-4A," and place it in your assignment folder.

6. Click back on the *Charge* tab in the *Transactions* module and complete the *Charge* screen for the same location, POS, provider, date, and diagnoses as in Activity 7-3. (**Note:** Because you are working in Mr. Smith's electronic chart, the previously entered diagnosis codes will be listed just above *Search Diagnosis*. In this screen you can now just place a check mark next to the diagnoses you want to select.) The provider has asked you to bill *Proc* code "99214." You know from prior billing and coding experience that 99214 is also a non-covered code for SNF charges. Once again, query the provider (because you cannot independently change codes). Upon questioning, the provider acknowledges he did not mean 99214, but meant to bill for an EKG. Knowing the diagnosis codes support the CPT® code for an EKG, you enter CPT® code "93000." If no amount pre-populates when you use the [Tab] key, enter "$46.50" into the *Fee* field.

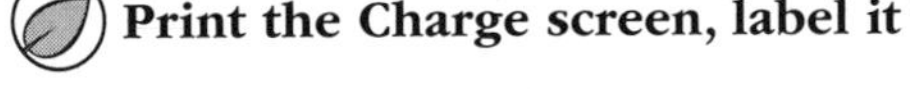

Print the Charge screen, label it "Activity 7-4B," and place it in your assignment folder.

7. Click on *Save* to save the charge.

ACTIVITY 7-5: Run a Journal

When you have finished entering data into your batch, you will run a journal to verify your batch and entry information. It is best practice to run a journal (as in Activity 4-7) prior to posting your batch to verify that you have entered all the financial transactions correctly in Optum™ PM.

1. Go to the *Reports* module > *Reports* tab > *Financial Reports* header > *Todays Journals* link (Figure 7-24).

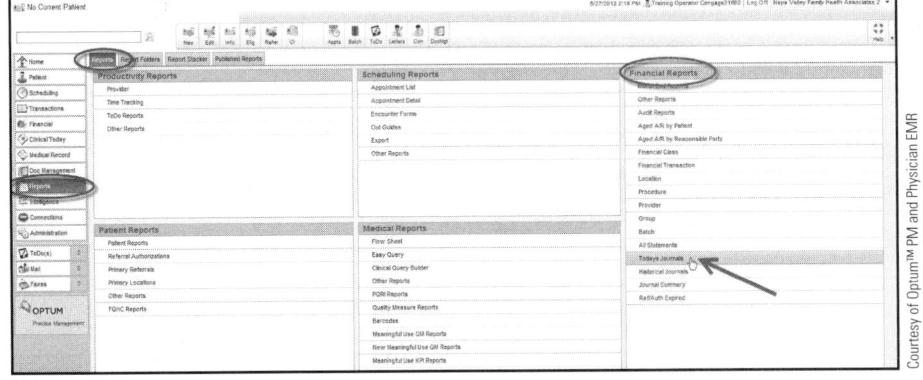

Figure 7-24 Todays Journals Link

2. Optum™ PM displays the *Todays Journal Options* screen. All of your group's open batches are listed in the *Todays Batches* box. You may need to click on the [+] sign to expand the *Batches* field (Figure 7-25).

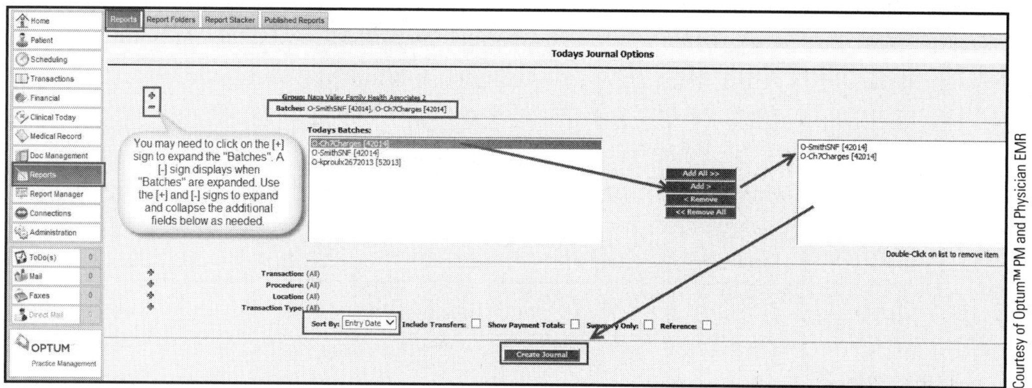

Courtesy of Optum™ PM and Physician EMR

Figure 7-25 Expand Journal Batch Options

3. Select a batch to include in the journal either by double-clicking on the batch name or by clicking on the batch and then clicking *Add >*. Optum™ PM adds the selected batches to the box on the right. Select batches "Ch7Charges" and "SmithSNF."
4. Scroll down to the bottom of the screen. From the *Sort By* drop-down list, select "Entry Date" (Figure 7-26).

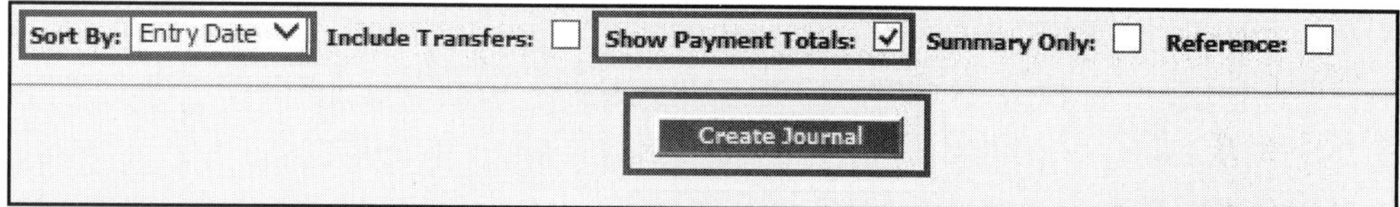

Figure 7-26 Sort By Entry Date

Courtesy of Optum™ PM and Physician EMR

5. Select the *Show Payment Totals* checkbox (see Figure 7-26).
6. Click *Create Journal*. Optum™ PM generates the journal (Figure 7-27).

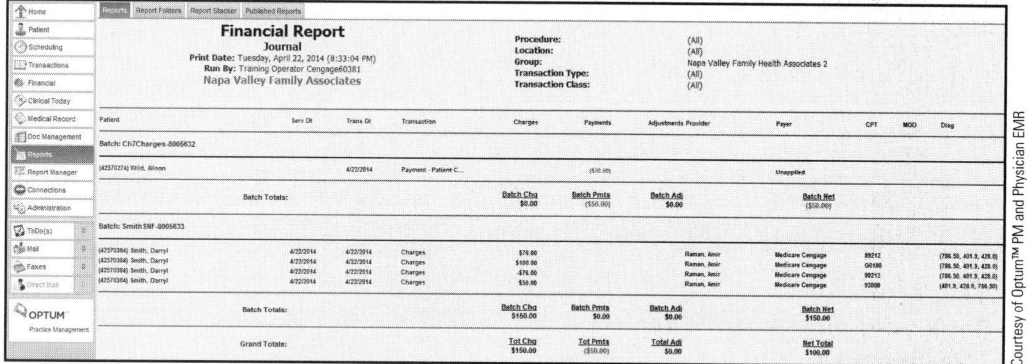

Courtesy of Optum™ PM and Physician EMR

Figure 7-27 Financial Report

7. To print, right-click on the journal and select *Print* from the shortcut menu.

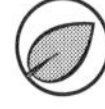 **Print the Journal, label it "Activity 7-5," and place it in your assignment folder.**

ACTIVITY 7-6: Post a Batch

Having generated a journal for the batch(es) you would like to post, review and identify any transaction errors that may have been made, and correct them prior to posting (using the steps outlined in Activity 7-4, Reversing a Charge). We will assume that there are no errors in the *Journal Report* created in Activity 7-5. Having balanced the money in your journal, post your open batch(es).

1. Go to the *Administration* module > *Practice* tab > *Financial* header > *Post* link (see Figure 7-28). Optum™ PM displays a list of all open batches for the group (see Figure 7-29).

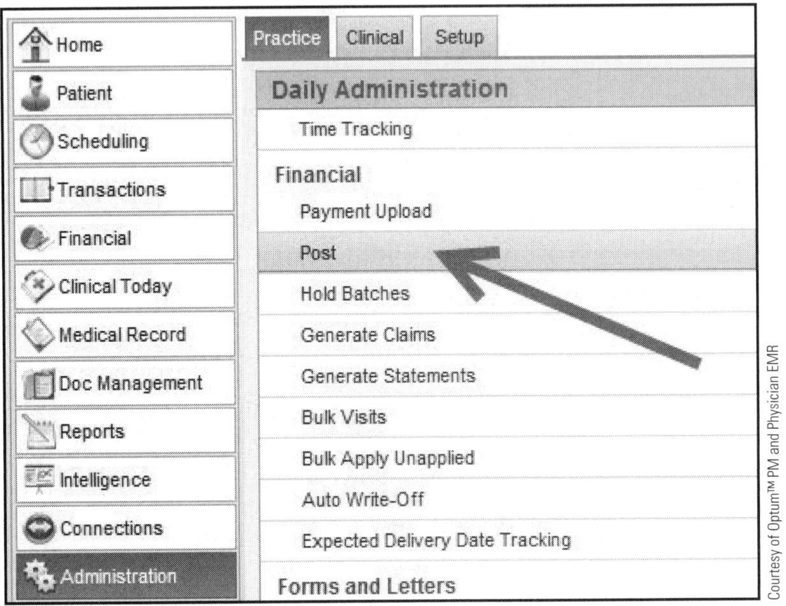

Courtesy of Optum™ PM and Physician EMR

Figure 7-28 Post Link from Practice Tab

ADMINISTRATIVE SPOTLIGHT

An alternate way to access and post batches is through the *Home* module > *Dashboard* tab > *Billing* header > *Open Batches* link.

2. Check the box next to the batch(es) you want to post, and then click *Post Batches*. Select the batch "Ch7Charges" (Figure 7-29). The batch "SmithSNF" should not be posted at this time.

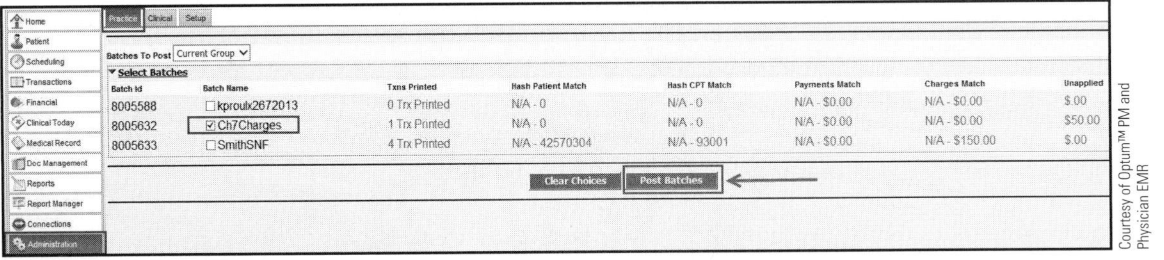

Courtesy of Optum™ PM and Physician EMR

Figure 7-29 Post Batches

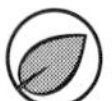 **Print the Post Batches screen, label it "Activity 7-6," and place it in your assignment folder.**

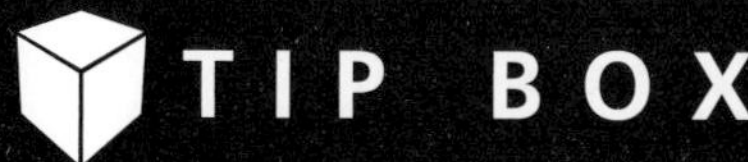

Although not required, it is recommended to only post a batch after a journal has been generated and balances verified. The total number of open batches for your group displays next to the *Open Batches* link.

ACTIVITY 7-7: Workflow for Electronic Submission of Claims

Claims can only be generated after your batch has been posted. You will simulate generating claims by following these steps because the *ClaimsManager* feature is not active in your student version of Optum™ PM. The claim will not actually generate, but you will be able to complete the steps.

1. Go to the *Administration* module > *Practice* tab > *Daily Administration* section > *Financial* header > *Generate Claims* link (Figure 7-30). Optum™ PM launches the *Generate Claims* application.

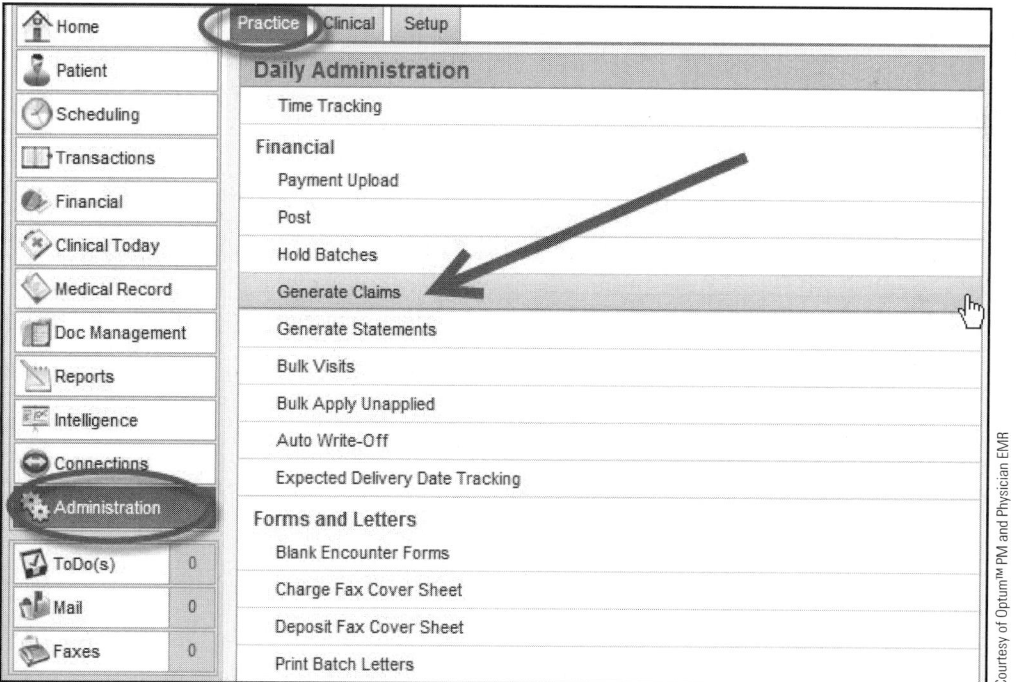

Figure 7-30 Generate Claims Link

2. Click *Generate Claims For This Group* (Figure 7-31). You will receive an error message (Figure 7-32) because the *ClaimsManager* feature of your student version is not active.

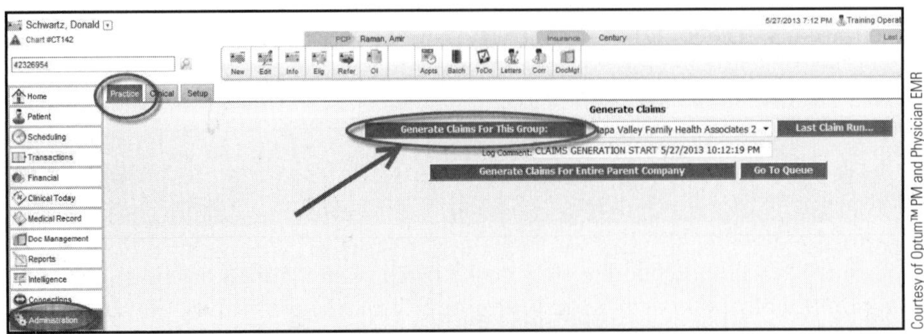

Courtesy of Optum™ PM and Physician EMR

Figure 7-31 Generate Claims for This Group

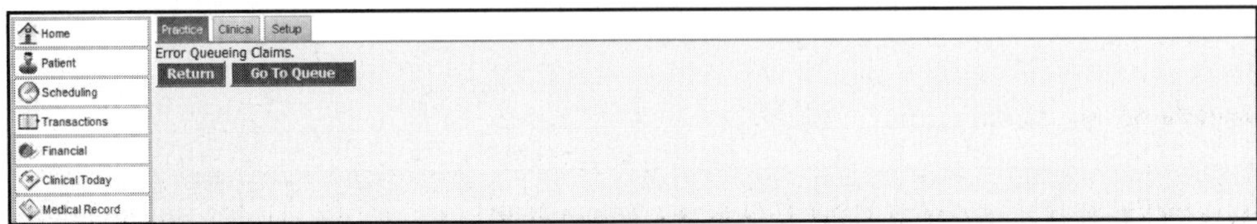

Figure 7-32 Error Queueing Claims

Courtesy of Optum™ PM and Physician EMR

3. In a live environment, your screen would look like Figure 7-33, which states "Claims are Queued for all Groups under this Parent Company." You would then click on *Go to Queue* and the report would generate. Figure 7-34 represents an example of the *Claims Queue* in a live environment, which displays the *Claims Worklist* (Figure 7-35).

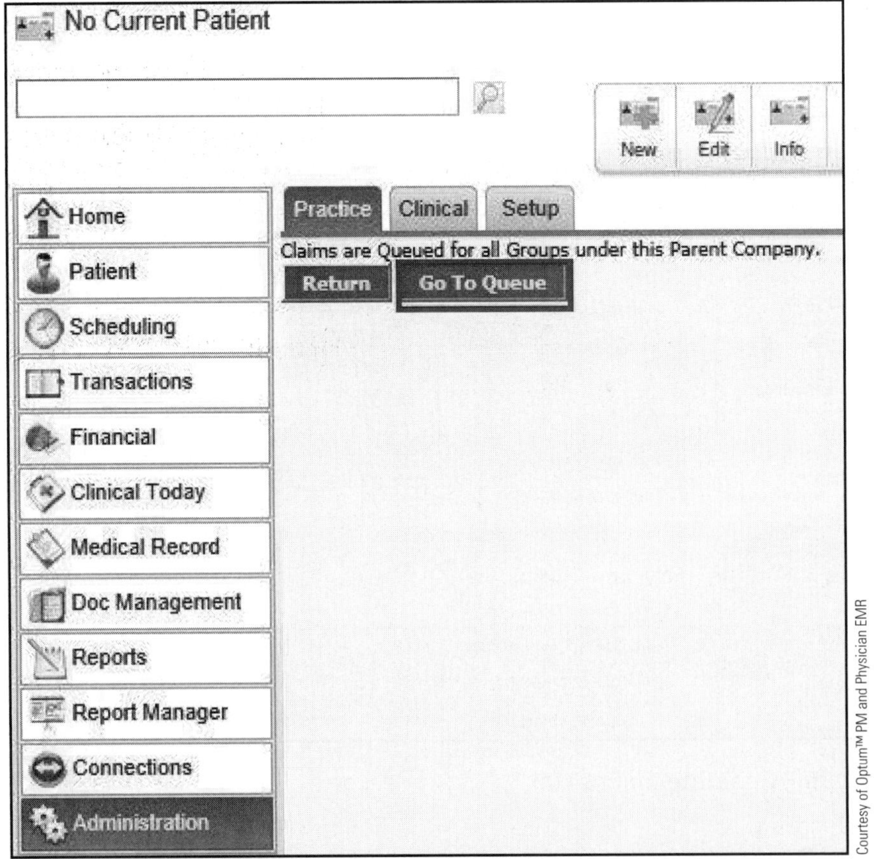

Courtesy of Optum™ PM and Physician EMR

Figure 7-33 Generated Claims

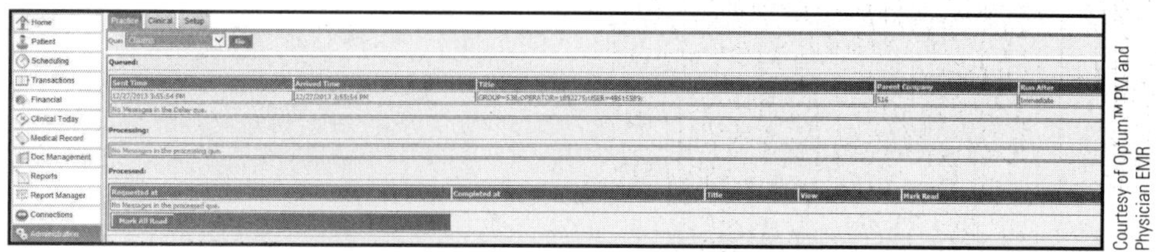

Courtesy of Optum™ PM and Physician EMR

Figure 7-34 Claims Queue

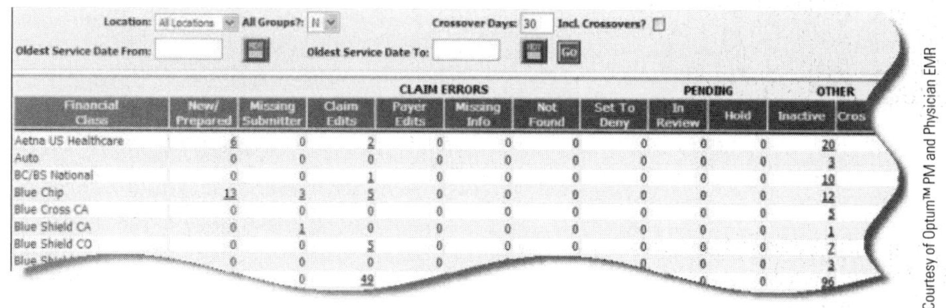

Courtesy of Optum™ PM and Physician EMR

Figure 7-35 Claims Worklist

4. Click back on the *Administration* module to clear the error message.

PM SPOTLIGHT

Claims wait in *Queue* to be processed at 5 p.m.

ACTIVITY 7-8: Apply Settings to Print Paper Claims

Although paper claims are rare, there are occasions when you will need to send one. In Optum™ PM, paper claims are generated by way of the method outlined in Activity 7-9. To print paper claims, you must first apply print settings. There are two ways to apply print settings in Optum™. For this activity, use the Optum™ *Dashboard*.

1. In Optum™ PM and Physician EMR, go to the *Home* module > *Dashboard* tab > *Billing* section > *Unprinted Paper Claim Batches* link. The application displays the *Print Options* window.
2. Click the *Print Options* button in the upper-right corner of the screen (see Figure 7-36).
3. Locate the desired claim form ("1500 CMS Paper Form") in the list and then enter the margin size for the form in the corresponding *Offset Top* field (enter "10") and *Offset Left* field (enter "10") if not already populated (Figure 7-36).

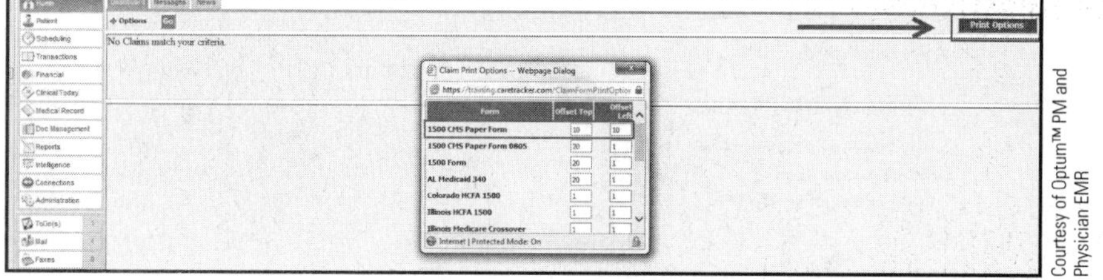

Courtesy of Optum™ PM and Physician EMR

Figure 7-36 Apply Settings to Print Paper Claims

Print the Claim Print Options window, label it "Activity 7-8," and place it in your assignment folder.

4. Scroll to the bottom of the dialog box and click *Update*. You must log out and then log back in to Optum™ PM and Physician EMR before the setting takes effect.

ACTIVITY 7-9: Generate a Paper Claim

1. Pull patient Darryl Smith into context.
2. Click the *OI* tab in the *Name Bar*.
3. Click on *Instant Claim* in the *First Clm* column (Figure 7-37) for each claim that you want to generate a paper claim for (select the charge you created in Activity 7-3 [G0180]). Optum™ PM displays the *Claims Summary* in the lower frame of the screen.

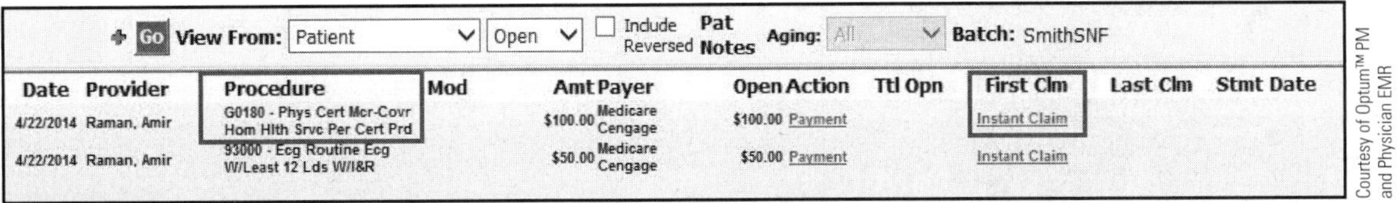

Courtesy of Optum™ PM and Physician EMR

Figure 7-37 First Clm Column

4. Place a check mark next to the claim you want to rebill to paper (select "G0180" and "93000"), and then click *Build Claim*. You will then note that the date you performed the activity is listed in the *First Clm* column.
5. Click on the date in the *First Clm* column (Figure 7-38) for which you want to generate a paper claim (select the charge you created in Activity 7-3 [G0180]). Optum™ PM displays the *Claim Summary* in the lower frame of the screen.

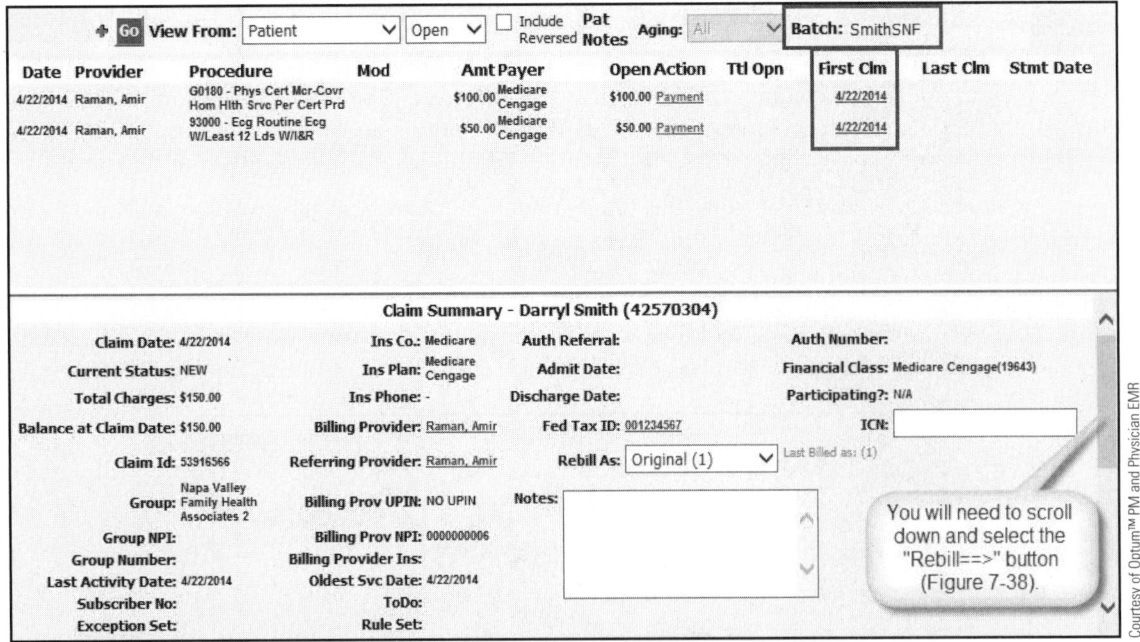

Courtesy of Optum™ PM and Physician EMR

Figure 7-38 First Clm Date

6. Scroll down and click the *Rebill To= = >* drop-down list at the bottom of the screen and select "Paper 1500." Click *Rebuild Paper* (Figure 7-39).

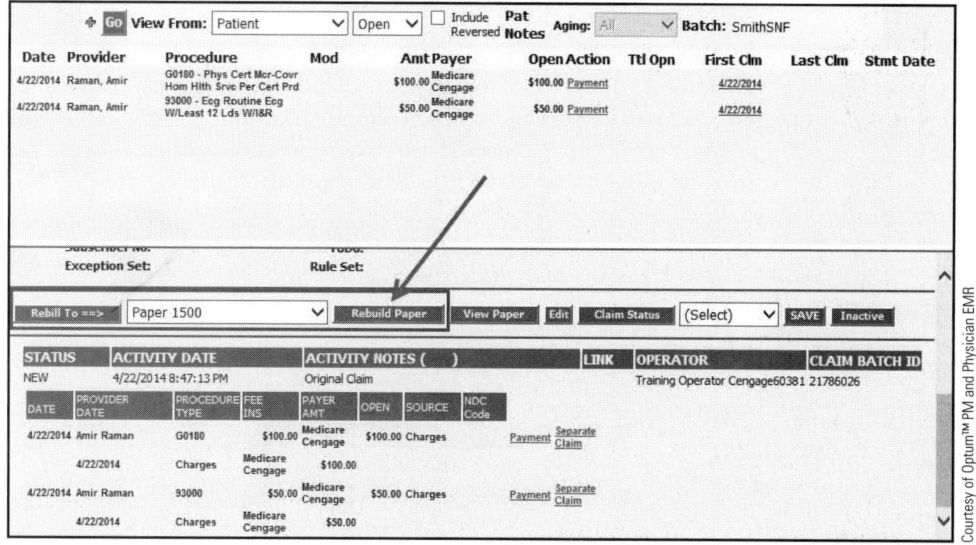

Courtesy of Optum™ PM and Physician EMR

Figure 7-39 Select Rebuild Paper Claim

7. In a live environment, Optum™ PM generates the *HCFA 1500 CMS Paper Form* in a new window. Your student version will not generate a paper 1500 form; instead, you will receive an error message on your screen (Figure 7-40). (**Note:** You can click "X" to close out of the error message and *Open Items* screens.)

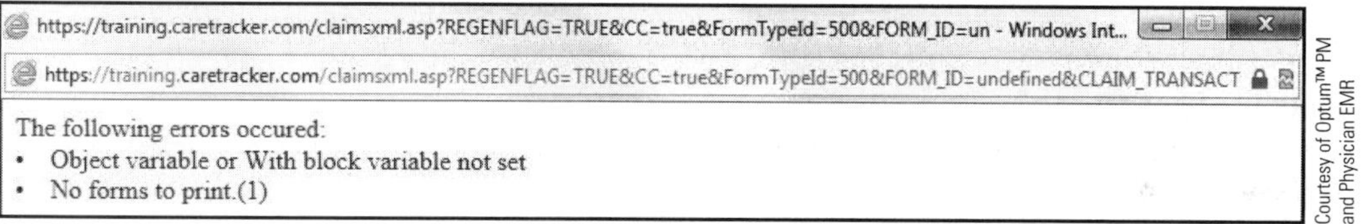

Courtesy of Optum™ PM and Physician EMR

Figure 7-40 Paper Claim Error Message

8. In a live environment your screen would look like Figure 7-41. To print the form, you would right-click on the form and select *Print* from the shortcut menu.

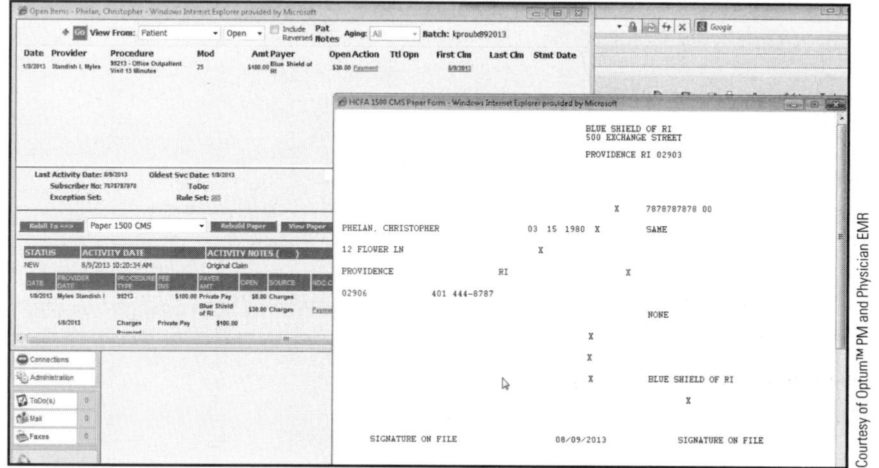

Courtesy of Optum™ PM and Physician EMR

Figure 7-41 Paper Claim to 1500

ACTIVITY 7-10: Process a Remittance

There is a normal flow of payment activity in Optum™ PM that begins when a patient pays his or her copayment. Copayments are entered in Optum™ PM when the patient checks in or checks out (depending on the office workflow). Next, a claim is sent to the insurance company. Remittances received electronically in Optum™ PM are identified in the *Electronic Remittances* application in the *Billing* section of the *Dashboard* (Figure 7-42). Optum™ PM matches the transactions on the electronic remittance to a specific patient, date of service, CPT® code, and charge amount.

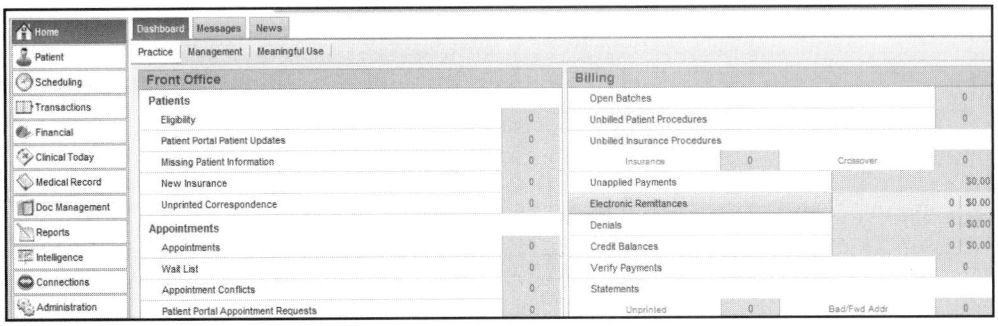

Courtesy of Optum™ PM and Physician EMR

Figure 7-42 Electronic Remittances Link

Electronic remittances should only be posted after the check is received from the insurance company. Using electronic remittances will change the process for posting payments. After payments have been posted electronically, you must work credit balances and denials as a separate process. Typically, credit balances and denials are handled as an EOB is processed.

Open Items is an application in the *Financial* module. There is an identical application accessed via the *Pmt Open Items* tab in the *Transactions* module, and this application can also be accessed as a window by clicking the *OI* button in the *Name Bar*. The *Open Items* application is used to view all dates of service and the associated procedures, financial transactions, and claims activity (Figure 7-43). In this application you can enter many different types of financial transactions including patient payments, insurance payments, third-party payments, transfer balances, refunds, and apply unapplied money. You can also view the procedure details of each procedure, enter denial descriptions, attach statement messages to appear on patient statements, view a claim history, potentially rebill a claim, view electronic responses received from insurance companies, and view EOBs attached to payments.

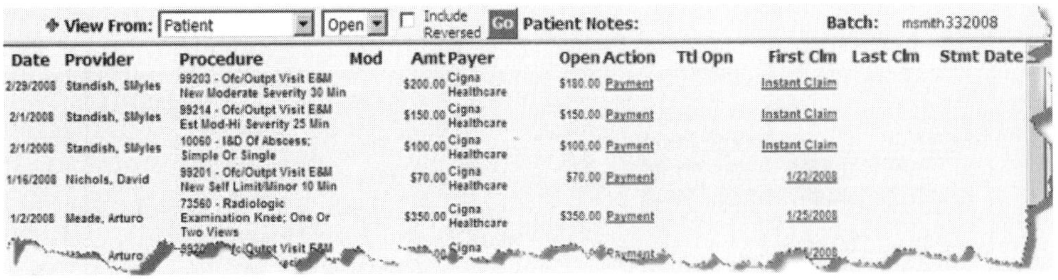

Courtesy of Optum™ PM and Physician EMR

Figure 7-43 Open Items

Before posting payments via *Electronic Remittances*, select one patient from the remittance, pull the patient into context, click the *OI* button on the *Name Bar*, and verify that the date of service is still open in Optum™ PM (see Figure 7-44).

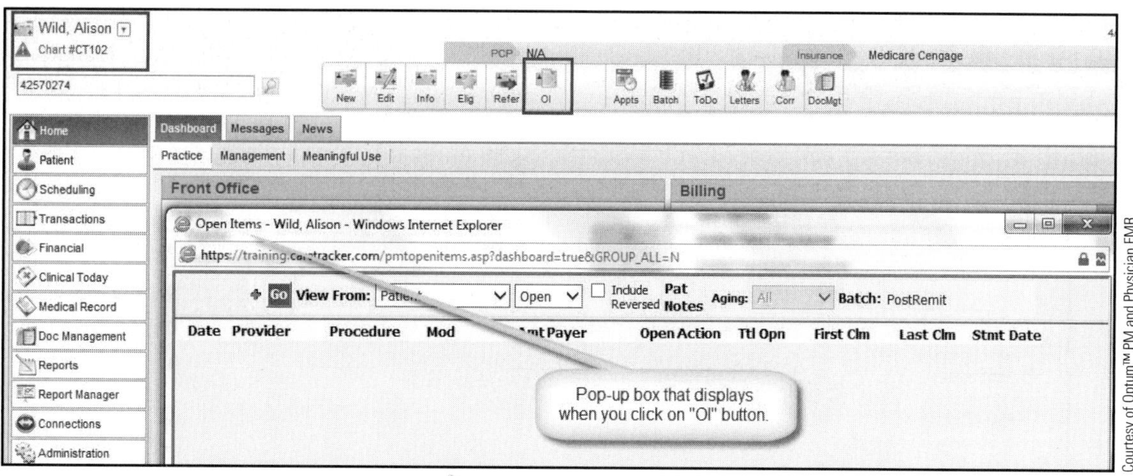

Figure 7-44 OI Electronic Remittance

To Process a Remittance:

1. Create a new batch and name it "PostRemit." Update the *Provider* to Alison Wild's provider and PCP (Dr. Raman), use *Location* "Napa Valley Family Associates," and use the same service and payment dates as the appointment you scheduled for her in Activity 4-1.
2. Pull patient Alison Wild into context.
3. Click on the *OI* button in the *Name Bar*.
4. All captured visits for the date entered will display. Find the date for which you want to process a remittance (select the appointment you created in Activity 4-1). Click on the *Payment* link in the *Action* column next to Procedure 99213. Optum™ PM displays the payment window in the lower frame of the screen (Figure 7-45). (**Note:** If you do not see Procedure 99213 listed in the *Open Items* window, follow the steps in the *Tip Box* on pages 126–127. Then, before continuing on to step 5, repeat Activity 7-9 and generate a paper claim for Procedures 99213, 90746, and 90471.)

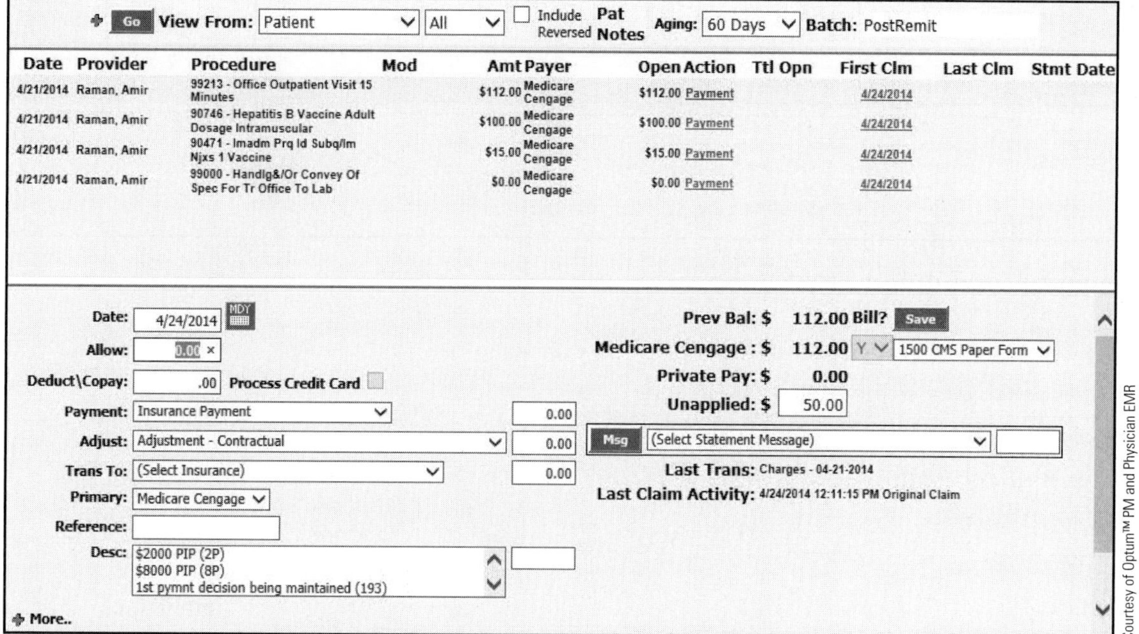

Figure 7-45 OI for Alison Wild

TIP BOX

Important!! If you do not see the charge in *OI* for the visit you entered in Activity 4-1, you will need to follow these instructions. Go to the *Home* module > *Dashboard* tab > *Visit* header > *Missing Encounters/Visits* link (Figure 7-46) and you will see that the *Visit* has not been saved (see Figure 7-47).

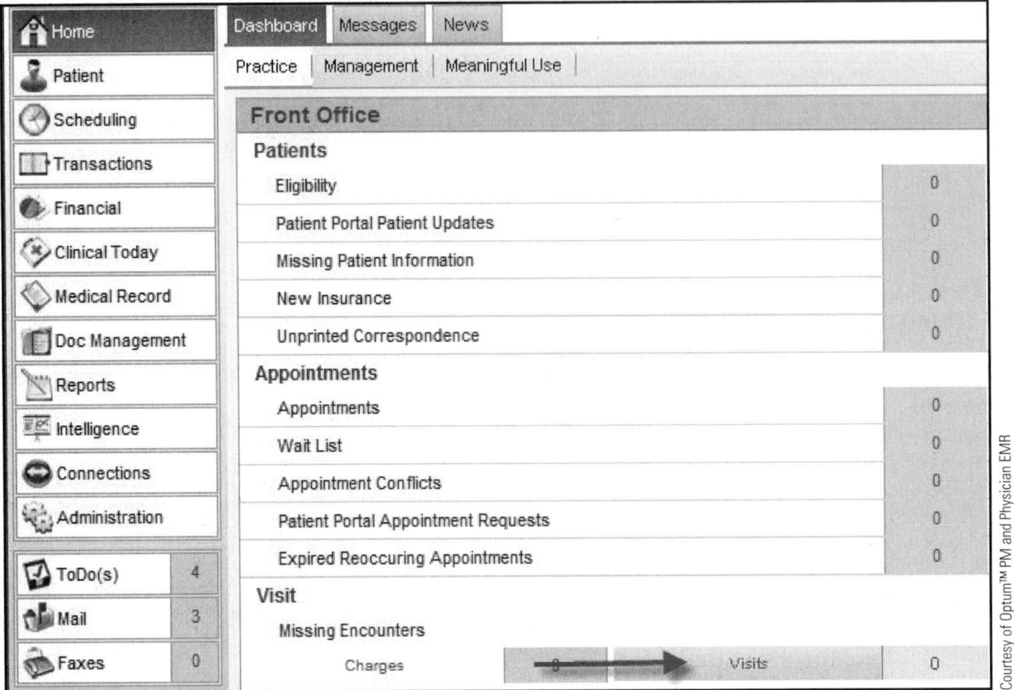

Figure 7-46 Missing Encounters/Visits Link

Courtesy of Optum™ PM and Physician EMR

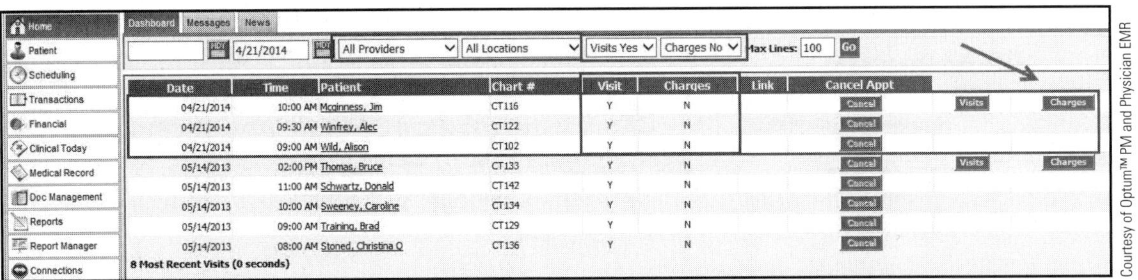

Figure 7-47 Visits Not Saved

Courtesy of Optum™ PM and Physician EMR

To save the *Charges*, set the fields as follows:

- Include the date of the patient encounter
- Select *All Providers*
- Select *All Locations*
- Select *Visits Yes*
- Select *Charges No*
- Click *Go*

(*Continues*)

Tip Box (*Continued*)

Scroll up and locate the date of service (DOS) for the patient you are working on. You will see the *Visits* and *Charges* buttons (see Figure 7-47). When you are working in *OI*, if more than one charge (e.g., multiple patient visits) appear on the same date, *Visits* will be saved for all patients. (**Note:** You may see visit information for patients other than those you are working on in the workbook. Ignore them for the time being as we focus on your current entries.)

- Click on the *Charges* button on the right side of your screen for the DOS.
- Click *Go* on the left side of your screen. The charges for all patient encounters on the DOS display.
- Scroll down and click *Save* on the bottom left of your screen. (**Note:** If more than one charge [e.g., multiple patient visits] appears on the date, the *Visits* will be saved for all patients.)
- **Important!!** You must wait until the "Transaction Saved" message appears before the charges will appear in the *Open Items* window.

5. In the payment window, enter the information from Alison Wild's EOB (Source Document 7-1 in Appendix A) for the *Visit* you created in Activity 4-1 and related charge you created in Activity 6-3. Enter the EOB information as listed below for procedure code 99213. Your completed screen should look like Figure 7-48 when you are done.

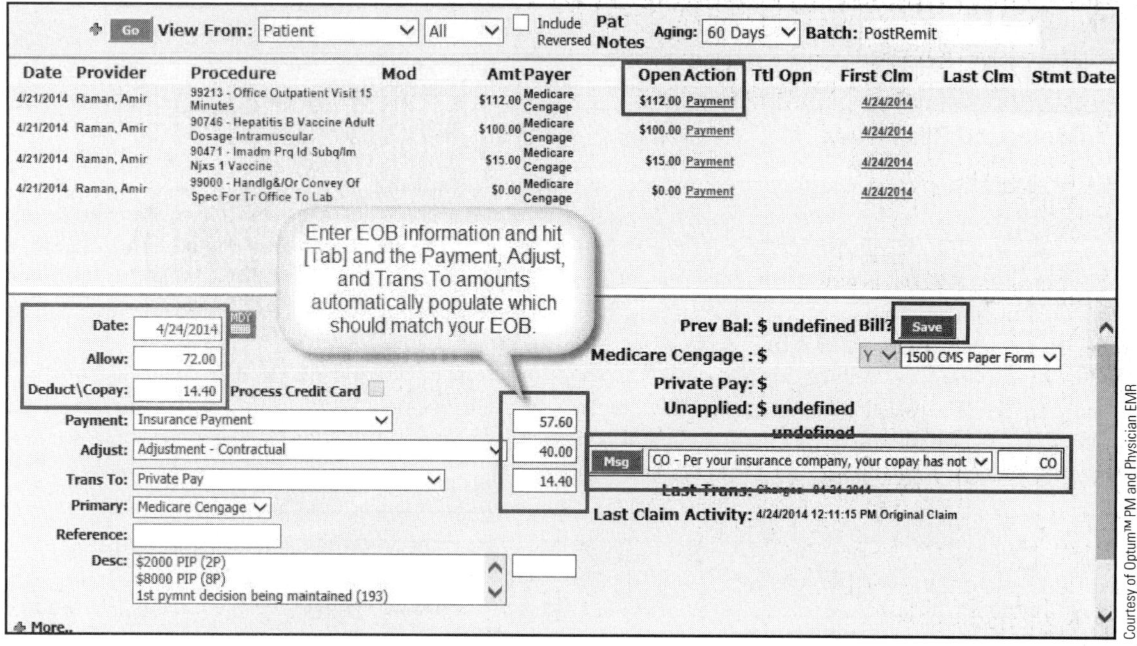

Figure 7-48 OI for Alison Wild

a. *Date:* This should match the date of the appointment you created in Activity 4-1 and Activity 6-3 *Visit* capture.

b. *Allow:* Enter the information from the *Amount Allowed* column on the EOB. Now hit the [Tab] key on your keyboard.

c. *Deduct/Copay:* Enter the information from the *Deduct/Coins/Copay* column on the EOB. Now hit the [Tab] key and this will populate the amount in the *Adjust* and *Transfer To* fields based on the information entered in the *Demographics* screen.

d. *Payment*: Confirm that "Insurance Payment" is selected.

e. *Adjust*: Confirm that "Adjustment – Contractual" is selected.

f. *Trans To:* Confirm that "Private Pay" is selected.

g. *Primary:* Confirm that "Medicare Cengage" is selected.

h. *Reference:* Leave blank.

i. *Desc:* Leave as is.

j. *Msg:* Enter "CO" in the blank box to the right of the drop-down menu and hit the [Enter] key.

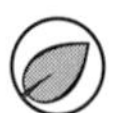

Print the Process Remittance (OI) screen, label it "Activity 7-10," and place it in your assignment folder.

6. Once you have entered the EOB information for 99213, click *Save*. Your transaction will be saved and the claim disappears.
7. Now repeat steps 5 and 6 for each additional billable procedure code on Ms. Wild's EOB (90746 and 90471). Once you have entered the remittance for all billable codes on the EOB, you will notice that each charge has been removed from your screen.
8. Close out of the *Open Items* window by clicking the "X" in the upper-right corner of the window.

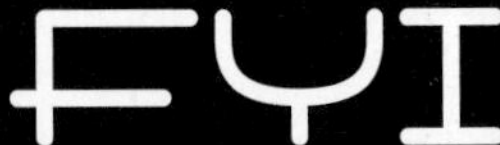

Enter a Denial and Remittance

Denials are claims that an insurance company has determined it will not pay, such as when a patient has not met his or her deductible or a service code has been submitted that is not a covered code by the insurance or is not supported by diagnosis codes. Because you have demonstrated excellent billing and coding skills by reviewing the A&Ps, querying providers for code errors, and performing eligibility checks to verify coverage, you do not have any denied claims to work. It is important to understand the cause of denials and the workflow to process denials and rebill as necessary.

The best practice for working denials is to do so separately from posting payments. This will improve efficiency in your practice. Your student version of Optum™ PM will not post *Denials* in your *Dashboard* because *ClaimsManager* is not active. The *Denials* screen can be accessed by going to the *Home* module > *Dashboard* tab > *Billing* header > *Denials* link (Figure 7-49).

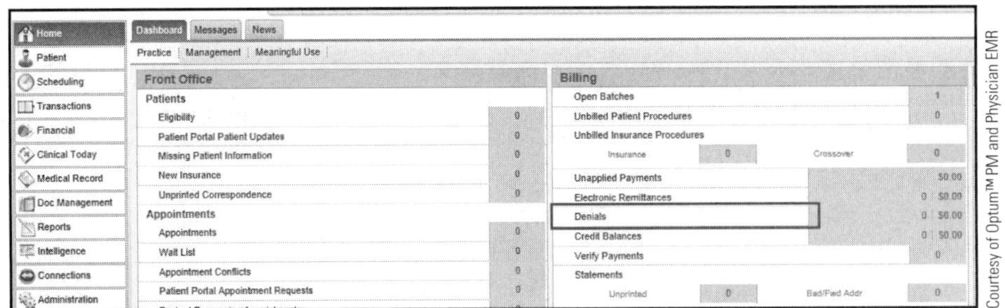

Courtesy of Optum™ PM and Physician EMR

Figure 7-49 Denials Link

To Enter a Denial and Remittance in a Live Environment:

1. With the patient in context, you would click on the *OI* button on the *Name Bar*.
2. All captured visits for the date entered will display. Scroll down to display the charge that has been denied.

(Continues)

FYI (*Continued*)

3. In the *Open Items* dialog box, click the *Payment* link under the *Action* header for the denied charge and enter the *Denial* information from the EOB (the amount that displays in the *Not Covered* column). (**Note:** If you were not currently working in a batch, you would be prompted to enter your batch information and redirects in the lower portion of the batch screen.)
   a. *Date*: Leave the date as entered.
   b. *Allow*: Leave blank.
   c. *Deduct/Copay*: Leave blank.
   d. *Payment*: Leave blank.
   e. *Adjust*: Select "Adjustment – Contractual."
   f. *Transfer To*: Use the drop-down and select "Private Pay." This will automatically populate the amount field to the right of *Trans To* as well as the *Prev Bal* and *Private Pay* fields.
   g. *Primary*: Leave blank.
   h. *Reference*: Leave blank.
   i. *Desc*: Type "96" in the blank box to the right of *Desc* and hit [Enter]. This will select "Non-Covered charge (96)."
   j. In the *Msg* tab, use the drop-down list and select "SEE BILLING NOTE."
   k. Click *Save*. Your transaction will be saved and the claim disappears.
4. If there were other charges on the EOB that were being paid by the insurance company, in the *Open Items* window you would click the *Payment* link under the *Action* header for the charge and enter the remittance information from the patient's EOB. (**Note:** Refer to step 5 in Activity 7-10 to process a remittance.)
5. You will have saved all the *Denial* and *Remittance* information from the EOB related to the charge (as noted in Figure 7-50). Once your transaction is saved (Figure 7-51), the claim disappears. (You may have to close out of the *OI* screen and reopen it before the claim disappears.) (**Note:** You must be sure to enter the charge in the period/year of the service as originally entered.)

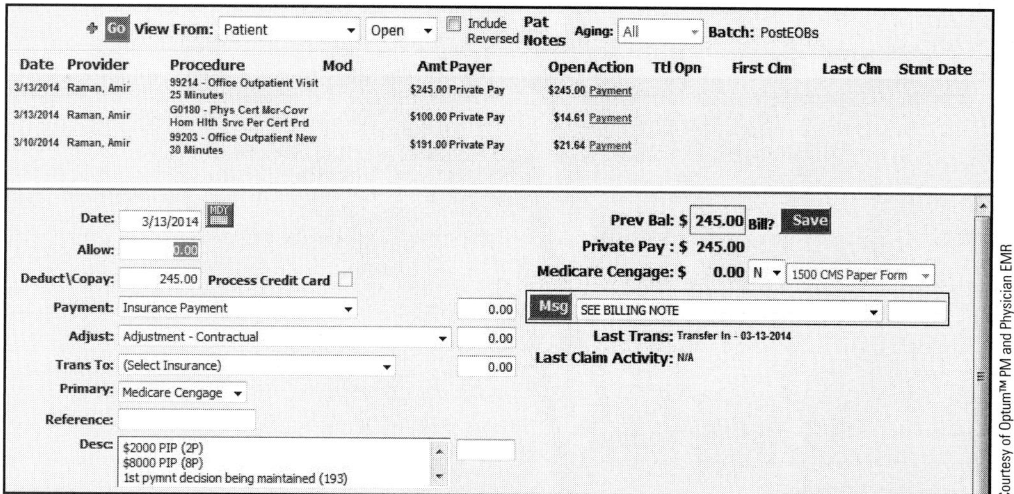

Figure 7-50 Denial Screen

(*Continues*)

FYI *(Continued)*

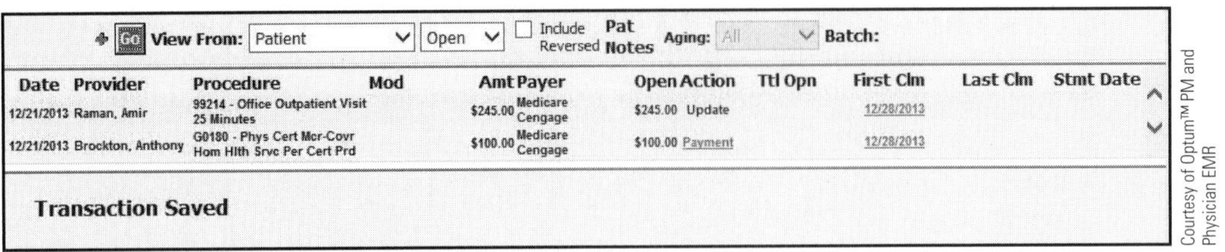

Courtesy of Optum™ PM and Physician EMR

Figure 7-51 Transaction Saved

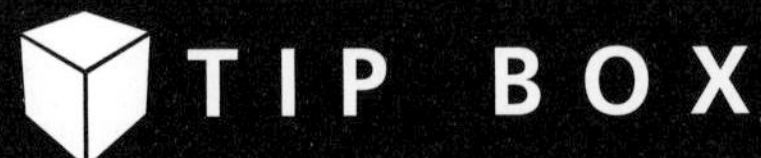

TIP BOX

Having entered the denial, the balance is transferred to private pay. (**Note:** It is important to remember that it takes 24 hours for *Denials* to display in the *Dashboard* in a live environment.) You can adjust your filters to set your display options. The *Dashboard* only shows *Denials* for the month.

PROFESSIONALISM CONNECTION

Although we have addressed patient and practice financial relations throughout this workbook, its importance cannot be overstated. For many patients and staff members, discussing the subject of money owed is touchy and uncomfortable. You must always address the topic in a calm and nonjudgmental way and comply with office policy, even if a patient requests special payment arrangements. Special requests should be documented and forwarded to the appropriate person or department, often the office manager, billing department, or managing provider. Never refer the patient directly to the provider to discuss billing and payment issues.

When asking for payment, use positive expressions. Practice your professionalism by role-playing with co-workers the following scenarios. Adjust the wording to your comfort level and to that of a service provider professional:

- When making an appointment by phone: "Copayment is expected at the time of service" or "Your office visit will be approximately $ ______. For your convenience we accept cash, checks, and credit card."
- For the patient checking in at the front desk: "Your copayment today will be $ ______."
- For patients checking out: "Your charges for today's office visit are $ ______. Would you like to pay by cash, check, or credit card?" or "I see your deductible has been met and/or insurance pays 80%. Your portion of the bill comes to $ ______. Would you like to pay by cash, check, or credit card?"

My challenge to you is to demonstrate how you would approach collection of payment in a positive and professional manner.

ACTIVITY 7-11: Work Credit Balances

Working credit balances by batch should be done immediately after a remittance has been posted in Optum™ PM. Credit balances are created when either a patient or an insurance company pays more money for a specific procedure for a specific date of service than what was billed. Credit balances can be identified by the *Credit Balances* link under the *Billing* section of the *Dashboard* in the *Home* module for a specific batch or group (Figure 7-52). After you post payments via electronic remittances, it is best practice to work credit balances for the batch you were working in before posting the batch.

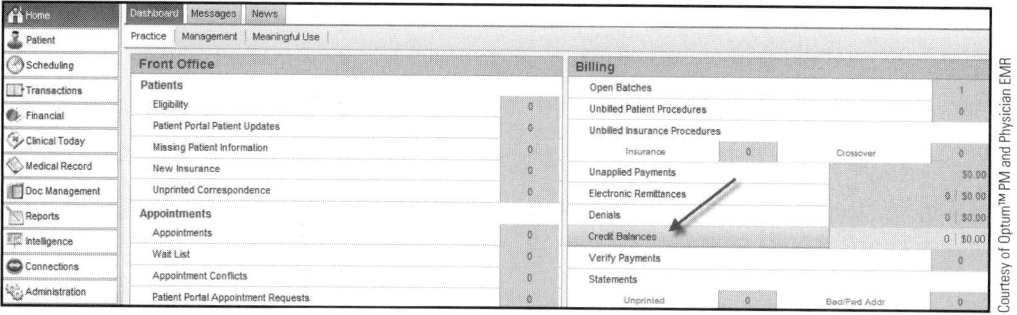

Courtesy of Optum™ PM and Physician EMR

Figure 7-52 Credit Balances Link

There are two ways to work credit balances: *by Batch* or *for Refunds* (Figure 7-53). Once you post the batch, this will create a charge on the patient's account. You can then post a payment to create the credit balance.

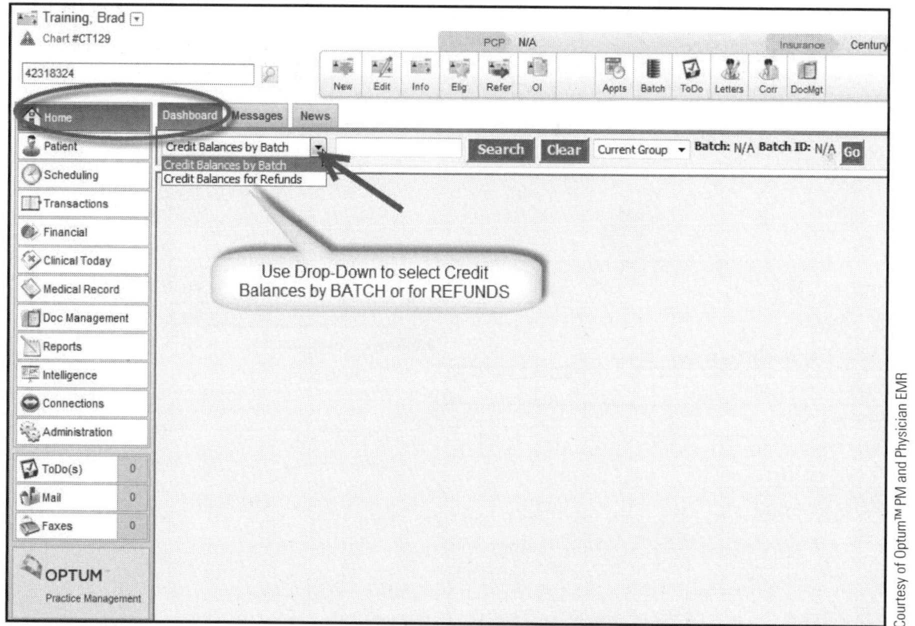

Courtesy of Optum™ PM and Physician EMR

Figure 7-53 Credit Balance by Batch or for Refunds

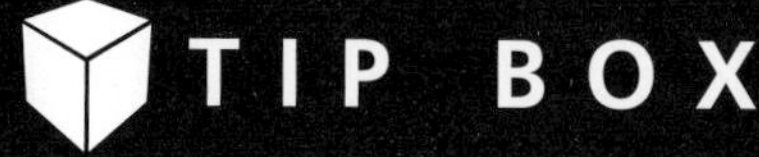

There is a big difference between a "Credit" and an "Unapplied Credit." A credit is an overpayment on account, and an unapplied credit is only a patient payment (not insurance) that has not been attached to a DOS.

To Work Credit Balances:

In order to work a Credit Balance, you must first have a credit in the patient's account.

1. Enter a patient's name to pull him or her into context in the *Name Bar* (select Alison Wild).
2. Using patient Alison Wild, create a new batch and name it "CredBal."
3. Click on the *OI* button on the *Name Bar*. Optum™ PM displays the *Open Items* application.
4. If you do not see a credit balance, you will need to post a payment to the patient's account first, following these instructions. (**Note:** The payment must be greater than the balance in the patient's account in *OI* in the *Amt Payer* column):
   a. Click on the *Payment* line in the *Action* column of her 99213 *Procedure* (which should be listed as "Private Pay" in the *Payer* column). The payment screen will display in the lower portion of the window.
   b. Using the *Payment* drop-down, select "Payment – Patient Cash (PATCSH)."
   c. In the amount field next to the *Payment* drop-down, enter a payment in the amount of $50.00 more than the OI balance of her account. In this instance, her OI balance displays as $14.40, so you would add $50.00 to that amount for a total entry of "$64.40." (**Note:** Do not enter the dollar sign.) You will see the *Private Pay* balance change to "$ −50.00."
   d. In the *Msg* drop-down select "Select Statement Message." Your screen should look like Figure 7-54.

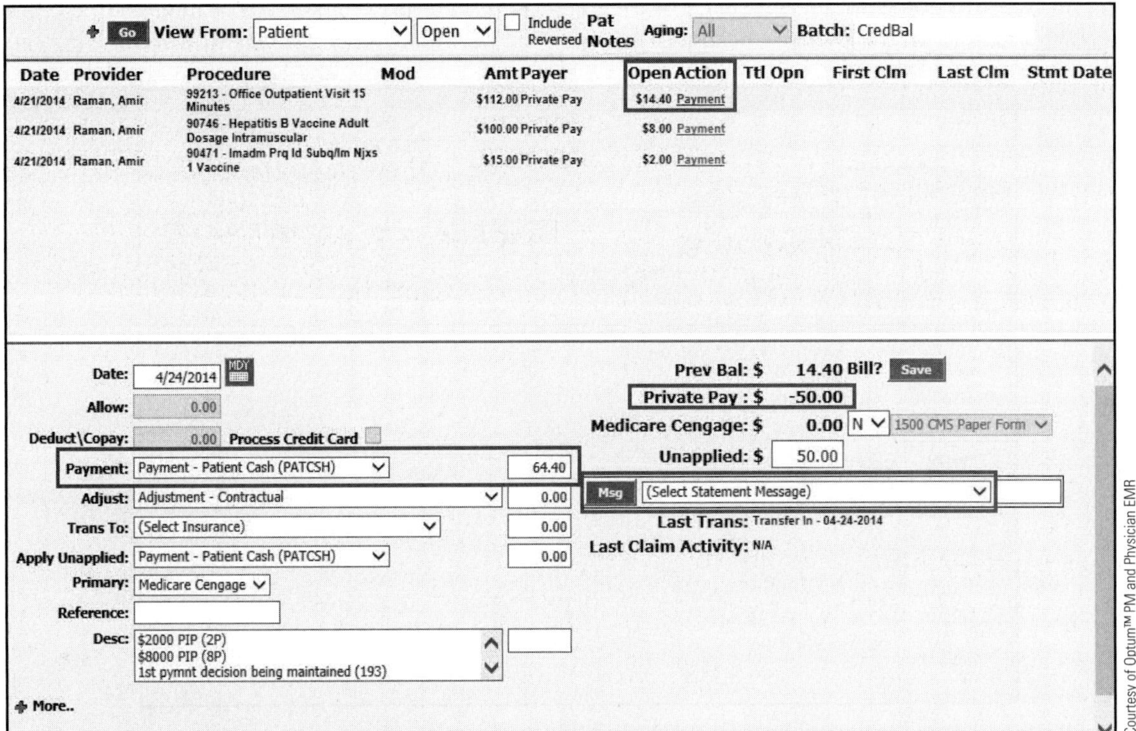

Courtesy of Optum™ PM and Physician EMR

Figure 7-54 OI Credit Balance Screen

   e. Click *Save*. To close the *Open Items* screen, click "X."
   f. Post the "CredBal" batch.
5. Go to the *Home* module > *Dashboard* tab > *Billing* header > *Credit Balances* link (see Figure 7-52).

6. Click on the *Search* button and Optum™ PM displays a list of batches in the *Provider Search* dialog box (Figure 7-55).

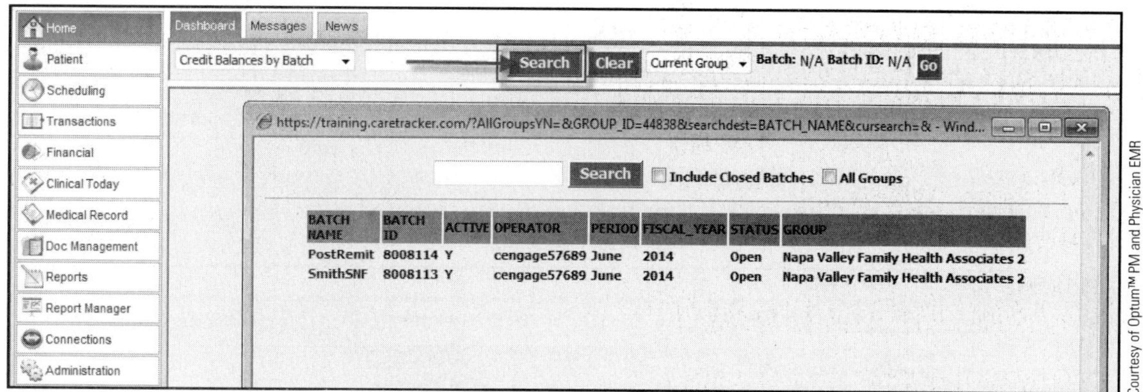

Courtesy of Optum™ PM and Physician EMR

Figure 7-55 Provider Search Dialog Box

a. If you had not posted your batch, in the *Provider Search* box you would click on the batch you want to view (select "CredBal"). Optum™ PM populates the *Batch* and *Batch ID* fields with the selected batch.

b. Since you did post your batch, in the *Provider Search* box you will need to select the checkboxes next to *Include Closed Batches* and *All Groups* and enter "Cr" or "Cred" in your batch name search field (Figure 7-56) and then click *Search*.

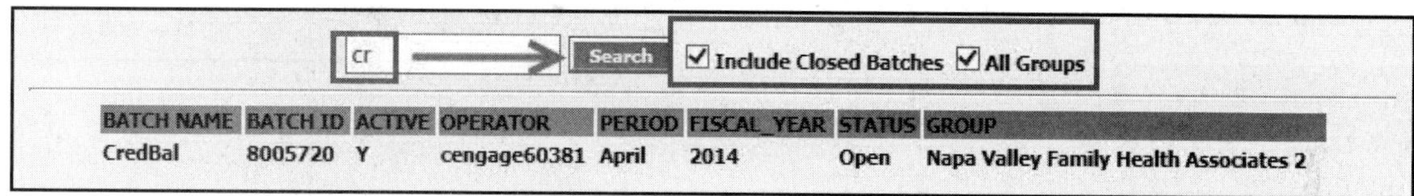

Figure 7-56 CredBal Search Criteria
Courtesy of Optum™ PM and Physician EMR

7. Click on the "CredBal" batch and it is pulled into context (Figure 7-57).

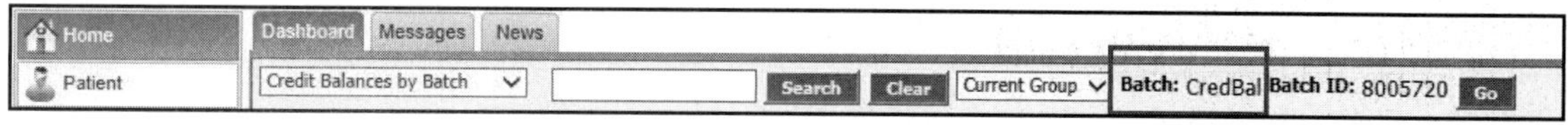

Figure 7-57 CredBal Batch in Context
Courtesy of Optum™ PM and Physician EMR

8. Click *Go* and Optum™ PM displays a list of credit balances including the patient's name, the financial class with the credit balance, the amount of the credit, and the patient's last transaction date.
9. Pull patient Alison Wild into context on the *Name Bar* if you have not already done so.
10. In the drop-down menu found directly under the *Dashboard* tab, change "Credit Balances by Batch" to "Credit Balances for Refunds." Since you posted the "CredBal" batch previously in this activity, you will be prompted to create a new batch. Name the new batch "CrBalRef."

PM SPOTLIGHT

If payments had been posted via electronic remittances, best practice would be to go into *Credit Balances* and search for the batch name associated with those payments, which will identify any credit balances created during the electronic payment process.

11. In the *Action* Column, use the drop-down and select "Refund-Patient (P)" (Figure 7-58). (**Note:** You may first need to adjust the *Date To* field to today's date and click *Go* for the screen to display.)

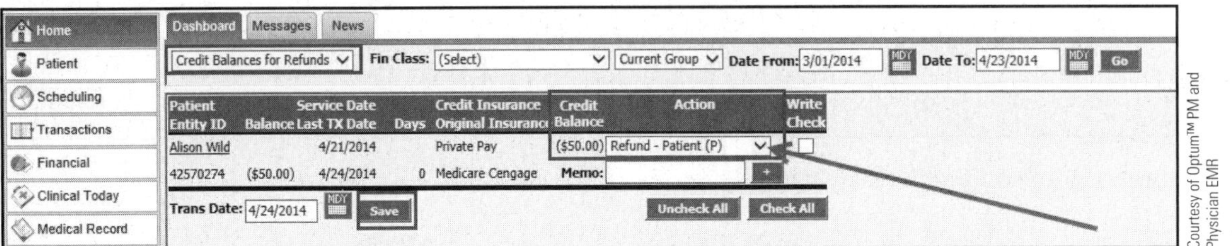

Courtesy of Optum™ PM and Physician EMR

Figure 7-58 Credit Balance Refund

12. Click *Save* (Figure 7-59).
13. The *Credit Balance Transfer* dialog box will display. Click on *Write Transactions* (see Figure 7-59).

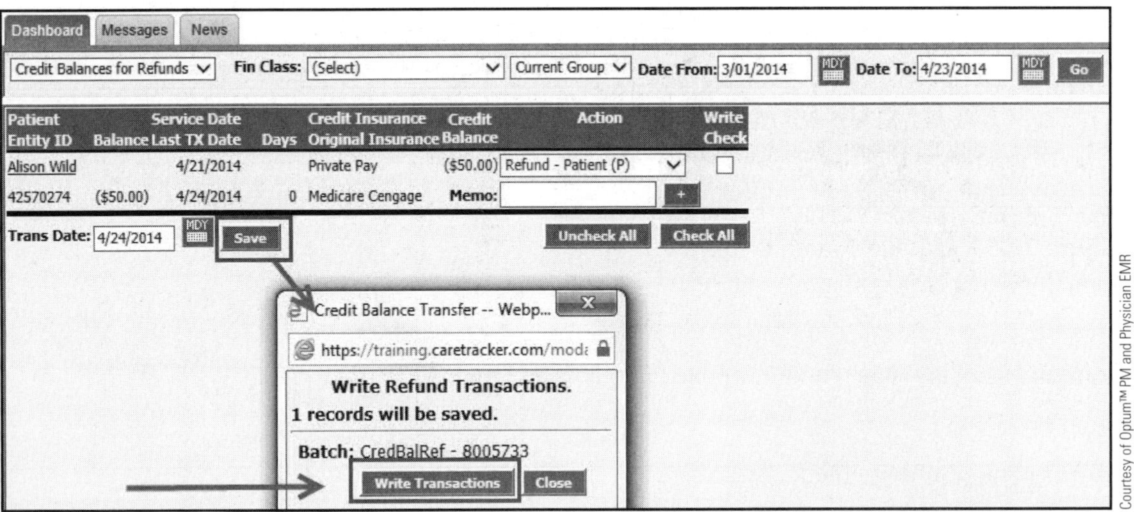

Courtesy of Optum™ PM and Physician EMR

Figure 7-59 Write Transactions

14. The *Credit Balance Transfer* dialog box will confirm that the transaction has been saved (Figure 7-60).

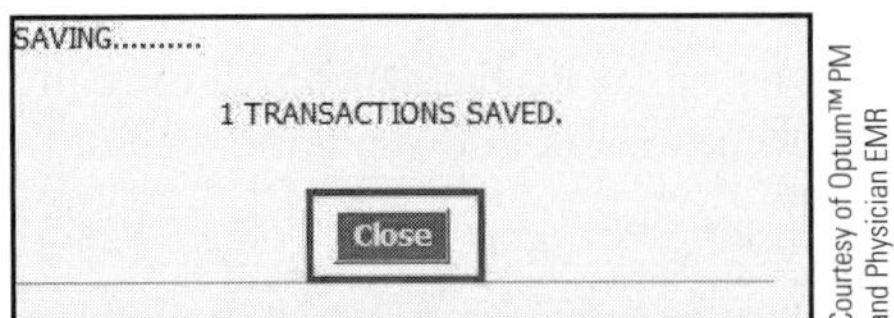

Courtesy of Optum™ PM and Physician EMR

Figure 7-60 Credit Balance Transfer Confirmation

15. Click *Close*, and the credit balance is removed from your screen.

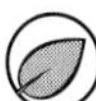

Print a screenshot of the Credit Balances for Refunds screen, label it "Activity 7-11," and place it in your assignment folder.

NVFHA MANAGER CHALLENGE

One of my primary responsibilities as office manager is to ensure the prompt receipt of payments and revenue flow to the medical office. As such, I will assume the role of coding and compliance officer for accurate and timely billing, directly supervising the medical assistant(s) in charge of capturing visits to charges and of reconciliation of the financial batch(es). If a claim is improperly coded, the claim will be rejected or, worse yet, could be interpreted as fraudulent. Today, more than ever, coding and billing for medical claims is often perceived as one of the most essential administrative duties performed. As office manager I will monitor the amount of claims rejected and look for trends that need adjustment.

An example would be if we find that a particular physician has more rejected claims than another, it may be possible that the physician is not using the most current codes, missing modifiers, or not providing the necessary supporting documentation. In addition, if we find a certain code is being rejected, we must track and trend the rejections and create an education plan for both providers and staff to avoid rejections that jeopardize timely payments to the practice for services rendered. The same would apply if the biller/coder had not included a code for a service provided. Commonly missed CPT® codes include handling charges for specimens and the fee for injections as well as the injectable (HCPCS code). In this instance it would be most beneficial to hold a coding workshop with providers and staff to show the trends of coding, the rejection of claims, and provide current updates and training to improve results. Keep your eyes open for rejected claims and missed codes. Consider the cause so corrective action can be taken. Present these findings to me and always use the claims scrubber software (*EncoderPro*) to ensure that the selected codes are appropriate and will be paid.

MINI-CASE STUDIES

Case Study 7-1

1. Before beginning Case Study 7-1, create a new batch and name it "Ch7MCSRemit."
2. Repeat Activity 7-9 and generate paper claims for all procedures listed for each patient. (**Note:** If a patient's charges are not showing on the *Open Items* window, follow the steps in the *Tip Box* on pages 126–127 to save all charges for the patient's date of service.)
3. For each patient, process the remittances (see Activity 7-10) for each encounter created. Process the remittances (EOBs) using Source Documents 7-2 and 7-3 in Appendix A.

   Patients:

   a. Alec Winfrey

   b. Darryl Smith
4. Upon completion, run a journal and review. **Do not** post the "Ch7MCSRemit" batch at this time.

Print the Journal after completing all the 7-1 case studies, label it "Case Study 7-1," and place it in your assignment folder.

(*Continues*)

MINI-CASE STUDIES (*Continued*)

Case Study 7-2

NVFHA MANAGER CHALLENGE

When Jim Mcginness checked in for his visit, the front desk clerk did not request a copy of his insurance card and did not verify his current information. Jim's employer had changed to a new Health Insurance plan since his last visit to NVFHA, and his claim will be rejected by his former insurance company because he was no longer covered by them.

a. How would you handle the situation?

b. How could it be avoided in the future?

c. Document all the steps required to be followed due to a failure to update information and copy the current insurance card. Describe the impact on the revenue cycle to the practice. Are there any other impacts? Would the patient lose faith in NVFHA and wonder if issues affecting his health care would also be compromised?

d. ***Hint:*** As best practice, run an eligibility check before generating the claim to the insurance and update information as necessary.

1. Perform an Eligibility Check before generating a claim. Although *ClaimsManager* is not active in your student version of Optum™, for this simulated activity you note that Jim's claim is denied. The original insurance recorded in his demographics returns an eligibility status of "ineligible" (current insurance no longer valid).
2. In this instance, you recall from Case Study 4-2 that Jim's insurance changed but was not updated at check-in. The normal workflow would be to call the patient to obtain updated insurance information and record it in his demographics. (**Note:** If the patient's visit had already been billed, rebill his visit to the correct insurance company if necessary.) Recall that you entered Jim's new insurance information in his *Demographics* in Case Study 6-1.
3. Repeat Activity 7-9 and generate paper claims for all procedures listed for Jim.
4. Process the Blue Cross Blue Shield remittance (EOB) (see Activity 7-10) for his encounter using Source Document 7-4 in Appendix A.
5. Upon completion, run a journal and review. **Do not** post the "Ch7MCS-Remit" batch at this time.

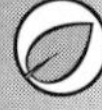 **Print the Journal, label it "Case Study 7-2," and place it in your assignment folder.**

Resources

The Optum PM and Physician EMR Help homepage represents a wealth of information for the electronic health record (https://training.caretracker.com/help/CareTracker_Help.htm).

American Medical Association

National Healthcare Association. (n.d.). *Certified Electronic Health Records Specialist (CEHRS™)*. Retrieved from http://www.nhanow.com/health-record.aspx

U.S. Department of Commerce, United States Census Bureau, American National Standards Institute. (2013). Retrieved from http://www.census.gov/geo/www/ansi/ansi.html

CHAPTER 8

ClaimsManager and Collections

LEARNING OBJECTIVES

1. Demonstrate understanding and use of the ClaimsManager feature.
2. Check status and work unpaid/inactive claims.
3. Generate patient statements.
4. Describe and identify components of the patient collection process including review of collection status and transfer of private pay balances.
5. Perform collection actions by creating and generating collection letters.

NVFHA MANAGER CHALLENGE

It cannot be overstated that all personnel, including office staff or collections agents, must act with the utmost professionalism during the collections process. Not only do numerous laws and regulations apply to the collections process, the sensitive nature of the relationship between provider and patient must be protected. Credit information of the patient is considered confidential and may not be released without the patient's expressed permission. Financial information regarding the patient is also confidential and must be protected according to law. Both in-person and telephone discussions should be conducted in an area that is out of view and hearing of other patients.

Credit arrangements and interest charges must be disclosed in writing. Enforcing the credit policy can be uncomfortable for both patients and staff. You must overcome any inhibitions regarding discussion of fees and payments. The success of the practice relies heavily on the medical assistant's ability to politely yet firmly ask for payment from patients. The first step in the collection process is to advise patients of the office policy regarding payment when they call to schedule an appointment. It is important that you remain calm, compassionate, and empathetic to patients. If you encounter a difficult patient, follow these steps to diffuse and resolve the matter:

1. Let the patient vent.
2. Express empathy to the patient. The tone of your voice goes a long way. Use a genuinely warm and caring tone to enhance the meaning of empathetic phrases.

(*Continues*)

NVFHA Manager Challenge *(Continued)*

3. Begin problem solving. Ask the patient questions to help clarify the situation and cause of the problem and double-check the facts.
4. Mutually agree on the solution. Be careful not to make a promise you cannot keep.
5. Follow up. You will score big points by following up with your patient to resolve the problem. This is sometimes referred to as service recovery.

You must demonstrate professionalism with every contact and treat each patient with the utmost respect. Your collection activities should be client-oriented and demonstrate the proper attitude and temperament with close attention given to protecting the goodwill established with your patient. Let me challenge you to role-play with your co-workers various collection scenarios that you might encounter. This will help with preparedness, conveying empathy, and noting the tone and inflection in your voice.

ACTIVITY 8-1: Work the Claims Worklist

Most claims are sent electronically in Optum™ PM. Any claims identified with a problem that would prevent them from being paid will show up on a *Claims Worklist* to be resolved. The *Claims Worklist* identifies the following:

- Newly prepared claims that will be transmitted during your next claim run
- Claims that cannot be transmitted electronically due to a missing submitter number
- Claims that cannot be transmitted from Optum™ PM because of missing information
- Claims that are not transmitted because of errors identified by *ClaimsManager*
- Claims that will not be accepted by a payer because of missing information
- Claims that you manually flagged as missing information or in review
- Claims that a payer does not have on file and claims with a denial status

Any claims flagged in any of the *Claims Worklist* columns, except *New/Prepared*, need follow up action, which typically requires you to add and/or edit information and rebill the claim. Optum™ PM performs an electronic claim status check and, based on its status, moves the claim to one of the *Claims Worklist* categories. You can also manually flag a claim to move it to a *Claims Worklist* category. The *Claims Worklist* is grouped into four main categories: *New/Prepared*, *Claim Errors*, *Pending*, and *Other* (Figure 8-1).

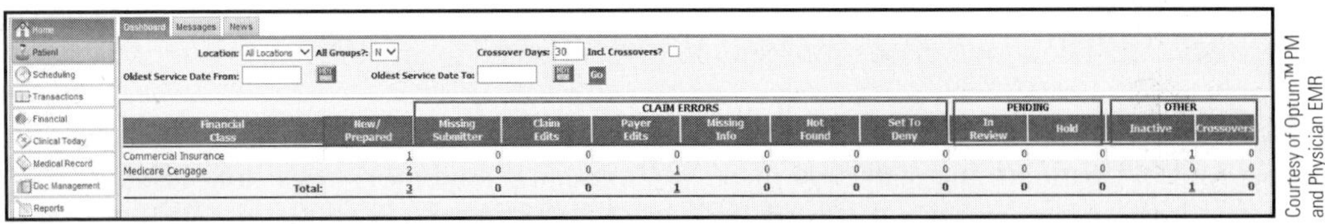

Financial Class	New/ Prepared	CLAIM ERRORS Missing Submitter	Claim Edits	Payer Edits	Missing Info	Not Found	Set To Deny	PENDING In Review	Hold	OTHER Inactive	Crossovers
Commercial Insurance	1	0	0	0	0	0	0	0	0	1	0
Medicare Cengage	2	0	0	1	0	0	0	0	0	0	0
Total:	3	0	0	1	0	0	0	0	0	1	0

Courtesy of Optum™ PM and Physician EMR

Figure 8-1 Claims Worklist Categories

The *Claim Summary* screen (see Figure 8-2) displays when an individual claim line is clicked. In this screen, actions can be performed on the selected claim only.

Having identified a problem (or problems) that would prevent a claim from being paid, you will now work the *Claims Worklist* to resolve the issue(s).

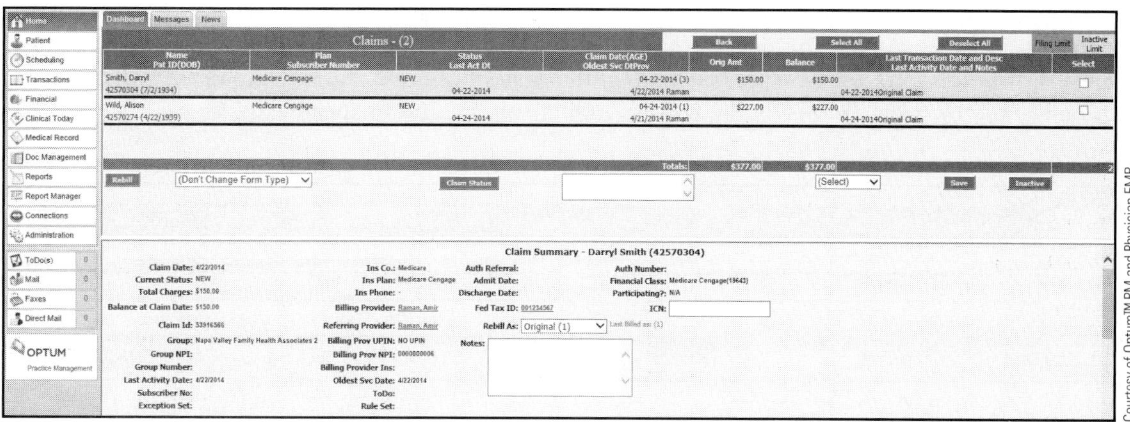

Figure 8-2 Claims Summary Screen

To Work the Claims Worklist:

1. Go to the *Home* module > *Dashboard* tab > *Billing* section > *Claims Worklist* link. There are three options: *Unbilled, Crossover,* and *Inactive* (Figure 8-3). Select *Unbilled.* This will take you to the *Claims Worklist* screen.

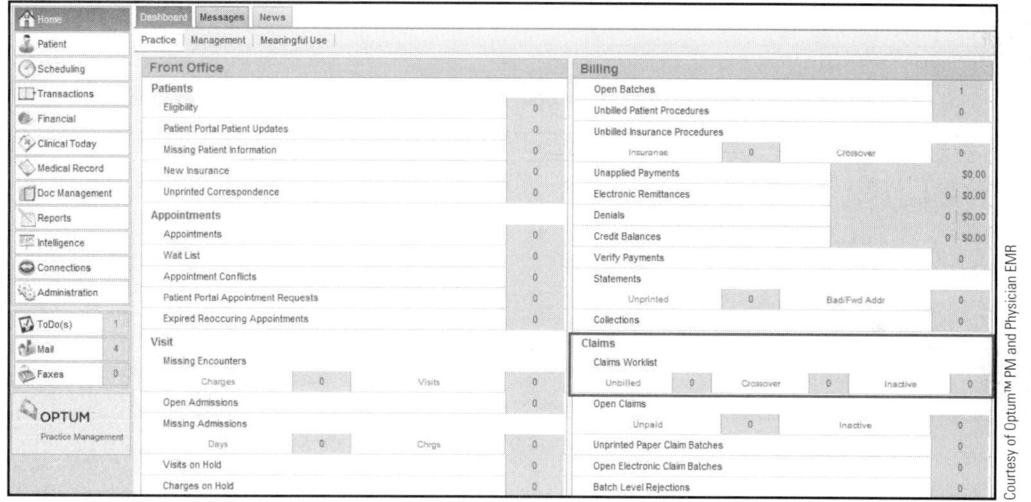

Figure 8-3 Claims Worklist Dashboard

2. The *Location* list defaults to "All Locations." You have the option to select a specific location if needed. (Leave as is.)
3. The *All Groups* list defaults to "N" for No. Select "Y" for Yes if you want to include claims for all groups. Select "Y."
4. Select the *Incl. Crossovers* checkbox to include crossover claims and enter "180" in the *Crossover Days* field.
5. (Optional) Enter a date range in the *Oldest Service Date From/To* boxes to view claims from a specific time period.
6. Click *Go.* The application displays a list of all claims broken down by financial class (Figure 8-4).

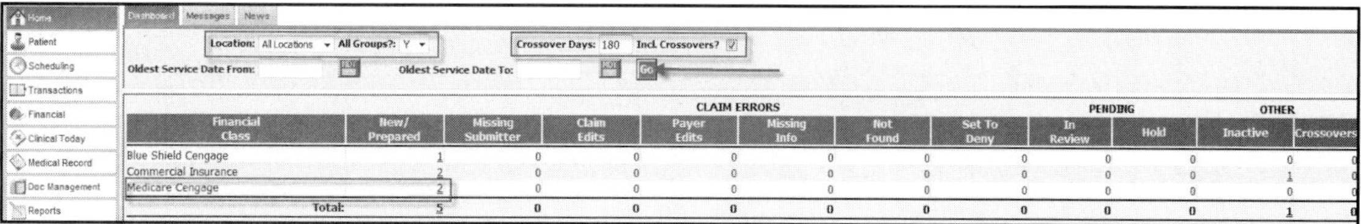

Figure 8-4 Claims by Financial Class

Courtesy of Optum™ PM and Physician EMR

7. Click on a number in the *New/Prepared* column for the corresponding financial class you need to work (select the column for "Medicare Cengage" [see Figure 8-4]). The *New/Prepared Claims* screen will display (Figure 8-5). (**Note:** You can also click the *Total* at the bottom of the column. Optum™ PM displays a claim line for all of the *Unbilled Claims* for the corresponding column and financial class.)

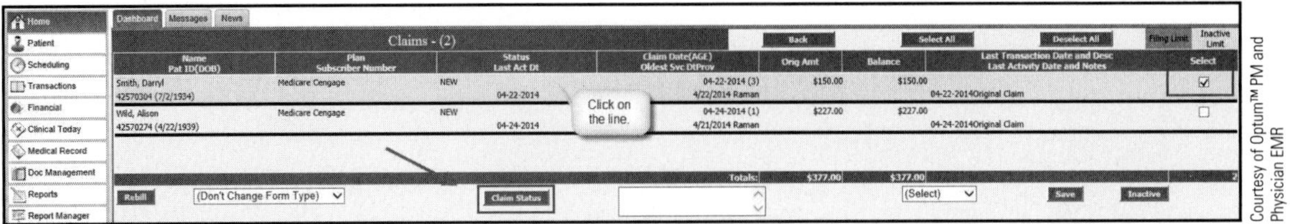

Courtesy of Optum™ PM and Physician EMR

Figure 8-5 New/Prepared Claims Screen

8. Select the checkbox in the *Select* column for each claim you want to work. Select the first claim for Darryl Smith and click the *Claim Status* button. (**Note:** You can select all of the claims by clicking *Select All.*) You will receive a pop-up (Figure 8-6) advising you of the claim's status (which displays "Processing. . . ."). **Do not** click the *Close* button in the pop-up *Claim Status* window as this will remove the claim from the *Unbilled Claims* screen. Rather, click on the "X" in the upper-right-hand corner to close out of the window.

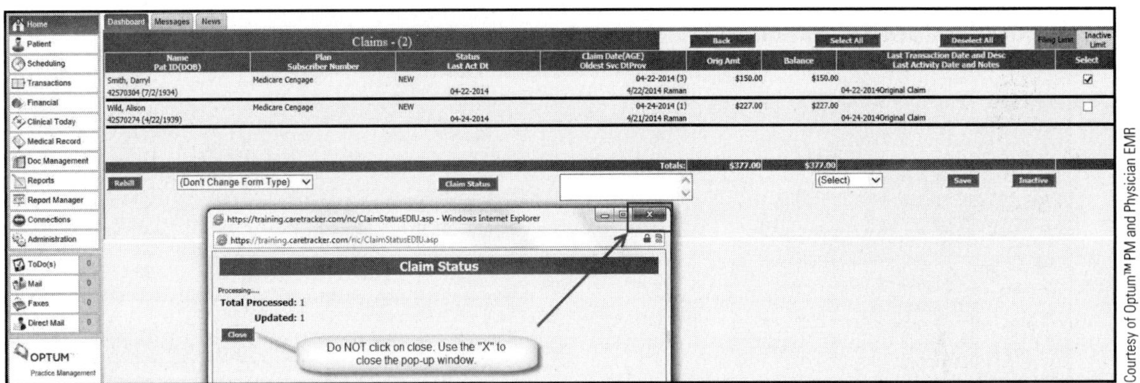

Courtesy of Optum™ PM and Physician EMR

Figure 8-6 Claim Status Pop-Up

9. To review, edit, check claim status, or rebill an individual claim, click in the claim summary line. The claim line now appears in yellow and the application displays the *Claim Summary* in the lower frame of the screen (see Figure 8-2). Look under the *Activity Notes* column to determine the inaccurate or missing claim information that, triggered by *ClaimsManager*, prevented the claim from being transmitted from Optum™ PM, prevented the claim from being accepted by a payer, or that caused the claim to be denied by the payer (Figure 8-7).

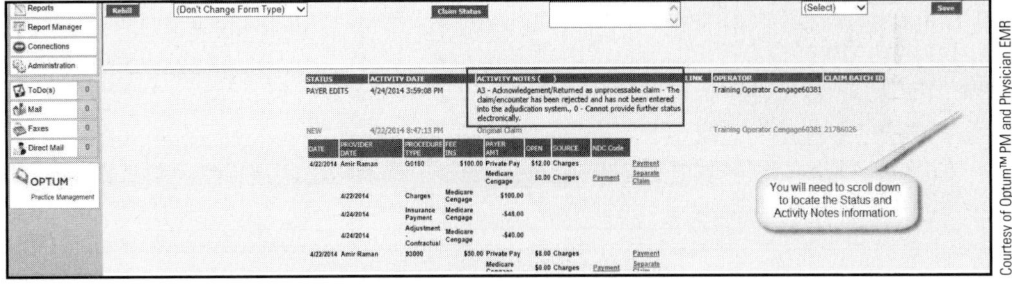

Courtesy of Optum™ PM and Physician EMR

Figure 8-7 Activity Notes

10. Perform the desired action on the claim(s):

   a. To edit claim information, such as diagnosis code or referring provider, scroll down and click *Edit* on the *Claim Summary* screen (Figure 8-8). The *Encounters* window displays the location, place of service, encounter specific claim information, referring provider, diagnosis code, and modifiers. Change the *Referring Provider* to "Dr. Shinaman" (you are choosing Dr. Shinaman as the referring provider because he was the last provider to visit Mr. Smith in the SNF) and then click *Save*. Once *Save* is clicked, you will briefly receive the "update" message noted in Figure 8-9. Your *Claim Summary* will now reflect the change to Referring Provider.

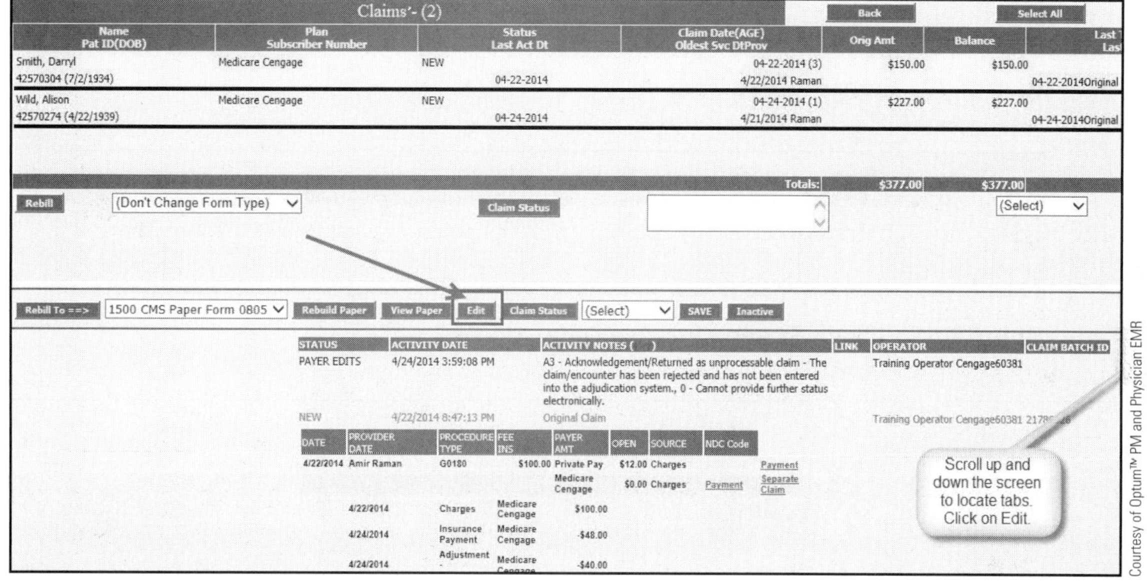

Figure 8-8 Edit Claim Summary

UpdateClaimTrxSummary(42398893,53913169,NOTES_HERE,50, ErrorCollection, N)
Claim Edited.
Claim Edited.

Figure 8-9 Update Claim Message

   b. To edit patient information, such as date of birth or subscriber number, click the *Edit* button in the *Name Bar*. Optum™ PM and Physician EMR opens the patient's demographics in a new *Patient Edit* window. Edit the patient information by adding mobile phone number 707-555-4321 to Mr. Smith's demographics.

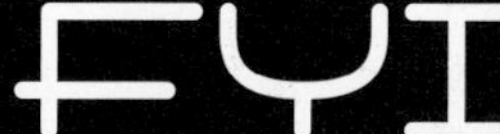

To inactivate a claim you would select the claim by placing a check mark in the *Select* column box. Click the *Inactive* button to inactivate a claim. A pop-up box appears. Enter the inactive date and then click *Accept* (see Figure 8-10). Your screen will refresh and the *Inactive* date appears in the *Last Transaction Date and Desc* column (see Figure 8-11).

(*Continues*)

FYI *(Continued)*

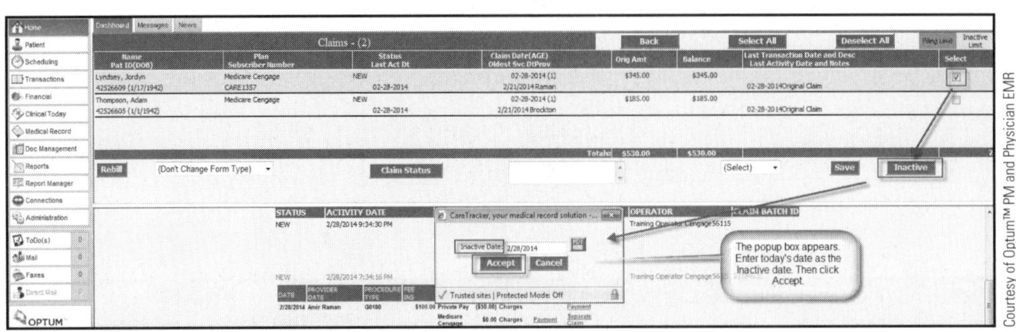

Courtesy of Optum™ PM and Physician EMR

Figure 8-10 Enter Inactive Date

Figure 8-11 Claims Screen - Inactive Date

Courtesy of Optum™ PM and Physician EMR

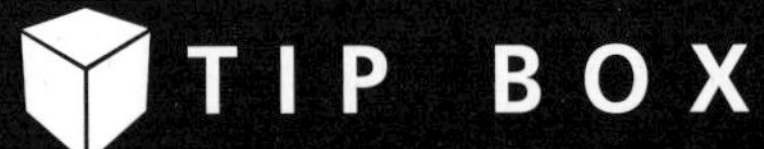

When the billing provider, dates of service, procedure codes, fee, units, servicing provider, or insurance need to be changed, the charge must be reversed from Optum™ PM via the *Edit* application in the *Transactions* module. The charge will then be put back into the system.

c. (FYI Only) Click the number link in the *Rule Set* field. The application displays descriptions of the rules for the insurance company where the claim is being submitted. Reviewing the rules can help you determine what claim information must be fixed.

d. (FYI Only) In the *Claim Summary*, select a claim frequency code from the *Rebill As* field to indicate why the claim is being resubmitted (if applicable). Each code is described in Table 8-1.

Table 8-1 Claim Frequency Codes

Code	Description
Insurance Default (I)	Rebills each claim with the default code that was set for the insurance on that claim.
Claim Default (C)	Rebills the claim with its current status.
Original (1)	First generation of claim. **Note:** This code is not used for rebilling.
Corrected (6)	Adjustment of a prior claim.
Replacement (7)	Replacement of a prior claim.
Void (8)	Void/Cancellation of a prior claim.

Courtesy of Optum™ PM and Physician EMR

11. Now select the same claim by clicking in the claim line (which will turn yellow) and checking the *Select* box. When all of the edits are complete, click *Rebill To*. Optum™ PM places the claim in the *New/Pending* category of the *Claims Worklist* and the claim will be transmitted during the next claim run. Scroll down the screen and, in the *Activity Notes* column, you will now see the activities completed (Figure 8-12).

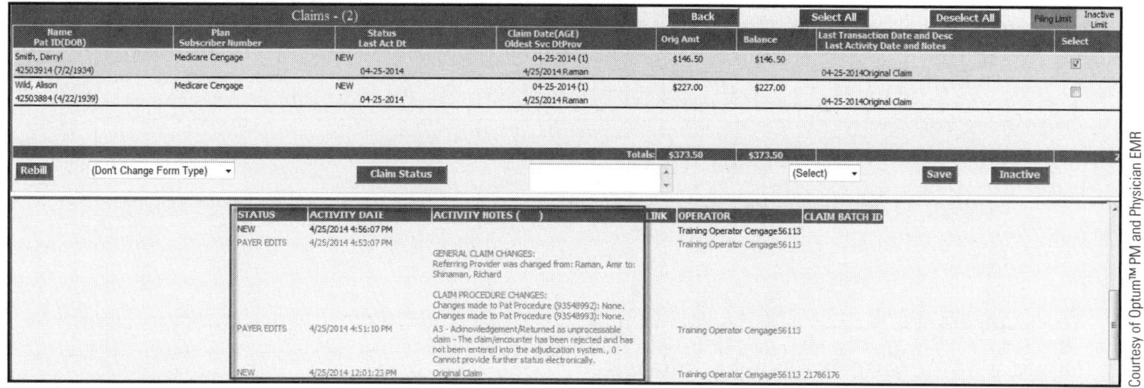

Courtesy of Optum™ PM and Physician EMR

Figure 8-12 Claims Status Activity Note

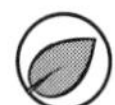

Print a screenshot of the Claim Status Activity screen, label it "Activity 8-1," and place it in your assignment folder.

ACTIVITY 8-2: Work Crossover Claims

A crossover claim is a claim that is automatically forwarded from Medicare to a secondary insurer after Medicare has paid its portion of a service.

1. Go to the *Home* module > *Dashboard* tab > *Billing* section > *Claims Worklist* link. Select *Crossover* from the three options. Optum™ PM opens the *Claims Worklist* application.
2. The *Location* list defaults to "All Locations." Leave as is.
3. The *All Groups* list defaults to "N" for No. Select "Y" for Yes to include claims for all groups.
4. Select the *Incl. Crossovers* checkbox. The *Crossover Days* field defaults to 30. (**Note:** You can adjust the crossover days to 180 if claims are not displaying for you.)
5. (Optional) Enter a date range in the *Oldest Service Date From/To* boxes.
6. Click *Go*. Optum™ PM displays a list of all claims organized by financial class (Figure 8-13).

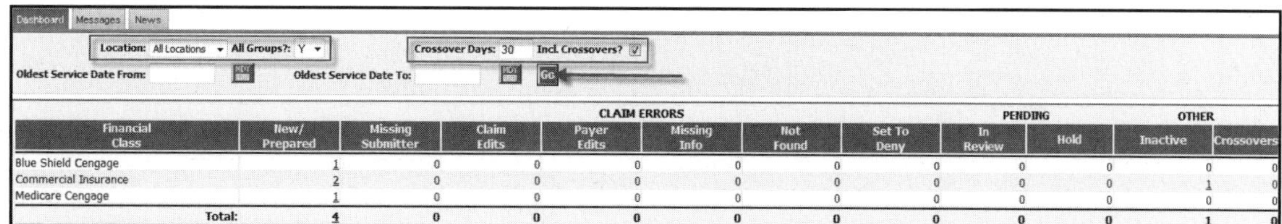

Financial Class	New/ Prepared	Missing Submitter	Claim Edits	Payer Edits	Missing Info	Not Found	Set To Deny	In Review	Hold	Inactive	Crossovers
			CLAIM ERRORS					PENDING		OTHER	
Blue Shield Cengage	1	0	0	0	0	0	0	0	0	0	0
Commercial Insurance	2	0	0	0	0	0	0	0	0	1	0
Medicare Cengage	1	0	0	0	0	0	0	0	0	0	0
Total:	4	0	0	0	0	0	0	0	0	1	0

Figure 8-13 Crossover Claims

Courtesy of Optum™ PM and Physician EMR

7. If there are crossover claims noted in the *Crossovers* column, click the number that corresponds to the financial class in which you want to work. Optum™ PM displays a list of crossover claims (Figure 8-14). There are no *Crossover Claims* for you to work here; however, in a live environment you would do the following:

    a. In the *Bill?* column, select the checkbox next to each claim you want to bill to secondary insurance. Alternatively, click *Check All* to bill all claims as crossover claims.

    b. Click *Set to Bill*. All crossover claims are saved as Secondary 1500 Forms under the *Unprinted Paper Claims* link for printing in the next bill run.

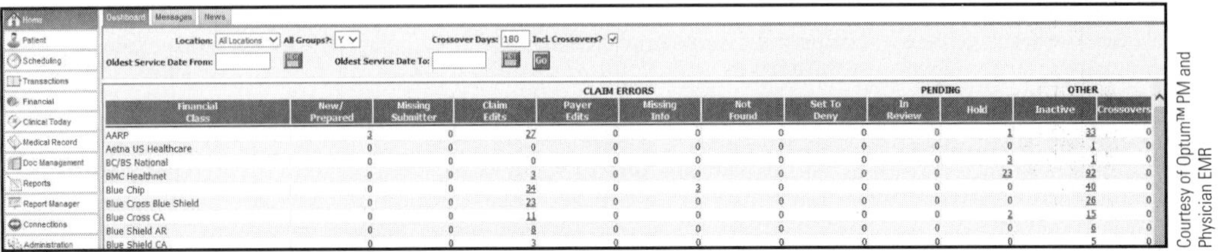

Courtesy of Optum™ PM and Physician EMR

Figure 8-14 Crossover Claims Displayed

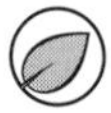

Print the Crossovers search screen, label it "Activity 8-2," and place it in your assignment folder.

ACTIVITY 8-3: Individually Check Claim Status Electronically

Optum™ PM automatically checks the status of unpaid claims every evening with specific payers and will check the status of all claims with an outstanding balance. When a check is complete, the claim's status is updated, attached to the claims, and if necessary will also be flagged in *Claims Worklist* if a status of "Not Found," "Set to Deny," or "In Review" is returned.

Typically, a manual claim status check is not necessary. However, if you need to manually check a claim status you do so individually or in a batch. Claim status for individual claims can be checked from any application in Optum™ PM where the *Claim Summary* screen displays.

1. Go to the *Home* module > *Dashboard* tab > *Billing* section > *Open Claims/Unpaid* link (Figure 8-15). Optum™ PM displays the *Open Claims* application.

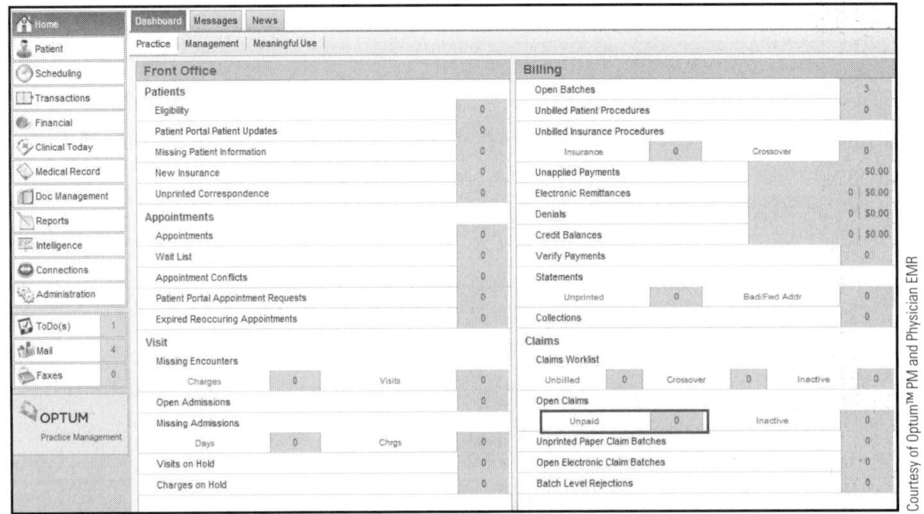

Courtesy of Optum™ PM and Physician EMR

Figure 8-15 Unpaid Claims Link

2. Select the desired filter options, as outlined next:
   a. *Status*: NEW
   b. *Age By*: Oldest Service Date
   c. *Financial Class*: Leave as is
3. Click *Go*. Optum™ PM displays the *Unpaid/Inactive* claims, broken down by financial class and by week. The total inactive claims for a financial class displays in the *Inactive* column. Totals for all unpaid claims for a financial class displays in the *Total* column, and for each week the total number of unpaid claims displays in the *Totals* row (Figure 8-16).

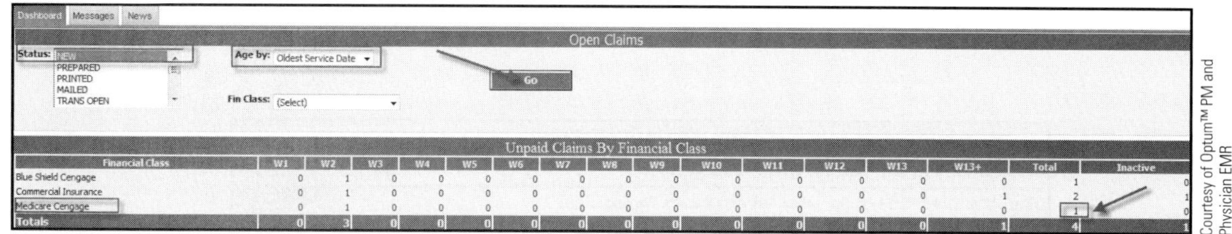

Courtesy of Optum™ PM and Physician EMR

Figure 8-16 Open Claims

4. Determine the unpaid/inactive claims for which you would like to electronically check claim status. Select the *Financial Class* "Medicare Cengage" and click on the corresponding number in the *Total* column. Optum™ PM displays a claim line for all corresponding *Unpaid/Inactive* claims with the patient's name, ID number, date of birth, subscriber number, the insurance plan for which the claim was transmitted, the claim status, last activity date on the claim, claim date, claim age, oldest service date on the claim, the provider on the claim, the original amount, balance remaining, and the last activity notes saved for the claim.
5. Place a check mark in the *Select* column, and then click on a claim summary line (select first claim). The line turns yellow and Optum™ PM displays the *Claim Summary* in the lower frame of the screen.
6. Scroll down the screen and you will be able to view the claim history (Figure 8-17). Click *Claim Status*. When the *Claim Status* window has finished processing, close out of it by clicking the "X" in the upper-right corner.

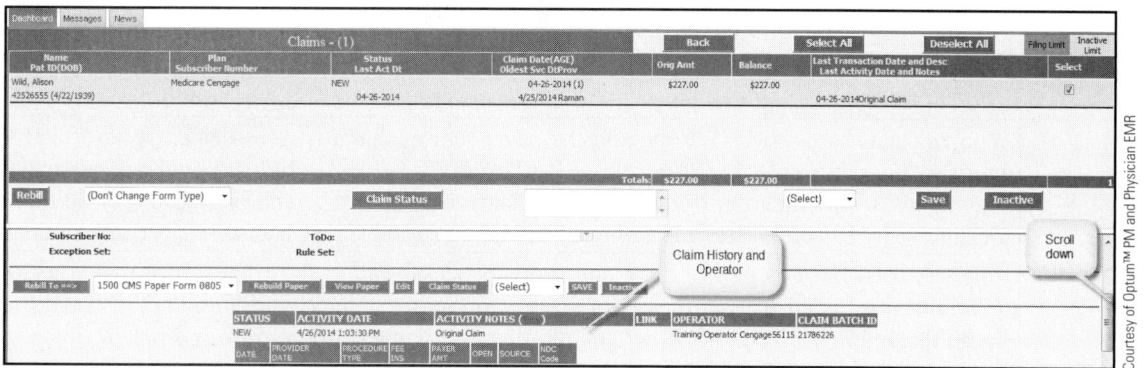

Courtesy of Optum™ PM and Physician EMR

Figure 8-17 Claim History

7. Re-select the claim and click on the *Claim Status* button above *Activity Notes* (Figure 8-18). Optum™ PM displays the *Claim Status History* window (Figure 8-19), which includes all previous status checks that have occurred, including the date of the status check, the operator who performed the check, the claim status category, and the *Claim Status* code.

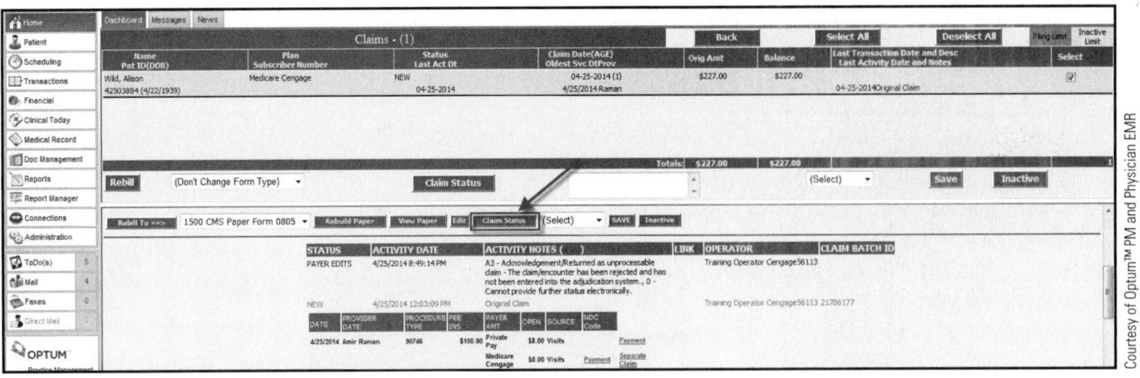

Courtesy of Optum™ PM and Physician EMR

Figure 8-18 Select Claim Status Button

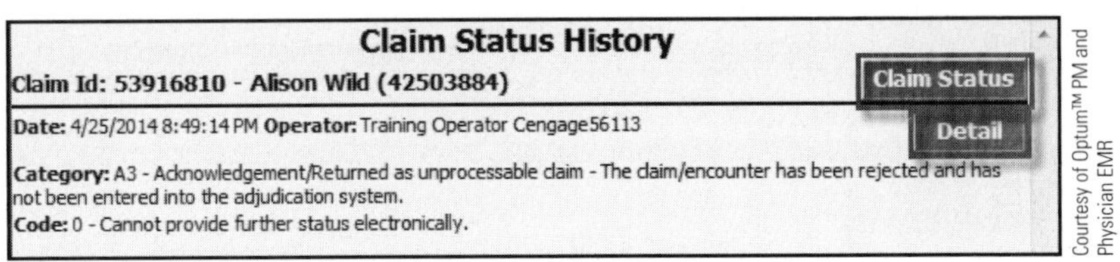

Courtesy of Optum™ PM and Physician EMR

Figure 8-19 Claim Status History

8. Click on the *Claim Status* button on the top right corner of the *Claim Status History* window to perform another claim status check. When the claim status is complete, the status of the current claim is automatically updated. Click on the "X" in the upper-right corner of the *Claim Status* window to close it. Possible statuses are included in Table 8-2.

Table 8-2 Possible Claim Statuses

In Process	When a claim status check is complete and the payer returns that it is "In Process," Optum™ PM sets the claim status to "In Process." When a claim is set to "In Process" its status will not be checked during a batch electronic claim status check for the next seven days. However, you can manually recheck the individual claim's status, overriding the seven-day period.
Finalized	When a claim status check is complete and the payer returns that it is "Finalized," Optum™ PM sets the claim status to "Finalized." A "Finalized" claim will have the details of the finalization listed under the *Activity Notes* section of the *Claims Summary* screen. After a claim has been set to "Finalized," no additional electronic claim status checks can be performed.
Set to Pay	When a claim status check is done and the payer returns that it is "Set to Pay," Optum™ PM will set the claim status to "Set to Pay." "Set to Pay" claims are going to be paid by the respective payer. These claims will remain in *Unpaid/Inactive* claims until they are paid or adjusted off in full. After a claim has been set to "Set to Pay," no additional electronic claim status checks can be performed.
Set to Deny	This will send back as part of the claim status process. Any of these messages that constitute a claim status denial will set the claim's status to "Set to Deny." In addition to these claims being flagged in the *Unpaids/Inactive* link, they are flagged in the *Claims Worklist* link as well because they have been denied and will require follow-up. After a claim has been set to *Set to Deny,* no additional electronic claim status checks can be performed.
Pending in Review	There are also *Claim Status* messages that will come back from the payer that the claim is "In Review." Any of these statuses will set the claim to *In Review. In Review* claims should be followed up on until they have been adjudicated by a payer.
Not Found	Any payer that has electronic claim status where the claim is not on file after seven days of the original claim date will be set to "Not Found" status.

Courtesy of Optum™ PM and Physician EMR

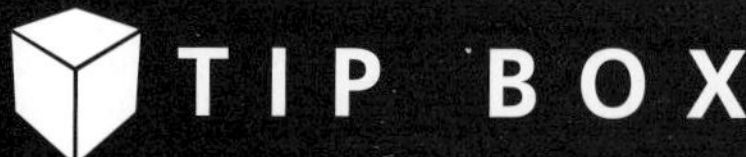

When a claim's status has been returned, except for "Set to Pay," the claim will be moved to the corresponding column on the *Claims Worklist* screen.

9. To view the details of the check, click on the *Detail* button and the *Claim Status Detail* dialog box displays (Figure 8-20). (**Note:** Since the *ClaimsManager* feature is not functional in your student environment, the *Claim Status Detail* dialog box will have the same default information for all patients.)

CLAIM STATUS DETAIL

Payer: UNITEDHEALTHCARE, Payor Identification = 87726
Submitter: Neuhauser, Andrew, Health Care Financing Administration National Provider Identifier = 1578547592
Provider: Neuhauser, Andrew, Health Care Financing Administration National Provider Identifier = 1578547592
Date of Birth: 8/14/1980, Gender: Female
Patient: JONES, KRIS, Member Identification Number = 846737659

Trace Number: 7046502X48141380
Effective Date: 4/23/2012
Total Claim Charge: $518.40
Claim Payment: $78.19
Adjudication Date: 1/11/2012
Claim Status Category: F1 = Finalized/Payment - The claim/line has been paid.
Claim Status Code: F1 = Cannot provide further status electronically.
Check Number: QG80686976
Payor's Claim Number: 3594671322 0073708217
Claim Statement Period Start: 12/19/2011 - 12/19/2011

Claim Status - Disclaimer

Patient claim status checks are submitted using current patient claim information and the results displayed are the payer response to the submitted information. CareTracker does not create or edit this information and only parses the payer response in a readable format. ALL benefit information is returned directly from the payer.

IEA02 = 114135855

Courtesy of Optum™ PM and Physician EMR

Figure 8-20 Claim Status Detail

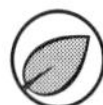 **Print the Claim Status Detail screen, label it "Activity 8-3," and place it in your assignment folder.**

ACTIVITY 8-4: Work Unpaid/Inactive Claims

Now that you have checked the claim status, begin working the unpaid/inactive claims. The steps are similar to checking a claim status, but you are now working the claim.

1. Go to the *Home* module > *Dashboard* tab > *Billing* section > *Open Claims/Unpaid* link.
2. Optum™ PM displays the *Open Claims* application. Enter the following:
   a. In the *Status* field, click on the status of the claims you want to view. Press the [Ctrl] key while clicking to select multiple statuses. Do not make a selection; leave as is.

b. In the *Age by* drop-down list select the age of claims to view. Select "Oldest Service Date."

c. (Optional) From the *Fin Class* drop-down list, select the financial class containing the claims you want to view. Leave as "(Select)."

d. Click *Go*. Optum™ PM displays the unpaid/inactive claims by financial class and by week.

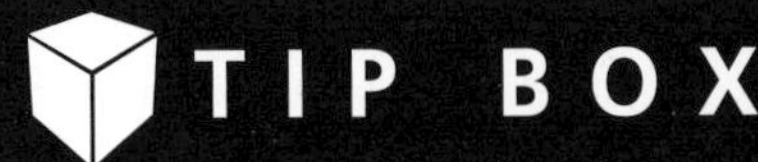

Unpaid Claims by Financial Class

- The *Inactive* column displays the total inactive claims for a financial class.
- The *Total* column displays the total unpaid claims for a financial class.
- The *Totals* row displays the total unpaid claims for each week.

3. Locate the claims you want to work and click on the corresponding number in the chart. Optum™ PM displays a claim line for each unpaid/inactive claim. Click the column headings to sort the columns. (**Note:** You cannot click on a zero total.) Select the number in the *Total* column for "Commercial Insurance."
4. When a number is clicked, a claim line for all corresponding *Unpaid/Inactive* claims displays with the patient's name, ID number, date of birth, subscriber number, the insurance plan for which the claim was transmitted, the claim status, last activity date on the claim, claim date, claim age, oldest service date on the claim, the provider on the claim, the original amount, balance remaining, and the last activity notes saved for the claim (Figure 8-21). Claims that have reached their *Filing Limit* will display in red.

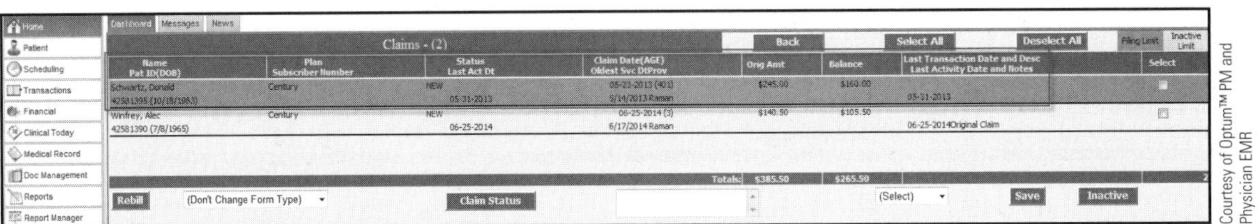

Figure 8-21 Unpaid/Inactive Claims

Courtesy of Optum™ PM and Physician EMR

5. To work claims in a batch:

a. (FYI Only) To work all claims, click *Select All* to select all of the claims and then click on the *Claim Status* button.

b. To review or work an individual claim, click on the claim summary line (select Alec Winfrey's claim). Optum™ PM displays the *Claim Summary* in the lower frame of the screen. You will need to scroll down on both the upper and lower screens to view all the claims and the *Claim Summary* information for the claim selected.

c. To change the location, place of service, encounter specific claim information, referring provider, diagnosis code, and modifiers, scroll down and click *Edit* on the *Claim Summary* screen (Figure 8-22) (click *Edit* in Alec Winfrey's claim). The *Encounters* window displays (see Figure 8-23), where you can make changes. (**Note:** Dates of service, procedure codes, fees, the insurance company, and the amount of the claim may not be edited from this window.)

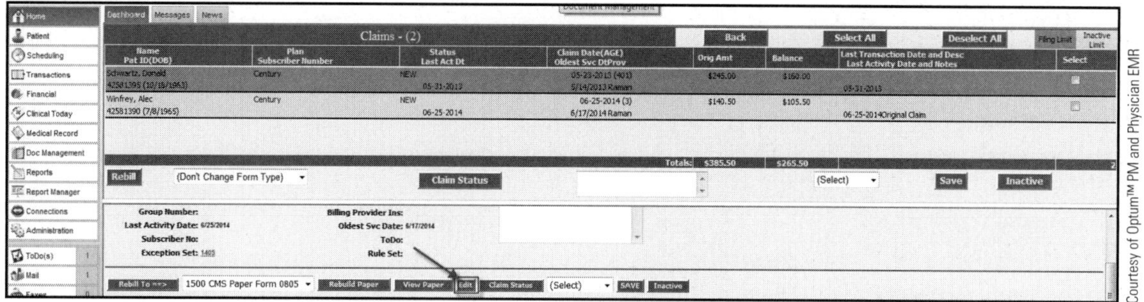

Courtesy of Optum™ PM and Physician EMR

Figure 8-22 Edit Claim Summary

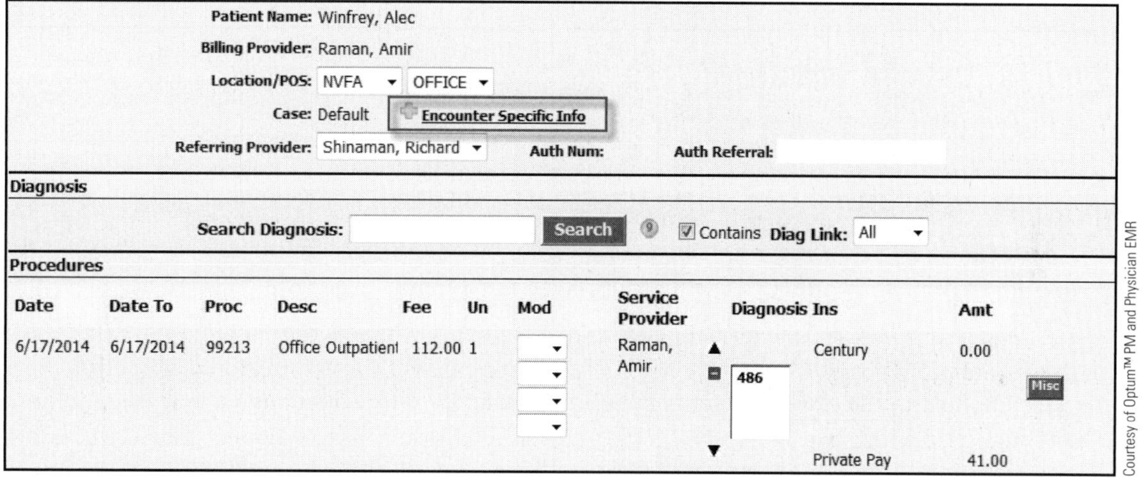

Courtesy of Optum™ PM and Physician EMR

Figure 8-23 Encounters Window

d. Click on the [+] sign next to *Encounter Specific Info* and a pop-up *Preferred Patient Case* dialog box will appear. In the *Claim Information* tab, use the drop-down arrow and select "Dr. Raman" as the *Supervising* and *Ordering Provider* (see Figure 8-24).

e. Click the *Save For Charge* button. The dialog box disappears and the screen returns to the *Encounters* dialog box.

f. Click the *Save* button and the *Encounters* dialog box will close.

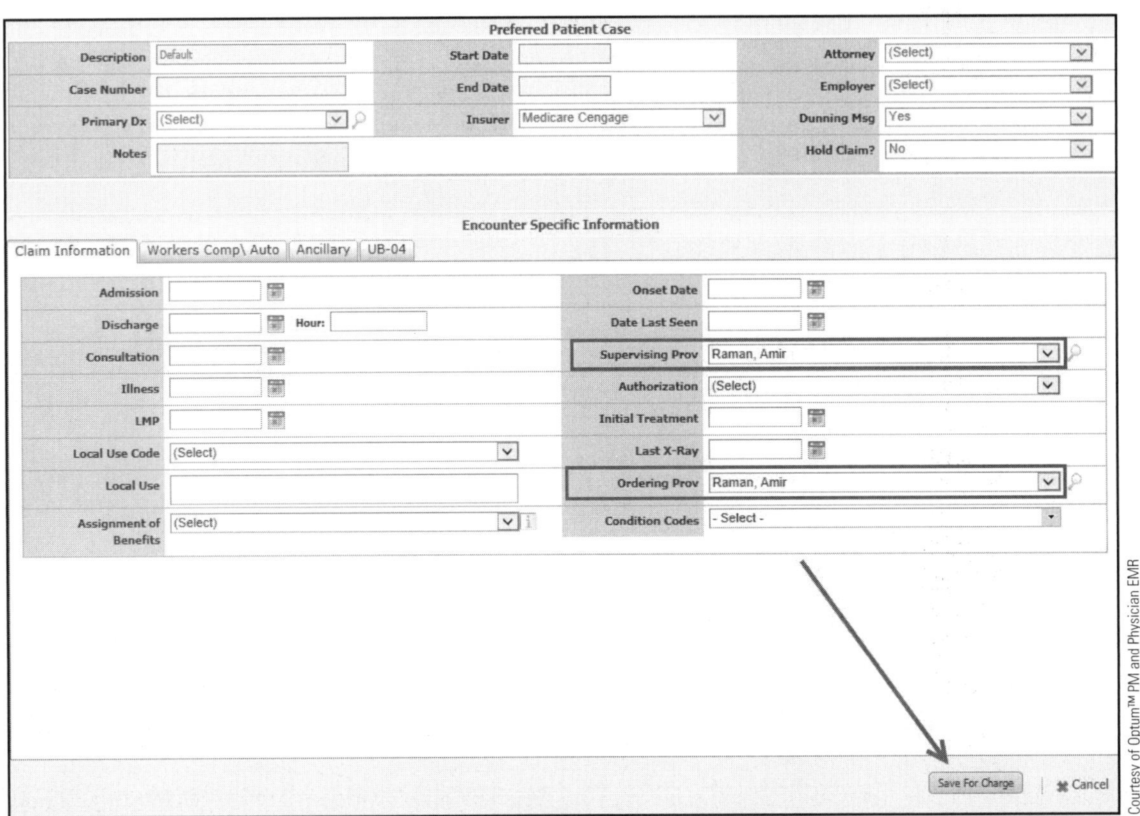

Courtesy of Optum™ PM and Physician EMR

Figure 8-24 Preferred Patient Case Dialog Box

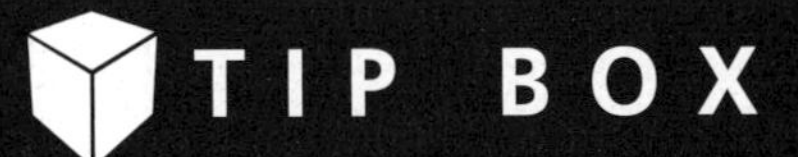

TIP BOX

If there is a number in *Rule Set*, click the number link next to *Rule Set* (Figure 8-25) to view descriptions of the rules for the insurance company. This can be helpful when determining the information that needs to be fixed. Click the *Key* link next to the *Activity Notes* heading to view a key for deciphering each missing information code (Figure 8-26).

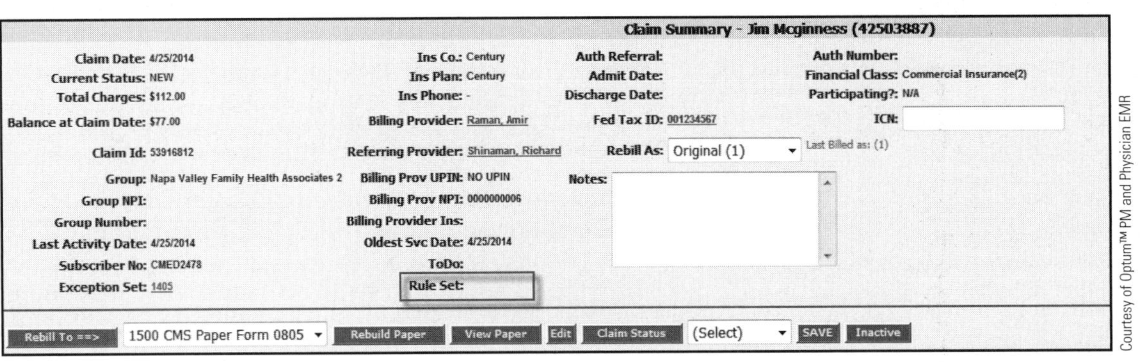

Courtesy of Optum™ PM and Physician EMR

Figure 8-25 Rule Set

(Continues)

Tip Box (*Continued*)

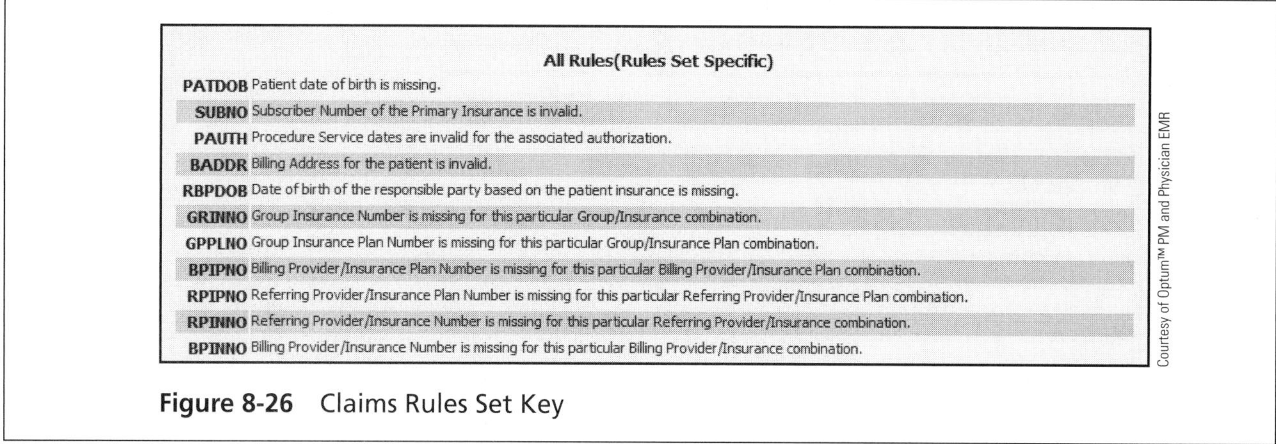

All Rules(Rules Set Specific)

PATDOB	Patient date of birth is missing.
SUBNO	Subscriber Number of the Primary Insurance is invalid.
PAUTH	Procedure Service dates are invalid for the associated authorization.
BADDR	Billing Address for the patient is invalid.
RBPDOB	Date of birth of the responsible party based on the patient insurance is missing.
GRINNO	Group Insurance Number is missing for this particular Group/Insurance combination.
GPPLNO	Group Insurance Plan Number is missing for this particular Group/Insurance Plan combination.
BPIPNO	Billing Provider/Insurance Plan Number is missing for this particular Billing Provider/Insurance Plan combination.
RPIPNO	Referring Provider/Insurance Plan Number is missing for this particular Referring Provider/Insurance Plan combination.
RPINNO	Referring Provider/Insurance Number is missing for this particular Referring Provider/Insurance combination.
BPINNO	Billing Provider/Insurance Number is missing for this particular Billing Provider/Insurance combination.

Courtesy of Optum™ PM and Physician EMR

Figure 8-26 Claims Rules Set Key

6. (FYI Only) To edit patient demographic information, click the *Edit* button on the *Name Bar*. Optum™ PM displays the patient's demographics in the *Patient Edit* window.
   a. You would edit the information as needed, and then click *Save*.
7. After editing the claim or patient information, click *Rebill To*. Optum™ PM will place the claim in the *New/Pending* category of the *Claims Worklist* screen and will transmit the claim during the next bill run (Figure 8-27).

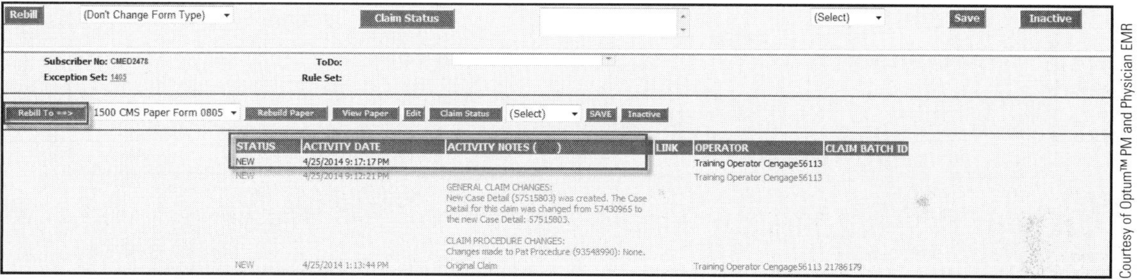

Courtesy of Optum™ PM and Physician EMR

Figure 8-27 Last Transaction Update

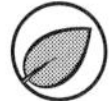 **Print a screenshot of the Unpaid/Inactive screen, label it "Activity 8-4," and place it in your assignment folder.**

ACTIVITY 8-5: Generate Patient Statements

Optum™ PM automatically generates patient statements each week. Statements are sent to responsible parties who owe a private pay balance. A statement will not be generated for a patient if the patient has an unapplied balance saved on his or her account that is equal to or greater than the patient's current balance amount.

1. Before beginning this activity, post the following batches: "CredBalRef," "PostRemit," "Ch7MCSRemit," and "SmithSNF."
2. With patient Alison Wild in context, go to the *Administration* module > *Practice* tab > *Daily Administration* section > *Financial* header > *Generate Statements* link (Figure 8-28). If a patient is in context, the application displays the option to generate statements for the parent company or the responsible party. You can generate statements for only the parent company when no patient is in context.

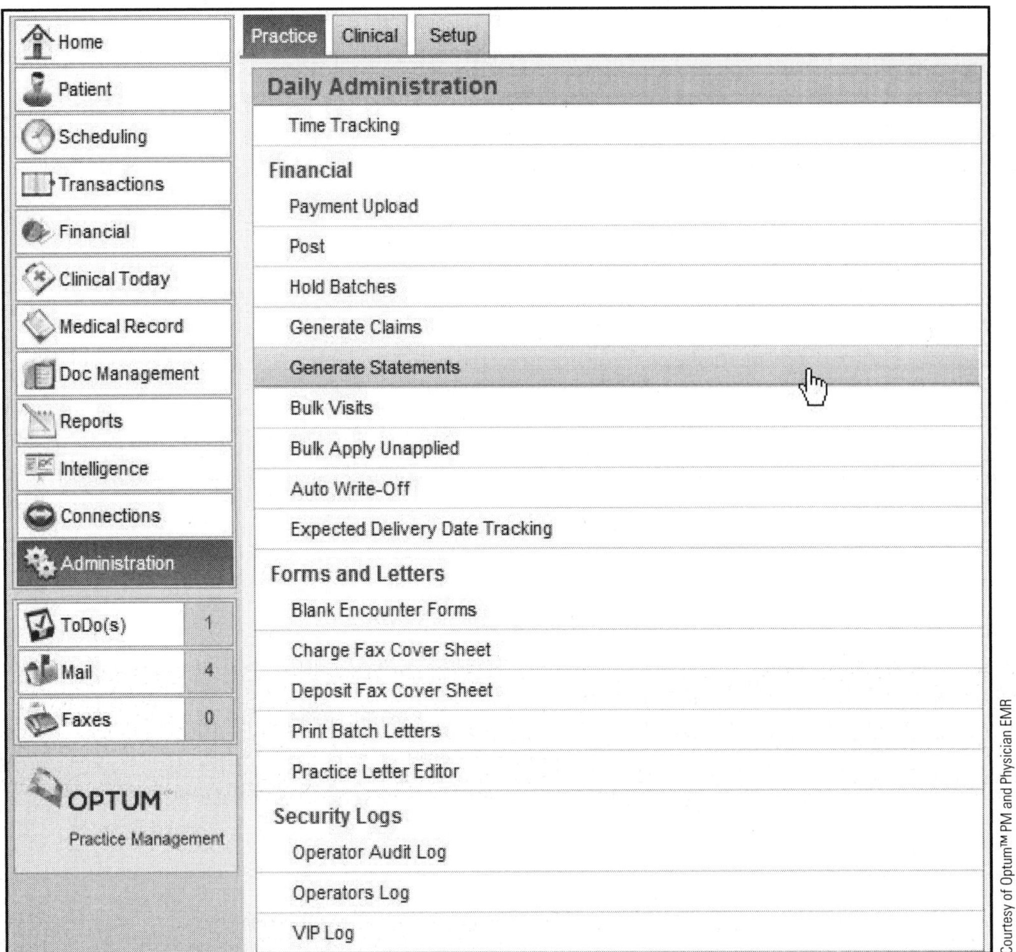

Courtesy of Optum™ PM and Physician EMR

Figure 8-28 Generate Statements Link

3. In the *Generate Statements for Responsible Party* field, select the responsible party for whom you want to generate statements (patient "Alison Wild") and then click *Go!* (see Figure 8-29).

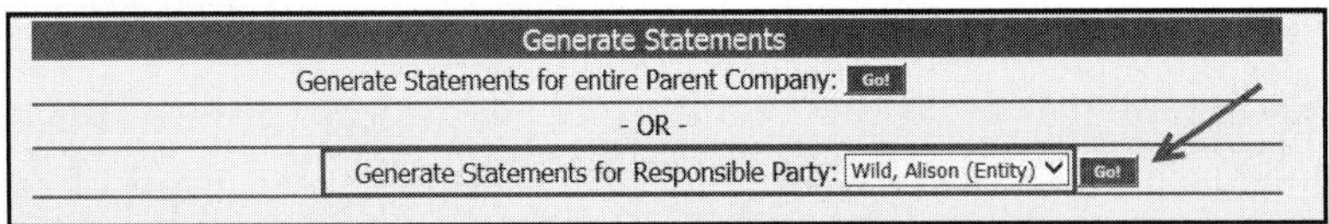

Figure 8-29 Generate Statements for Responsible Party – Alison Wild

Courtesy of Optum™ PM and Physician EMR

4. The application schedules the statements to be printed. Your screen will look like Figure 8-30. (**Note:** Patient statements will not be generated by Optum™ PM until 5 p.m. (Figure 8-31) regardless of the time of day you request statements to be produced.)

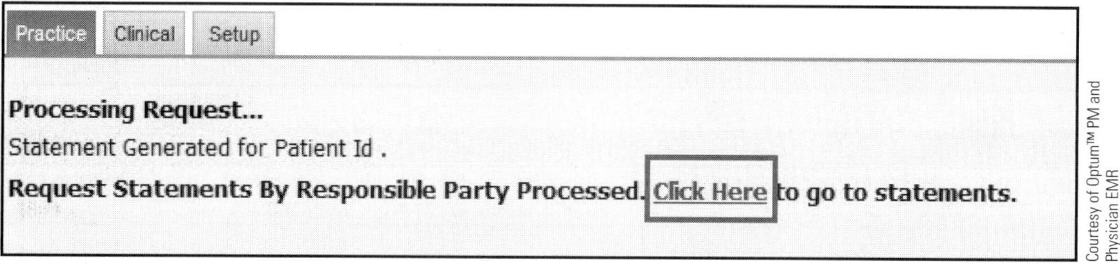

Courtesy of Optum™ PM and Physician EMR

Figure 8-30 Statement Generated

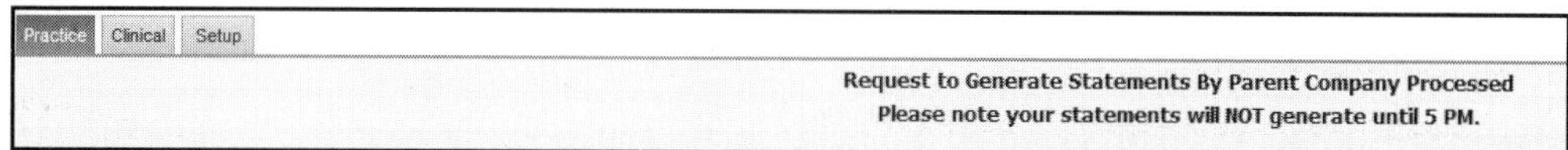

Figure 8-31 Statements Generate at 5 p.m.

Courtesy of Optum™ PM and Physician EMR

PM SPOTLIGHT

If no statements are displaying, recheck after 24 hours (or after 5 p.m. on the date the activity is performed). Continue with your activities, and repeat Activity 8-5 in 24 hours.

5. Click on the blue "Click Here" prompt (see Figure 8-30) to go to the statements. Your screen will now look like Figure 8-32. (**Note:** If no results are showing, change the *Date Range* to "All Dates.")

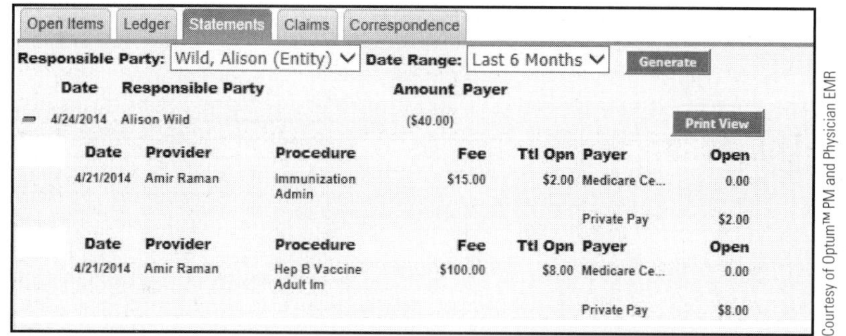

Courtesy of Optum™ PM and Physician EMR

Figure 8-32 Statements Display

6. Click on the *Print View* button. The patient's statement will display in a new window (see Figure 8-33).
7. Print the statement by right-clicking on the screen and selecting *Print* from the drop-down menu.

Napa Valley Family Associates	ACCOUNT #	36409-42503884	STATEMENT DATE	4/25/2014
	LAST PAYMENT	$14.40	STATEMENT TOTAL	$40.00

Statement - Page 1

DATE OF SERVICE	PATIENT	DESCRIPTION OF SERVICES	PROCEDURE CODE	SERVICING PROVIDER	AMOUNT	PATIENT AMT DUE
4/25/2014	Wild, Alison (42503884)	Hepatitis B Vaccine Adult Dosage Intramuscular	90746	Raman, Amir	$100.00	**$8.00**
		Per Your Insurance Company, Your Copay Has Not Been Paid In Full. The Balance Is Your Responsibility. Thank You.				
		Transaction 04/25/2014, Insurance Payment			-$32.00	
		Transaction 04/25/2014, Adjustment - Contractual			-$60.00	
4/25/2014	Wild, Alison (42503884)	Imadm Prq Id Subq/Im Njxs 1 Vaccine	90471	Raman, Amir	$15.00	**$2.00**
		Per Your Insurance Company, Your Copay Has Not Been Paid In Full. The Balance Is Your Responsibility. Thank You.				
		Transaction 04/25/2014, Insurance Payment			-$8.00	
		Transaction 04/25/2014, Adjustment - Contractual			-$5.00	

MAKE CHECKS PAYABLE TO: Napa Valley Family Associates	PLEASE PAY THIS AMOUNT	$40.00

TO ENSURE PROPER CREDIT, PLEASE DETACH AND RETURN BOTTOM PORTION WITH YOUR PAYMENT

Napa Valley Family Associates
101 Vine Street
Napa, CA 94558

707- 555-1212 Ext:

ACCOUNT #	36409-42503884	STATEMENT DATE	4/25/2014
AMOUNT ENCLOSED $		STATEMENT TOTAL	$40.00

☐ CHECK BOX AND ENTER ADDRESS OR INSURANCE CORRECTIONS ON THE REVERSE SIDE

☐ IF PAYING BY CREDIT CARD, FILL OUT THE INFORMATION ON THE REVERSE SIDE

ADDRESSEE:
ALISON WILD
1022 BARSOW
VALLEJO, CA 94503

REMIT TO:
NAPA VALLEY FAMILY ASSOCIATES
101 VINE STREET
NAPA, CA 94558

Figure 8-33 Patient Statement

Statement - Page 2

IF ANY OF THE INFORMATION HAS BEEN CHANGED SINCE YOUR LAST STATEMENT, PLEASE INDICATE...

ABOUT YOU:

YOUR NAME (Last, First, Middle Initial)		
ADDRESS		
CITY	STATE	ZIP
TELEPHONE ( )	MARITAL STATUS ☐ Single ☐ Married	☐ Divorced ☐ Widowed
EMPLOYER'S NAME	TELEPHONE ( )	
EMPLOYER'S ADDRESS	CITY	STATE ZIP

IF PAYING BY CREDIT CARD, FILL OUT BELOW

☐ AMERICAN EXPRESS	☐ MASTERCARD ☐ VISA
CARD NUMBER	
CHARGE THIS AMOUNT	EXPIRATION DATE
SIGNATURE	CARDHOLDER NAME

ABOUT YOUR INSURANCE:

YOUR PRIMARY INSURANCE COMPANY'S NAME		EFFECTIVE DATE
PRIMARY INSURANCE COMPANY'S ADDRESS		PHONE
CITY	STATE	ZIP
POLICYHOLDER'S ID NUMBER		GROUP PLAN NUMBER
YOUR SECONDARY INSURANCE COMPANY'S NAME		EFFECTIVE DATE
SECONDARY INSURANCE COMPANY'S ADDRESS		PHONE
CITY	STATE	ZIP
POLICYHOLDER'S ID NUMBER		GROUP PLAN NUMBER

Courtesy of Optum™ PM and Physician EMR

Figure 8-33 *(Continued)*

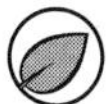

Print the patient statement, label it "Activity 8-5," and place it in your assignment folder.

ACTIVITY 8-6: View and Reprint a Patient Statement Using the Financial Module

The *Statements* application in the *Financial* module (Figure 8-34) allows you to view and reprint statements that have been generated for the patient in context. A statement can be reprinted by clicking on the *Print View* button next to the appropriate statement line. When *Print View* is clicked, the patient's statement displays in a new window, and by right-clicking on top of it the statement can be printed.

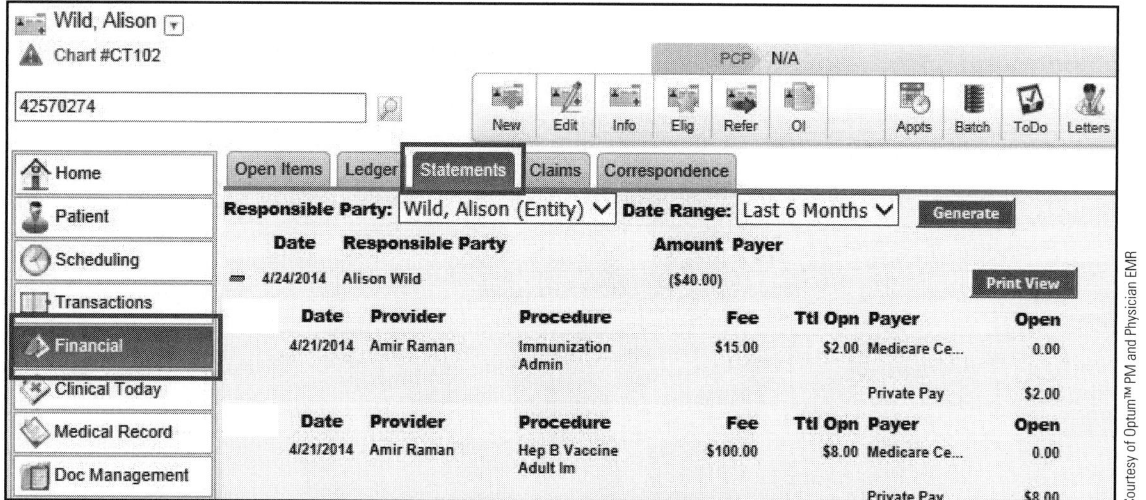

Courtesy of Optum™ PM and Physician EMR

Figure 8-34 Statements Application in Financial Module

1. Pull patient Alison Wild into context.
2. Click the *Financial* module. Click *Go*. The *Open Items* for the patient display (Figure 8-35). (**Note:** You can also access the open items by clicking the *OI* button on the *Name Bar*.)

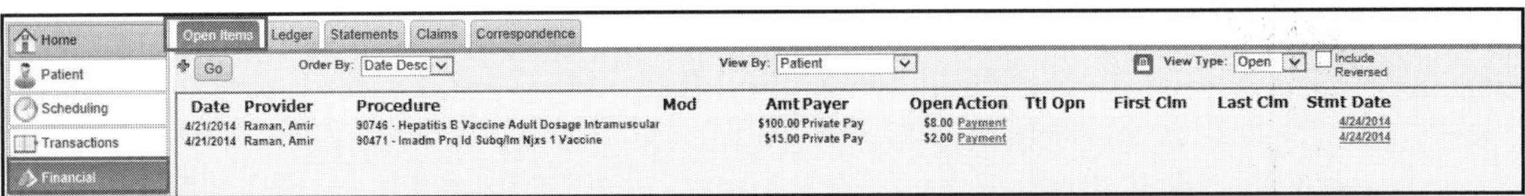

Figure 8-35 Financial Open Items

Courtesy of Optum™ PM and Physician EMR

3. Click the *Statements* tab. Optum™ PM opens the *Statements* application (see Figure 8-34).
   a. The *Responsible Party* list defaults to the responsible party set in the patient's demographic. Leave as is. (**Note:** You can select a different responsible party or "(All)" responsible parties, if applicable.)
   b. The *Date Range* list defaults to "Last 6 Months." Use the drop-down next to *Date Range* and select "All Dates."
4. Click *Generate*. Optum™ PM generates a list of the patient's statements and displays a processing message in the lower frame of the screen.
5. Select the *Click Here* link in blue. The application displays the list of statements.

TIP BOX

Click on a statement line to view the statement details in the lower frame of the screen. Click the *plus sign* [+] next to a statement line to view the procedure details included in the statement. Click on a procedure line to view the complete procedure details (Figure 8-36).

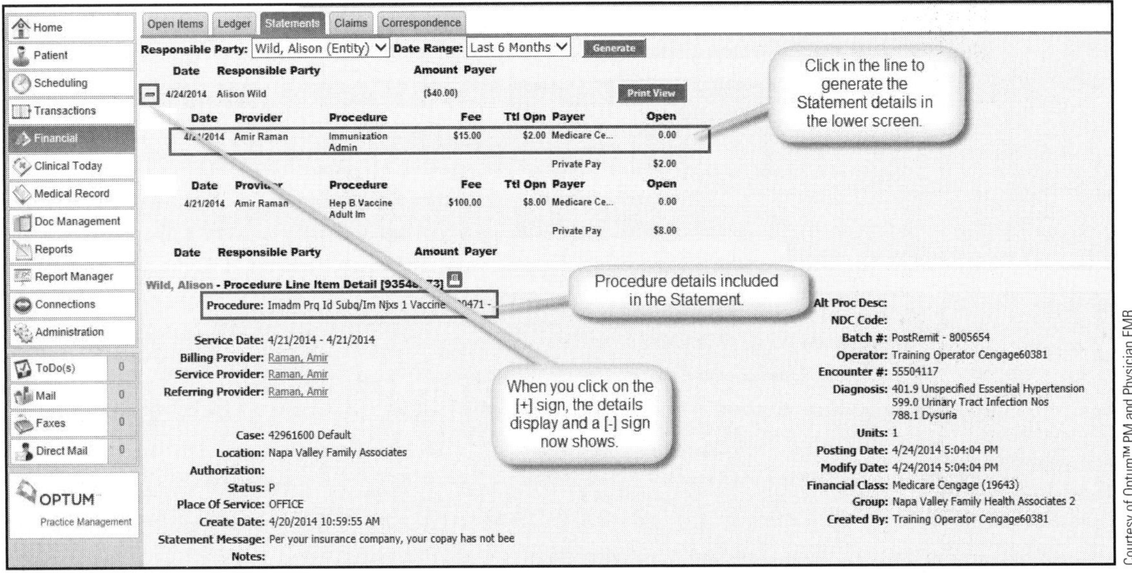

Figure 8-36 View Procedure Details

6. Click *Print View* next to the statement you want to print. Select the most recent statement. The application displays the statement in a new window. (**Note:** It may take a few moments to display.)
7. Right-click on the statement, and then select *Print* from the shortcut menu.

Print the statement, label it "Activity 8-6," and place it in your assignment folder.

8. Close the statement window when the statement has printed.

ACTIVITY 8-7: Transfer a Balance

The *Collections* application is accessed from the *Home* module > *Dashboard* tab > *Practice* tab > *Billing* section > *Collections* link (Figure 8-37). Seven collection statuses are available in Optum™ PM: New, Open Collections, Review, Collections Actual, Collections Pending, Collections Pending – NS, and Hold (see Figure 8-38).

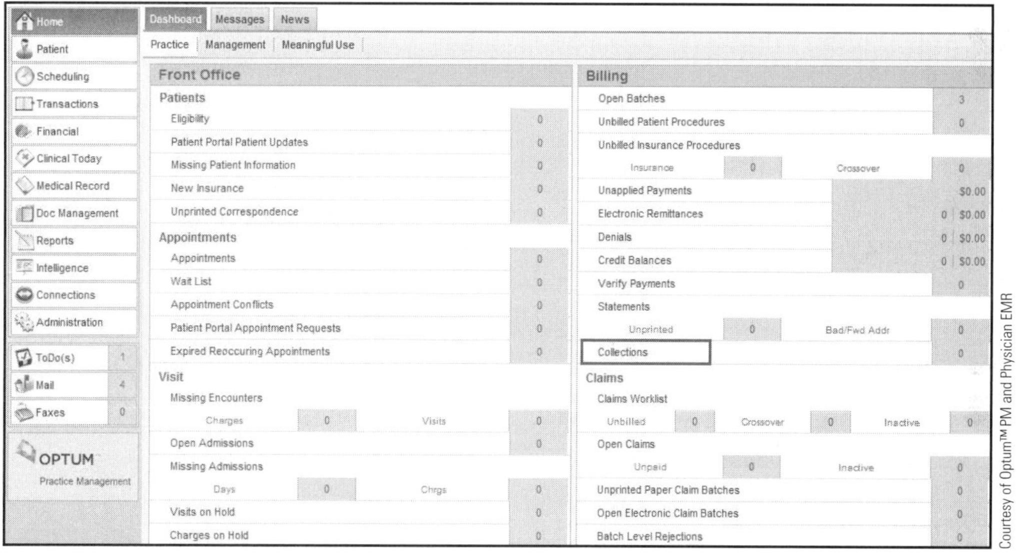

Courtesy of Optum™ PM and Physician EMR

Figure 8-37 Collections Link

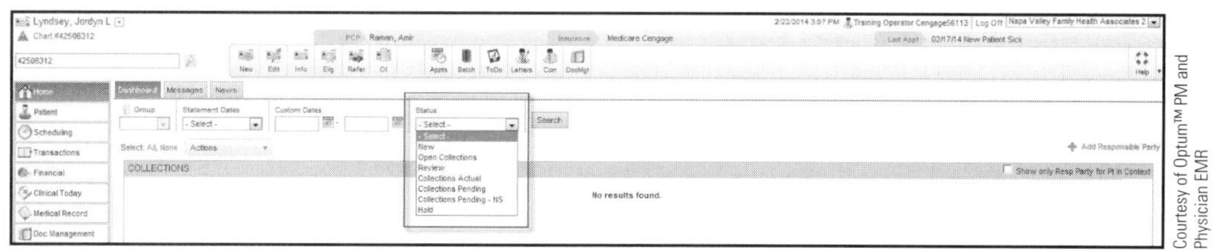

Courtesy of Optum™ PM and Physician EMR

Figure 8-38 Seven Collection Statuses

The *Collections* application in Optum™ PM allows you to focus collection efforts on patients with balances at least 30 days overdue. You can determine whether patients are identified by the collections system immediately or after their balance is 30, 60, 90, or 120 days overdue. Optum™ PM automatically moves patients into *Collections* when their overdue balance reaches the aging level assigned in the group settings and automatically removes patients from *Collections* when their overdue balance is paid. Operators can also move patients in and out of *Collections* manually. In *Open Items*, you can add a patient to *Collections* by clicking the *Add Responsible Party* link in the *Collections* work area or by transferring a balance to *Collections*.

Patients manually added to *Collections* are flagged with an asterisk (*) next to their name in the work area. Patients manually added to *Collections* must be removed from *Collections* manually as well. When manually adding a patient to *Collections*, Optum™ PM pulls the patient into context and filters the *Collections* list to show the responsible party for that patient.

To Transfer a Balance:

1. Go to the *Home* module > *Dashboard* tab > *Practice* tab > *Billing* section > *Collections* link. Optum™ PM displays a list of collection statuses and the number of patients in each status.
2. If there is no patient listed, click the *Add Responsible Party* link in the far upper-right corner of the screen. In the *Add Manual Collection* window click the *Search* icon and enter the name of the patient you are searching for (Alison Wild). Click on the patient name in the *Results* window. The patient name now populates in the *Add Manual Collection* window. Click *Save*.
3. Click the *Edit* icon next to the balance you want to transfer to a new financial class. Optum™ PM displays the *Edit* window (Figure 8-39).
   a. In the *Transfer To* line:
      - *Insurance*: Leave blank (-Select-)
      - *Overdue*: Leave blank (-Select-)
      - *Trans Date*: Use today's date

   b. *Letter*: Leave blank (-Select-)

   c. *Change Status*: Select "Open Collections"

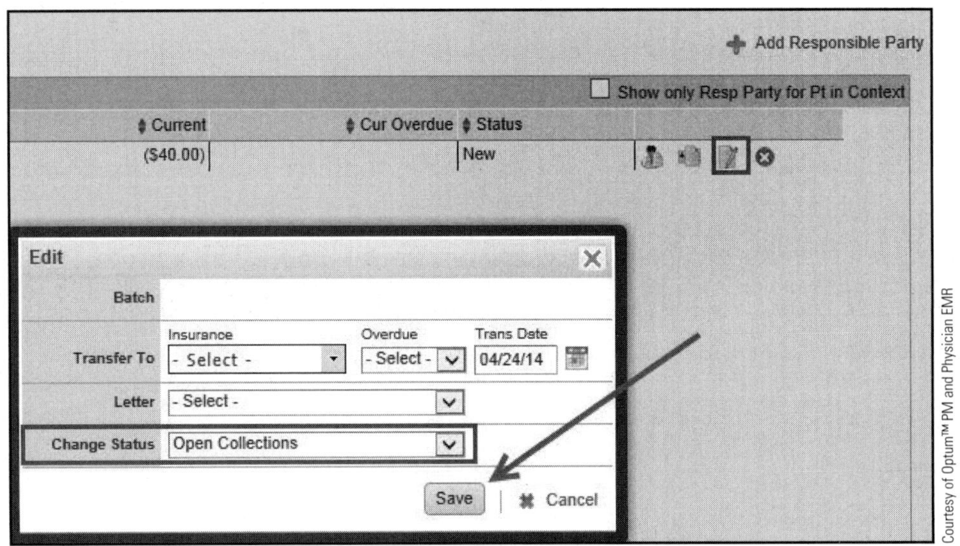

Figure 8-39 Edit Collections Dialog Box

4. Click *Save*. Optum™ PM updates the patient's status in the *Collections* application, transfers the outstanding balance to the selected financial class, and adds the selected "Transfer To" financial class to the patient's *Demographics* record. Click "Close" to close the dialog box.

Print a screenshot of the Balance Transfer screen, label it "Activity 8-7," and place it in your assignment folder.

TIP BOX

You can add the *Collections Pending Statement, Collections Pending No Statement, Collections Actual* financial classes, or your collection agency name to the *Insurance Plans* "quick pick" list in the *Quick Picks* application in the *Administration* module.

PROFESSIONALISM CONNECTION

Collection letters should do two things: retain customer goodwill and help you get paid. One way to know if the letter is working is based on the response received. A good letter will generate multiple responses (phone calls and/or payments). If you send a batch of letters and there is no response, it may be time to revise your collection letters and/or procedure. Any correspondence from the medical office is a reflection of the practice, so keep it professional.

Your letter is intended to persuade someone to send you money; therefore, the wording and tone are critical, especially if this is a patient you want to continue to do business with. Enclosing an envelope for payment is always a good idea. If you can include postage on the payment envelope, that is even better. The easier you make it for the customer to make the payment, the better your chances are of getting paid. If you cannot include a prepaid return envelope (due to high cost), propose an alternative form of payment (i.e., credit/debit card). Always remember to close the letter with an appropriate salutation.

Review the "Global Collection Letters" available in the templates provided and see if they fit with the "message" you want to send to the patient along with the appropriate "image" of the practice. How would you feel if you received one of the generic "collections" letters? How could you customize the language to accomplish the goal of collecting money due, yet keeping the relationship with the patient intact?

ACTIVITY 8-8: Create a Custom Collection Letter

The *Global Collection Letters* application contains the following letters, which are available to all users in Optum™ PM.

- "Collections 1": Explains that the account is overdue and lists the overdue balance.
- "Past Due": Explains that the overdue balance or a portion of the balance is more than 60 days past due.
- "Delinquent": Explains that the overdue balance or a portion of the balance is more than 90 days past due.
- "Final Notice": Tells the patient that her overdue balance or a portion of her balance is more than 120 days past due. This is the final written notice the patient will receive, and, if payment is not received, the account will be sent to *Collections*.
- "75 Collection": States that if the overdue balance is not paid in full, the billing office will continue with its collection policy, which may include using a collection agency.
- "Collection Payment Plan": Informs the patient that she can set up a weekly or monthly payment plan to pay off the overdue balance. On a "Collection Payment Plan" letter, the patient can also indicate if she has insurance that covered the services for which she has an overdue balance. When a patient indicates that he or she has insurance to cover the services, the patient must also complete the insurance section on the back of a statement.

You can also create custom collection letters in the *Letter Editor* application in the *Administration* module. Group-specific collection letters are built in the *Practice Letter Editor* in the *Administration* module. After creating a custom collection letter, you must add the letter to your *Form Letters Quick Picks* via the *Quick Picks* application in the *Administration* module. This will allow you to access the letter in the *Collections* module.

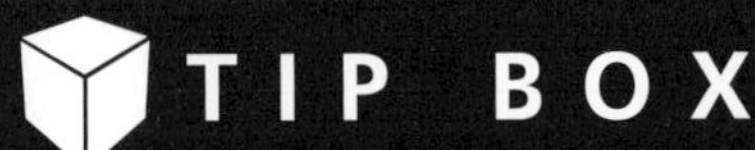

When you create a group-specific collection letter, the top portion of the letter by default includes patient information, such as name, address, and so on. The only portion of the letter you need to build in the *Letter Editor* is the text you want to appear in the letter.

To Create a Custom Collections Letter:

1. Go to the *Administration* module > *Practice* tab > *Forms and Letters* header > *Practice Letter Editor* link (Figure 8-40).

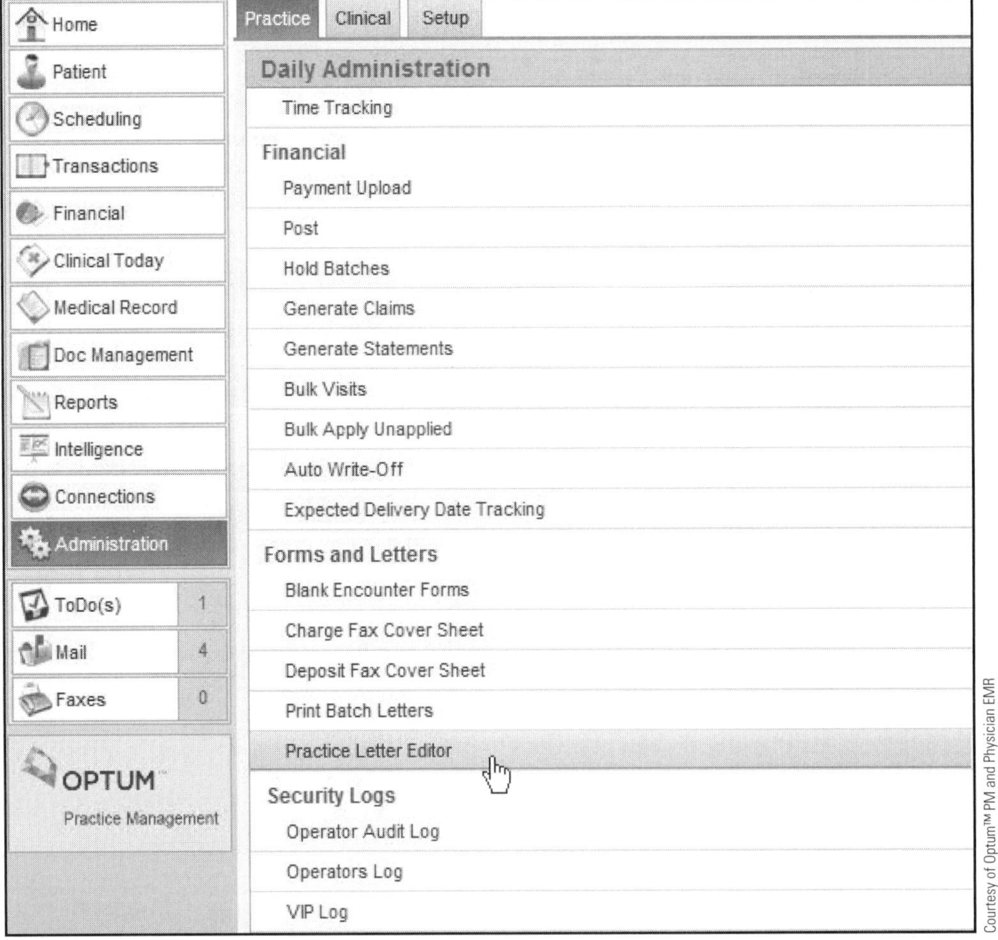

Figure 8-40 Practice Letter Editor Link

2. From the *Letters* drop-down list, select "Create New Letter" (see Figure 8-41). The application displays the *New Letter* window (see Figure 8-42).
3. Enter a descriptive name for the form letter in the *Letter Name* field. Enter "RTA Fee Letter."

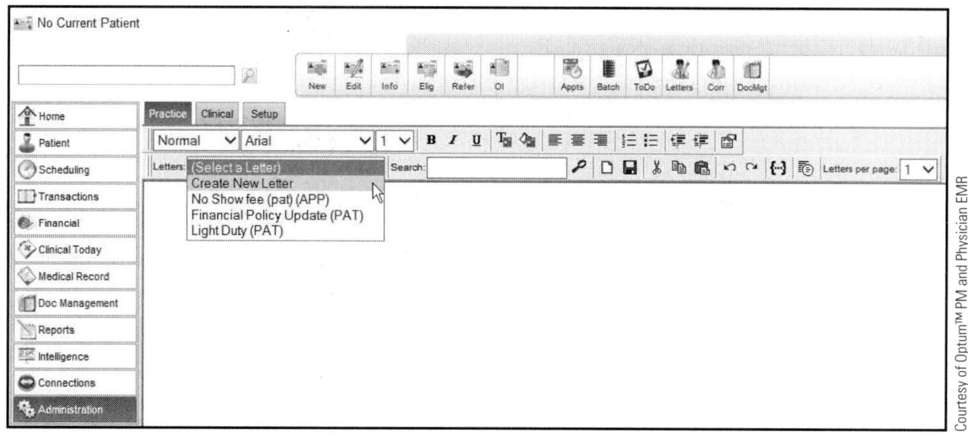

Figure 8-41 Create New Letter

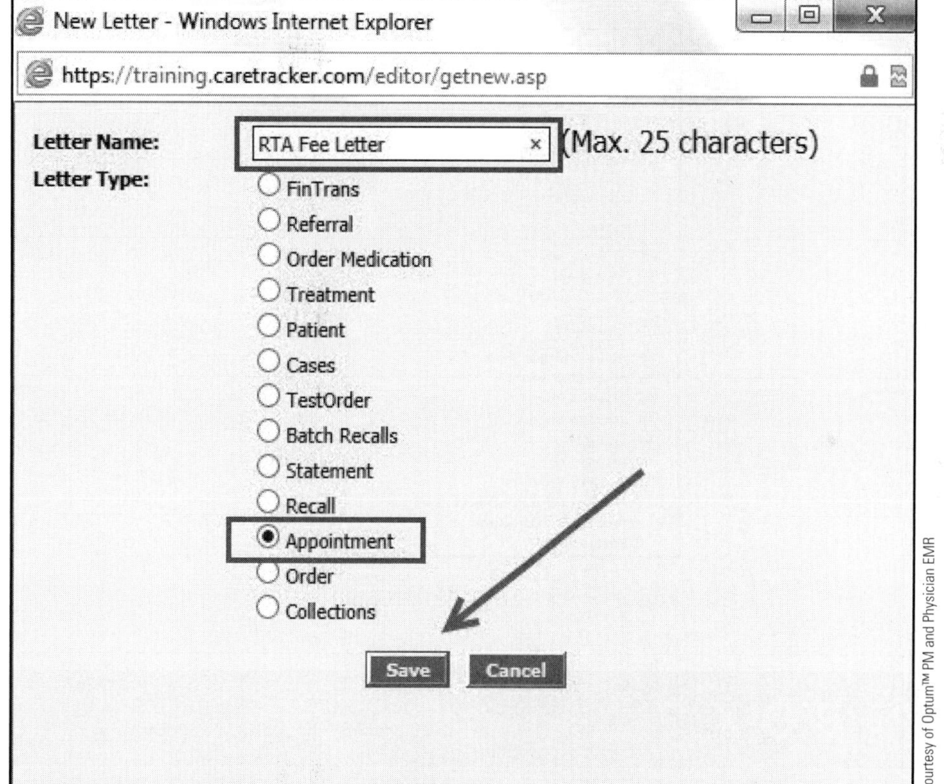

Figure 8-42 New Letter Window

4. In the *Letter Type* field, select the radio button next to the type of form letter you are creating (select "Appointment") and then click *Save* (see Figure 8-42). The application closes the *New Letter* window and pulls the new letter name and type into the *Letters* field (see Figure 8-43). (**Note:** It may take a few moments for the screen to refresh.)

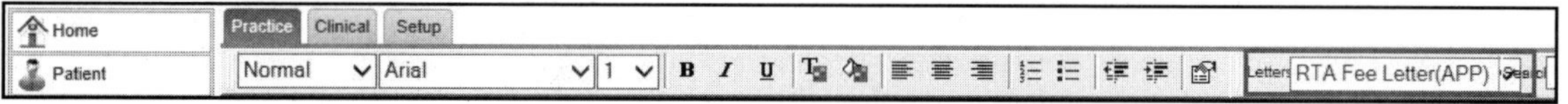

Figure 8-43 Letters Field

Courtesy of Optum™ PM and Physician EMR

5. Enter the text from Figure 8-44 to appear in the form letter and insert data fields where necessary using the *Select Field* {··} icon. Select data fields from the drop-down list in the *Select Field* list (see Figure 8-45) to complete your letter. (For example, for the first line of the letter, select "Current Date - Long" from the *Special Fields* section in the *Select Field* list.) Be sure to format the letter as you would like it to appear.

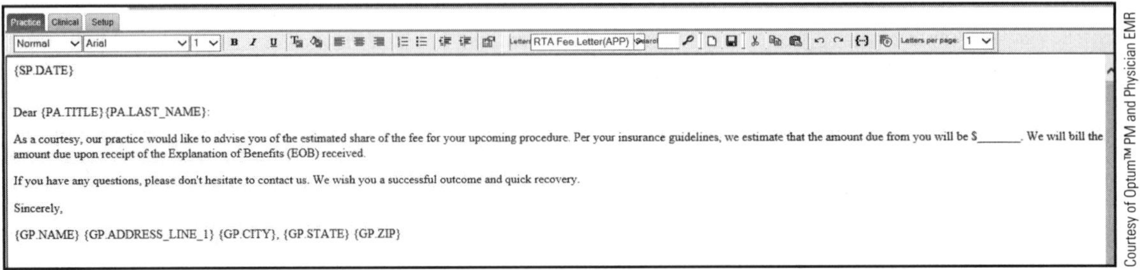

{SP.DATE}

Dear {PA.TITLE}{PA.LAST_NAME}:

As a courtesy, our practice would like to advise you of the estimated share of the fee for your upcoming procedure. Per your insurance guidelines, we estimate that the amount due from you will be $_______. We will bill the amount due upon receipt of the Explanation of Benefits (EOB) received.

If you have any questions, please don't hesitate to contact us. We wish you a successful outcome and quick recovery.

Sincerely,

{GP.NAME} {GP.ADDRESS_LINE_1} {GP.CITY}, {GP.STATE} {GP.ZIP}

Courtesy of Optum™ PM and Physician EMR

Figure 8-44 RTA Fee Letter

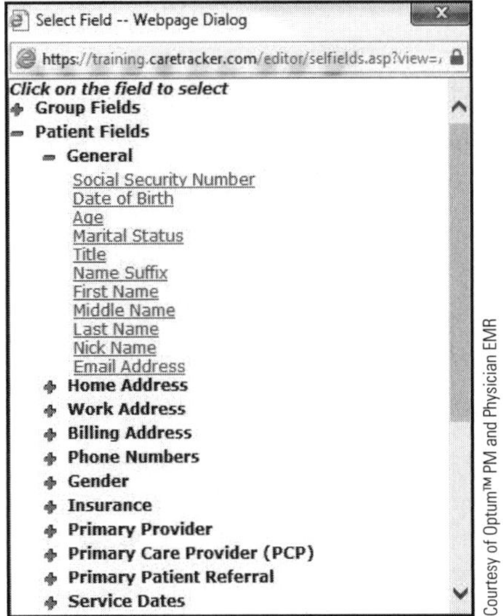

Courtesy of Optum™ PM and Physician EMR

Figure 8-45 Select Field List

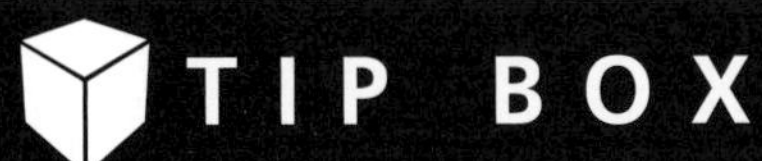

The *Letter Editor* is preset to double space when you hit the [Enter] key to enter a new line of text. For single spacing, hold the [Shift] key down as you press the [Enter] key.

6. Click the *Save File* icon when you are finished with your form letter. (As a best practice, you should click *Save* periodically while building your letter.)

Print the screen that displays the Custom Collection Letter, label it "Activity 8-8," and place it in your assignment folder.

ACTIVITY 8-9: Add a Form Letter to Quick Picks

After creating a new form letter, you must add it to your *Quick Picks* to make it available for use in Optum™ PM and Physician EMR.

1. Go to the *Administration* module > *Setup* tab > *Financial* header > *Quick Picks* link.
2. From the *Screen Type* drop-down list, select "Form Letters" (see Figure 8-46).

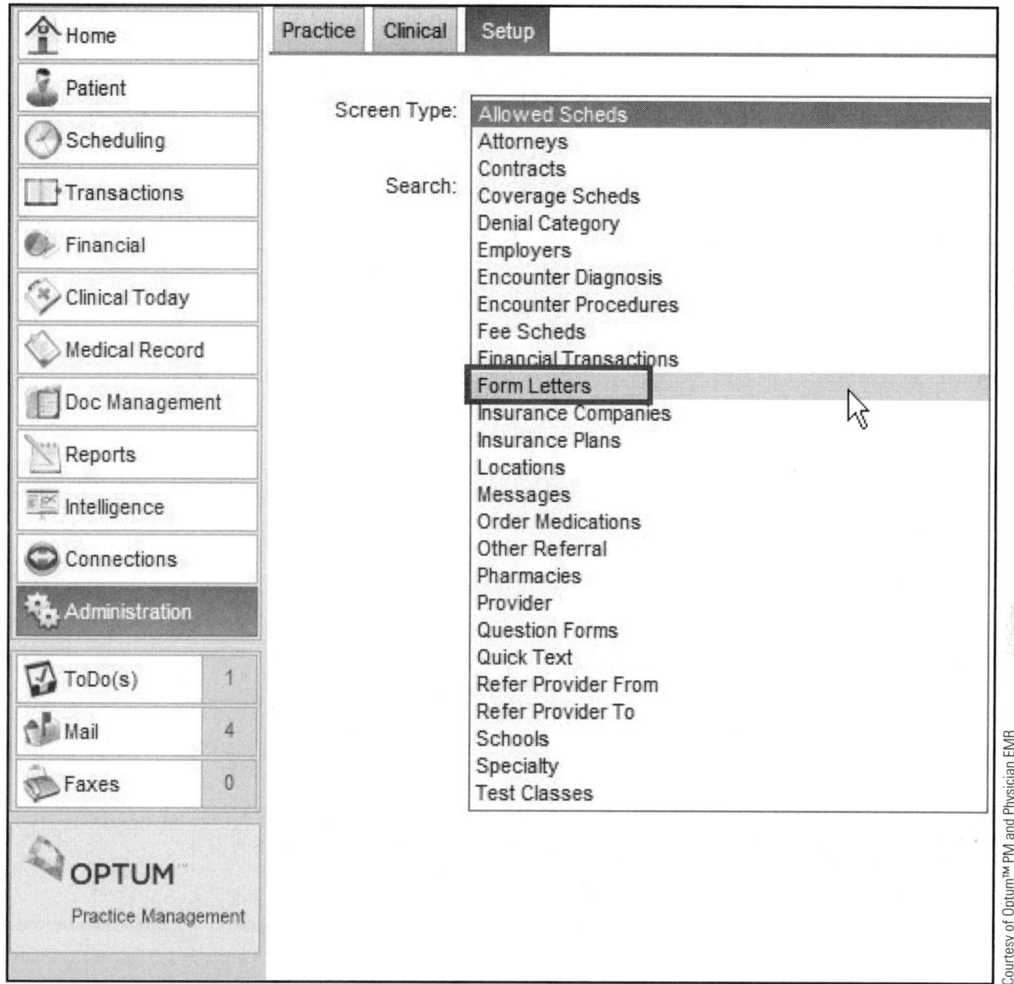

Figure 8-46 Screen Type - Form Letters

3. Enter the name of the new form letter you created in Activity 8-8 in the *Search* field (enter "RTA"), and then click the *Search* icon. The application displays a pop-up of all of the letters that match the search criteria (see Figure 8-47).
4. Click on the form letter you want to add to your *Quick Pick* list (select "RTA Fee Letter"). You will receive a pop-up *Success* box stating "Quick Pick information has been updated." Click *Close* on the *Success* box (see Figure 8-48).

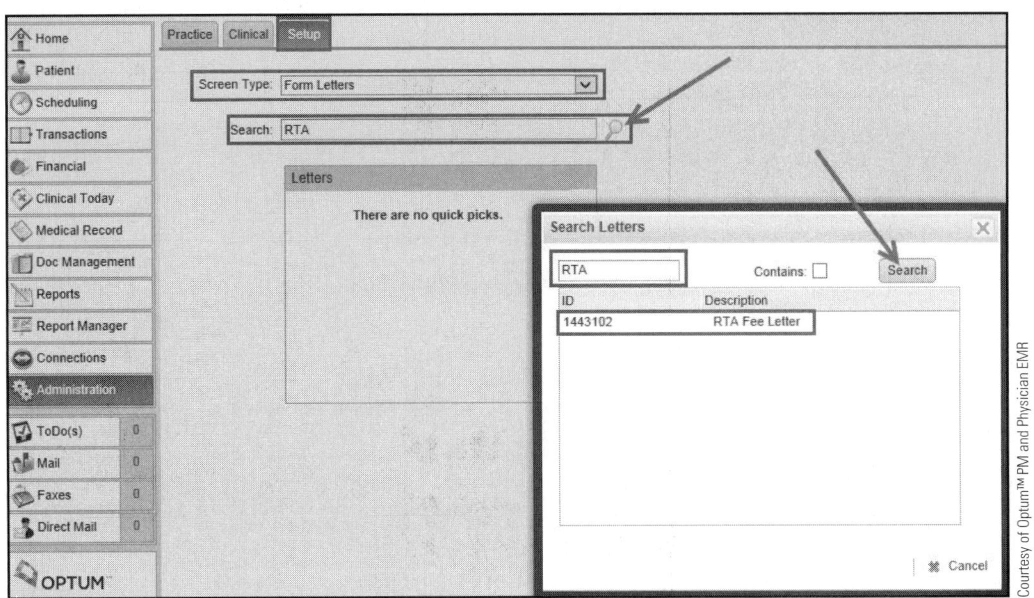

Figure 8-47 Search Letters Window

5. The application adds the letter to the *Quick Picks* list where it will be available to generate for patients (Figure 8-48).

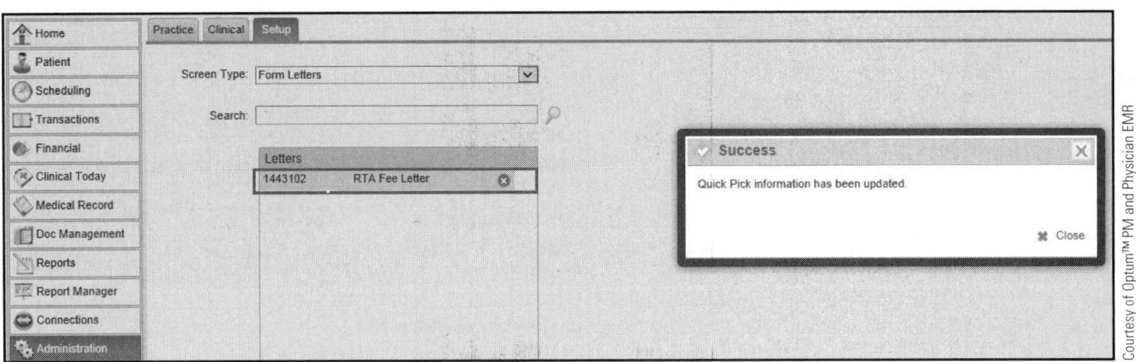

Figure 8-48 Quick Picks Letters

Print a screenshot of the Quick Picks list screen, label it "Activity 8-9," and place it in your assignment folder.

ACTIVITY 8-10: Generate Collection Letters

To generate collection letters, use one of two options: Optum™ PM and Physician EMR's global collection letters, or build a custom collection letter specific to your practice. After collection letters have been generated, they must be printed from the *Print Batch Letters* application in the *Administration* module. Generated collection letters are saved in the patients' record in the *Correspondence* application of the *Financial* module.

1. Go to the *Home* module > *Dashboard* tab > *Billing* section > *Collections* link. Optum™ PM displays a list of collection statements.

2. To search *Collections*, select an option from one or more of the following search fields and then click *Search* (Figures 8-49 and 8-50).
   - *Group* – This field is only available when statements for the company are set up by group.
   - *Statement Dates* – This allows you to view a week's worth of statements.
   - *Custom Dates* – Enter a custom date range in the fields provided.
   - *Status* – Select the status of the collection statements you want to view.

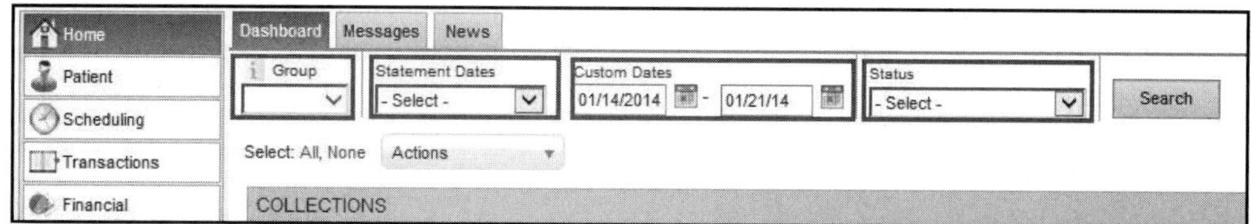

Figure 8-49 Search Collections Fields

Courtesy of Optum™ PM and Physician EMR

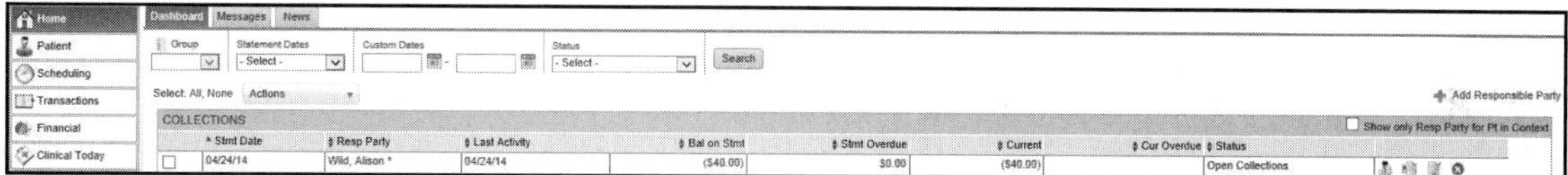

Figure 8-50 Search Collections Results

Courtesy of Optum™ PM and Physician EMR

3. Use the filters at the top of the page to view statements by *Group, Status,* or date range. For this activity, in the drop-down list in the *Status* field, leave as "(-Select-)."
4. Click the name in the line of the *Resp Party* column (Alison Wild) to view the *Statement Details* (Figure 8-51). It is helpful to review this information when determining a status change and/or deciding what action to take on a patient's balance. Close the *Statement Details* dialog box.

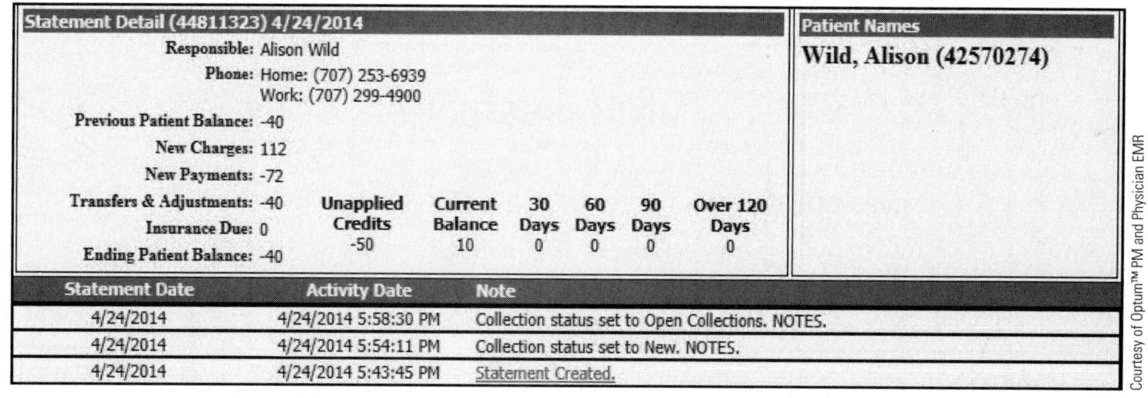

Courtesy of Optum™ PM and Physician EMR

Figure 8-51 Statement Details

5. Click the *Edit* icon next to the statement line for which you want to generate a collection letter. Optum™ PM displays the *Edit* box.
6. From the *Letter* list, select the letter you want to generate. Select "Past Due 60 1st."
7. If needed, select a new status from the *Change Status* list. (Leave blank.)

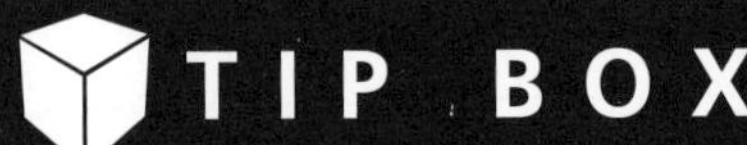

To generate letters for multiple patients, select the checkbox next to each patient for whom you want to generate a letter and then click *Actions* > *Edit*.

8. Click *Save*. Generated collection letters can be printed from the *Print Batch Letters* application in the *Administration* module (Figure 8-52). You will receive an error message because you are not able to print batch letters in your student version of Optum™ due to the *ClaimsManager* feature not being functional.

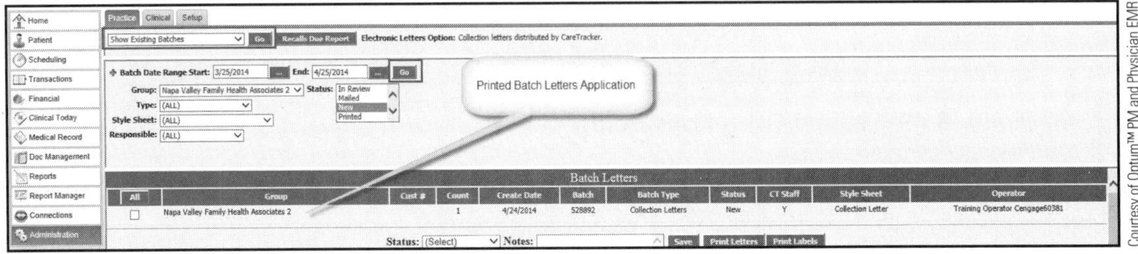

Courtesy of Optum™ PM and Physician EMR

Figure 8-52 Print Batch Letters Application

Print a screenshot of the Batch letters screen, label it "Activity 8-10," and place it in your assignment folder.

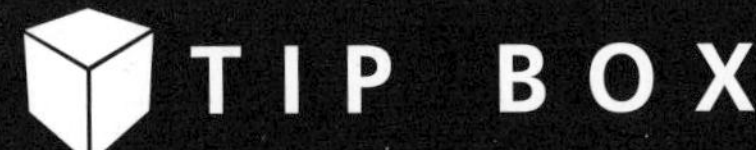

If you do not print the collection letters, Optum™ PM and Physician EMR will automatically print the letters to send out to the patient the next day.

MINI-CASE STUDIES

Complete all case studies for the following patients. (**Note:** Prior to completing case studies, post any open batches.)

a. Alec Winfrey

b. Darryl Smith

Case Study 8-1

1. Prior to beginning Case Study 8-1, create a new batch and name it "Ch8MCS."
2. Repeat Activity 8-5 and generate statements for both patients noted above. (**Note:** After pulling a patient into context, you may need to refresh your screen for the patient to appear in the *Responsible Party* field.)

Print the Generated Statements, label them "Case Study 8-1A" and "Case Study 8-1B," and place them in your assignment folder.

Case Study 8-2

Repeat Activity 8-7 and transfer the balance for both patients.

Once all balances have been transferred, print the screen showing all Transferred Balances, label it "Case Study 8-2," and place it in your assignment folder.

Case Study 8-3

Repeat Activity 8-10 and generate collection letters for both patients. (Select "Past Due 60 1st.")

Print the Batch Letters screen showing the Collection Letters generated, label it "Case Study 8-3," and place it in your assignment folder.

Case Study 8-4

1. Run a journal for your batch. Review and make any corrections if necessary.
2. Post the batch.

Print the screens of the Journal and Open Batch(es), label them "Case Study 8-4A" and "Case Study 8-4B," and place them in your assignment folder.

Case Study 8-5

NVFHA MANAGER CHALLENGE

Earlier in the chapter we touched on the subject of service recovery. In this case study, consider how you would address an issue such as billing a wrong insurance because at check-in, the patient's information was not updated and the new insurance card was not scanned. If your tone in words (written or verbal) is accusatory or harsh, you would certainly alienate the patient. Therefore, it is important to accept responsibility for the error and sincerely apologize. Often a practice sends an apology letter along with a gift card to the patient as a gesture of goodwill.

Repeat Activity 8-8 and create a custom "Service Recovery" letter as discussed in the Manager's Challenge to use when the practice needs to apologize and retain goodwill. Use *Letter Type* "Patient."

Print the screen showing the Service Recovery Letter created, label it "Case Study 8-5," and place it in your assignment folder.

Case Study 8-6

Repeat activity 8-9 and add the custom "Service Recovery" letter created in Case Study 8-5 to *Quick Picks*.

Print the Quick Picks screen showing the Service Recovery Letter generated, label it "Case Study 8-6," and place it in your assignment folder.

Resources

The Optum PM and Physician EMR Help homepage represents a wealth of information for the electronic health record (https://training.caretracker.com/help/CareTracker_Help.htm).

American Medical Association

National Healthcare Association. (n.d.). *Certified Electronic Health Records Specialist (CEHRS™)*. Retrieved from http://www.nhanow.com/health-record.aspx

CHAPTER 9

Applied Learning for the Paperless Medical Office

NVFHA MANAGER CHALLENGE

Congratulations on completing Chapters 1 through 8 of *The Paperless Medical Office for Billers and Coders: Using Optum™ PM and Physician EMR*. You are now expected to use all the information you have learned from the workbook activities and related case studies to complete this final chapter. It is up to you to prove that you are now prepared to work in the EHR and demonstrate proficiency by completing the following Applied Learning Case Study. Good luck!

Case Study 9-1: Gretchen O'Toole

Gretchen O'Toole is an established patient who calls the office this morning to schedule an appointment with Dr. Brockton, her primary care provider. She says she wants to see Dr. Brockton regarding her diabetes management because she has not been feeling well the past few weeks. Gretchen has not been in to see Dr. Brockton since the office converted to electronic records, but she is registered in the database. Search the database confirming her DOB, current address, phone number, and insurance, and then schedule the appointment for her.

Step 1: Search the Database and Schedule an Appointment

1. Search the database confirming the patient's DOB, current address, phone number, and insurance. Because this is her first visit since the practice converted to the EMR, you need to update and confirm that she has signed the HIE, NPP, and Consent forms. If you notice any other outstanding or missing information in her demographics, update it at this time.
2. Schedule an appointment for Gretchen with Dr. Brockton, using the first available morning slot.
   - *Appointment Type:* Follow-up
   - *Complaint:* Follow-up; Diabetes management
   - *Location:* NVFA

Step 2: Enter Payment and Check In Patient

When Gretchen arrives for her appointment, view her *At-A-Glance* patient information and confirm that she is still insured with Century Med PPO and has a $35.00 copay. Before accepting Gretchen's payment, create a new batch.

1. Accept and enter Gretchen's cash payment for her copay and print a receipt for her.

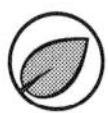 **Label the printed receipt "Case Study 9-1A."**

2. Check Gretchen in for her visit with Dr. Brockton.

Step 3: Patient Workup

To begin EMR activities, edit your operator preferences in the *Batch* for clinical workflows with Dr. Brockton as the provider.

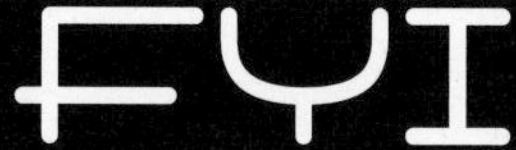

Background Information About Gretchen O'Toole

Gretchen was diagnosed with type 2 diabetes mellitus approximately 20 years ago—around the same time she was diagnosed with hypertension. She has been very compliant over the years and remains on an oral hypoglycemic. She is here for a routine follow-up appointment exam after discovering at a local church health fair that her cholesterol is elevated and wants to discuss the findings with the doctor.

1. *Transfer* Gretchen to Exam Room #1.
2. Ms. O'Toole is being seen today for diabetes management and hypertension. Because Gretchen is now ready to see Dr. Brockton, create a progress note for her. Refer to Table 9-1 while completing the progress note. (**Note:** Select progress note template "IM OV Option 4 (v4) w/A&P.")

Table 9-1 Gretchen O'Toole Progress Note Information

Tab	Entry
CC/HPI	*Chief Complaint*: Select "Established Patient" and "Follow-Up Visit" boxes
	Other complaints box: Enter "Wants cholesterol checked. Had blood test (finger stick) at a church health fair. Result was elevated. Does not recall reading"
	History of Present Illness box: Enter "Pt. here for an F/U exam for diabetes and hypertension. Pt. states she checks her blood sugar in the morning when she first gets up and 2 hours after each meal. 'Readings have stayed below 130 mg/dL.' Last A1c was in October of last year, result 6.4. Pt. also states that home blood pressure readings have been running between 140 and 160 on the systolic side and between 85 and 95 on the diastolic side. Pt. has some tingling in her toes but not often. Regularly sees an ophthalmologist for eye care. Overall, pt. states that she feels very good!"
Skip the HX, ROS, PE, TESTS, and PROC Tabs	(No entry)
ASSESS	*Diagnoses:* DM, Type 2, Diabetic Peripheral Neuropathy (250.60 and 337.1); Hypertension (401.9)
	Assessment box: Enter "Overweight (278.02)"

Table 9-1 (*Continued*)

PLAN	*Additional Plan Details* box: 1. EKG 2. Hemoglobin A1c/Hemoglobin total in blood 3. Glucose Blood Test - Global 4. Lipid panel with direct LDL in serum or plasma 5. Have patient follow up with podiatrist 6. Rx: MetFORMIN HCI Oral Tablet 850 mg. Sig: One 850 mg tablet twice a day, 180 tabs. 4 refills 7. Rx: Micardis Oral Tablet 40 mg. Sig: One 40 mg tablet daily, 90 tabs, 4 refills, take in the evening 8. Patient Education Materials: a. PERIPHERAL NEUROPATHY b. HIGH BLOOD PRESSURE-ESTABLISHED 9. 3-month follow-up appointment 10. Referral to Podiatrist: Dr. William R. Todd, DPM in Napa, CA
***Remember to *Save* the progress note.**	

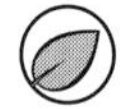

When you have completed Step 3: Patient Workup, print the patient's Chart Summary and label it "Case Study 9-1B."

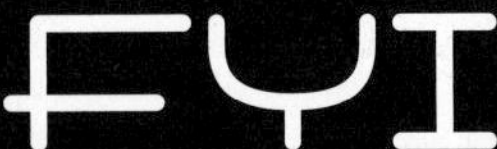

Completing the Visit by Entering Lab Orders

Before Gretchen leaves the office, the clinical medical assistant will add a *Recall* for her CPE one year plus one day from today's date, and complete the *Orders* and *Referral* in the *Plan* section of the progress note. As the biller and coder, you will not be entering the lab orders, recall, or referral and will instead move on to capturing the visit.

Step 4: Capture the Visit and Sign the Note

Now that all of the orders as indicated in the progress note are completed, capture the *Visit* and sign the progress note (review the A&P to be sure you capture all billable items).

1. Capture the *Visit* by entering:
   a. *CPT® code(s)*: 99213; 82962; 80061; 36415; 93000; and 99000

      Source: Current Procedural Terminology © 2013 American Medical Association.

   b. *ICD-9 code(s)*: 250.60; 337.1; 401.9; and 278.02

2. Sign the progress note.

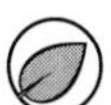 **Print the signed progress note and label it "Case Study 9-1C."**

3. Schedule a follow-up appointment as indicated in the A&P.

Step 5: Verify Charges and Generate a Claim

Verify charges for Gretchen's *Visit* and then generate a claim.

1. Using the batch you created at the beginning of the case study, run a journal and verify charges.

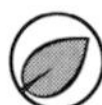 **Print the Journal and label it "Case Study 9-1D."**

2. Generate the claim.

Step 6: Process Remittance (EOB) and Transfer to Private Pay

1. Create a new batch to record Gretchen's EOB.
2. Refer to Gretchen's EOB (Source Document 9-1 in Appendix A) and process the remittance. (**Hint:** Be sure to save all charges and build all claims first.)
3. Run a journal to verify charges.

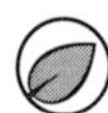 **Print the Journal and label it "Case Study 9-1E."**

Step 7: Work Claims and Generate Patient Statement

1. Work the *Claims Worklist.*
2. Post all open batches.
3. Generate a patient statement for Gretchen.

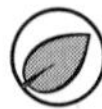 **Print the Statement and label it "Case Study 9-1F."**

Case Study 9-2: Transfer to Collections

It has now been more than 60 days since you generated a statement for Gretchen and her payment has not been received. Create a new batch for collection activities.

1. Manually transfer Gretchen's account to *Collections.*
2. Generate a collection letter appropriate to the office policy for accounts older than 60 days.

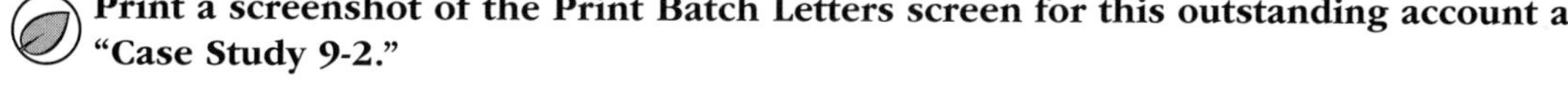

Print a screenshot of the Print Batch Letters screen for this outstanding account and label it "Case Study 9-2."

3. Run a journal and post the batch.

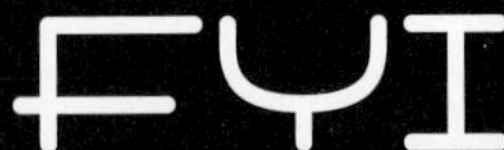

Operator Audit Log

The *Operator Audit Log* maintains an audit trail of all actions performed in Optum™ PM and Physician EMR by each operator. This log is helpful to monitor each operator's usage. As a billing and coding professional, the audit log is a powerful tool in monitoring usage and entries that affect compliance. The steps to view an *Operator Audit Log* are as follows:

1. Click the *Administration* module. The application opens the *Practice* tab.
2. Click the *Operator Audit Log* link under *Security Logs* (Figure 9-1). The application launches the *Operator Audit Log*.

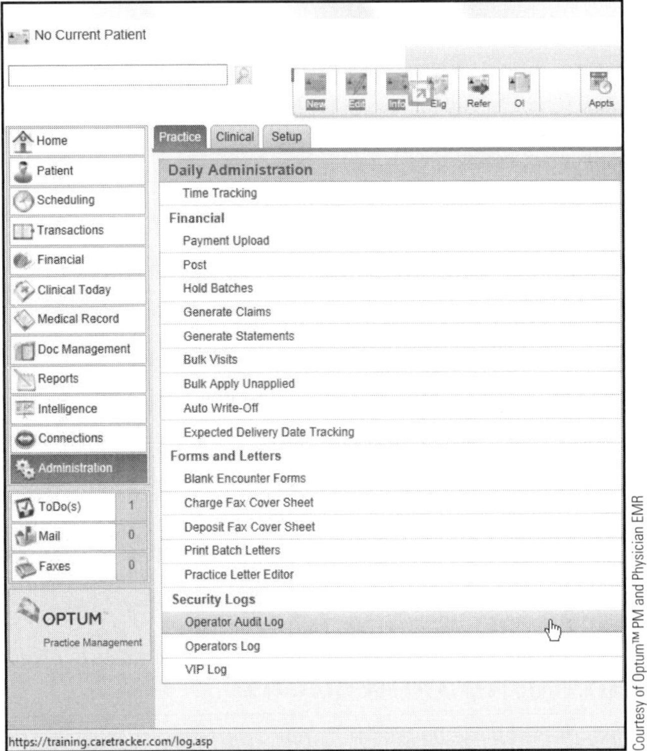

Courtesy of Optum™ PM and Physician EMR

Figure 9-1 Operator Audit Log

3. From the *Operator* list, select the operator for whom you want to generate an audit log "(Current Operator)." To see a log of all operator activities, you would choose "-Select-".
4. From the *Type* list, select the type of activity for which you want to view a log. Choose "-Select-" to view a log of all activities.
5. The *From/To Date* boxes default to the previous seven days to include in the audit log. Leave as is.
6. Click *Show Log*. Optum™ PM displays the log in the bottom half of the screen (Figure 9-2).

(*Continues*)

FYI *(Continued)*

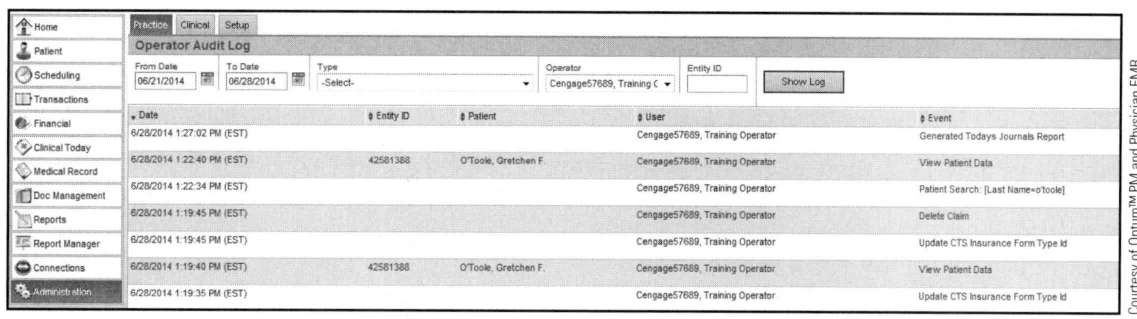

Courtesy of Optum™ PM and Physician EMR

Figure 9-2 Operator Log

VIP Patient Log

In addition to the *Operators Audit Log*, there is also a tool for viewing the VIP log. There are many reasons to flag a patient as a VIP. Doing so allows you to restrict operator access to the patient's demographic information. Any operator may flag a high-profile patient as a VIP, but only operators assigned either the "VIP Patient Access" or the "VIP Patient Access Break Glass" override in their profile can access a VIP demographic. Each time an operator accesses a VIP patient demographic, Optum™ PM and Physician EMR creates an entry in the *VIP Patient Log*. The log lists the patient name, the operator who accessed the record, and the date and time the record was accessed. The steps to view the *VIP Patient Log* are as follows:

1. Click the *Administration* module. Optum™ PM displays the *Practice* tab.
2. Click the *VIP Log* link under the *Security Logs* section. The application displays the *VIP Patient Log* (Figure 9-3).

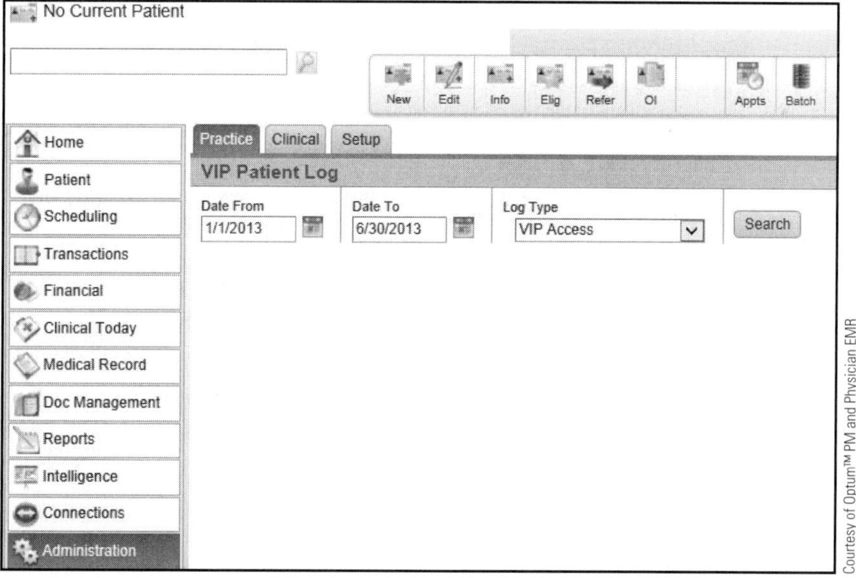

Courtesy of Optum™ PM and Physician EMR

Figure 9-3 VIP Patient Log

3. Select the date range in the *Date From* and *Date To* fields.
4. Select the *Log Type* to view:
   a. VIP Access: displays operators with *VIP Patient Access* override included in their profile.
   b. VIP Break Glass Access: displays the activity of users with the *VIP Break Glass* override included in their profile.

(Continues)

FYI *(Continued)*

5. Click *Search*. Optum™ PM displays the log (Figure 9-4).

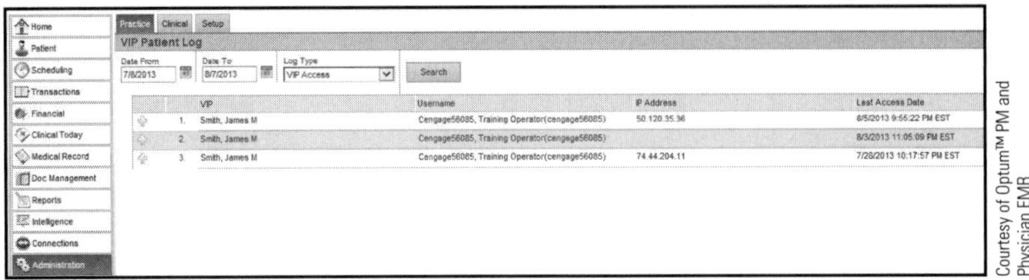

Courtesy of Optum™ PM and Physician EMR

Figure 9-4 VIP Patient Log Created

6. Click the plus sign next to the patient's name to expand the log and view additional details (Figure 9-5).

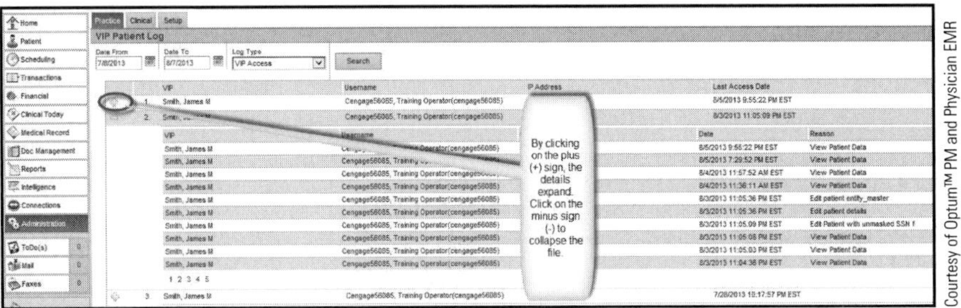

Courtesy of Optum™ PM and Physician EMR

Figure 9-5 VIP Patient Log Expanded

Case Study 9-3: Close the Fiscal Periods and Fiscal Years

Having completed the activities in this workbook and the applied learning case studies, close any open fiscal periods and fiscal years. Follow the instructions in Activity 2-6 (Open a Fiscal Period) and the FYI Box instructions to Close a Fiscal Period.

Warning!! Once a fiscal period or fiscal year is closed, it cannot be reopened. Be sure you have completed all activities and assignments in this workbook prior to closing. (**Note:** You may want to wait until the end of the semester so that you can review your assignments with your instructor or make any necessary changes to the activities.)

1. Access *Open Fiscal Period(s)/Open Fiscal Year(s)*. Write down a list of all open periods.
2. Review *Open Batches* and run a *Journal* for any open batches.
3. Review your *Open Batches*, *Journal*, and *Open Fiscal Period(s)/Open Fiscal Year(s)* with your instructor.
4. Upon confirmation that all activities have been completed as assigned and that any open batches have been posted, close all the fiscal period(s) and fiscal year(s).

NVFHA MANAGER CHALLENGE

Dear Student:

Congratulations on completing *The Paperless Medical Office for Billers and Coders: Using Optum™ PM and Physician EMR* activities, your first step toward becoming a "super-user" of electronic health records! As office manager, I screen applicants for open positions within the practice. In addition, I maintain a network with local hospitals' human resources departments and refer from the candidate pool for open positions for which the medical assistant is qualified.

Once a job opening is posted and applications and résumés are received, I will begin the screening process. The following qualifications and characteristics are some of the ways applicants will be evaluated:

- Education (certification or degree from accredited program)
- Experience (total length of each place of employment related to job opening)
- Quality of application and résumé (grammar, spelling, punctuation)
- References (verify with former employers)
  - Length of employment
  - Eligible (or not) for re-hire
  - What would provider say about the applicant? (best and worst qualities)
  - What would co-workers say about the applicant? (best and worst qualities)
  - Attendance and punctuality
  - Attention to detail; accurate data entry
  - Teamwork behavior
  - Work ethic and habits

If you have a chance to extern as a biller and/or coder, it would be very important to accept such a position because most practices that prepare their own coding and billing prefer experience. Having completed this workbook, you can list on your application and résumé that you have completed training and are a "super-user" of Optum™ PM and Physician EMR. In addition, many practices outsource their billing to a private firm. Finding extern positions and employment with such a business will also give you the valued hands-on experience that is so desirable. In addition, with the transition from ICD-9 to ICD-10, it is even more important to demonstrate your knowledge and ability to use an electronic code verification system such as Optum™. This affords the extern a good opportunity to observe the needed billing and coding skills as well as demonstrate good work ethic and habits. Many times an externship position can lead to employment within the practice or private billing firm.

How would you rate your qualifications and characteristics? How will the information you learned from this workbook enhance your capabilities to obtain the desired position you are seeking? Have you created your résumé and portfolio yet? If not, it would be good practice to begin documenting your achievements. It has been our pleasure to have you as a "Student MA" here at NVFHA. Congratulations and best wishes on a successful career!

Sincerely,

Takari Miata

Takari Miata, Office Manager

Napa Valley Family Health Associates

APPENDIX **A**

Source Documents

Source Document 7-1: Explanation of Benefits

MEDICARE CENGAGE

Medicare Cengage
P.O. Box 234434
San Francisco, CA 94137

Date: MM/DD/YYYY (Appt. date used in Activity 4-1)
Payment Number: 1334557
Payment Amount: $ 97.60

AMIR RAMAN, D.O.
Napa Valley Family Health Associates (NVFHA)
101 Vine Street
Napa, CA 94558

Account Number	**Patient Name**				**Subscriber Number**		**Claim Number**			
Dates of Service	**Description of Service**	**Amount Charged**	**Not Covered**	**Prov Adj Discount**	**Amount Allowed**	**Deduct/ Coins/ Copay**	**Paid to Provider**	**Adj Reason Code**	**Rmk Code**	**Patient Resp**
CARE1357	**Wild, Alison**									
(Appt. date used in Activity 4-1)	99213	$112.00	$0.00	$ 40.00	$ 72.00	$14.40	$57.60	45*		$14.40
(Appt. date used in Activity 4-1)	99000	$ 0.00	$0.00	$ 0.00	$ 0.00	$ 0.00	$ 0.00	45*		$ 0.00
(Appt. date used in Activity 4-1)	90746	$100.00	$0.00	$ 60.00	$ 40.00	$ 8.00	$32.00	45*		$ 8.00
(Appt. date used in Activity 4-1)	90471	$ 15.00	$0.00	$ 5.00	$ 10.00	$ 2.00	$ 8.00	45*		$ 2.00
TOTALS		**$227.00**	**$0.00**	**$105.00**	**$122.00**	**$24.40**	**$97.60**			**$24.40**

Amount Allowed (45*) = Charges exceed your contracted/legislated fee arrangement
Amount Allowed (20*) = Not a covered code

Source Document 7-2: Explanation of Benefits

CENTURY MEDICAL PPO - CENGAGE

Century Medical PPO
PO Box 87542
San Jose, CA 95101

Date: MM/DD/YYYY (Appt. date used in Activity 4-1)
Payment Number: 212311
Payment Amount: $0.00

AMIR RAMAN, M.D.
Napa Valley Family Health Associates (NVFHA)
101 Vine Street
Napa, CA 94558

Account Number	Patient Name				Subscriber Number		Claim Number			
Dates of Service	**Description of Service**	**Amount Charged**	**Not Covered**	**Prov Adj Discount**	**Amount Allowed**	**Deduct/ Coins/ Copay**	**Paid to Provider**	**Adj Reason Code**	**Rmk Code**	**Patient Resp**
CMED2478	**Winfrey, Alec**									
(Appt. date used in Activity 4-1)	99213	$112.00	$0.00	$36.00	$76.00	$76.00	$0.00	22*		$76.00
(Appt. date used in Activity 4-1)	71020	$ 13.50	$0.00	$ 3.50	$10.00	$10.00	$0.00	22*		$10.00
(Appt. date used in Activity 4-1)	36415	$ 15.00	$0.00	$ 5.00	$10.00	$10.00	$0.00	22*		$10.00
(Appt. date used in Activity 4-1)	85025	$ 0.00	$0.00	$ 0.00	$ 0.00	$ 0.00	$0.00	45*		$ 0.00
TOTALS		**$140.50**	**$0.00**	**$44.50**	**$96.00**	**$96.00**	**$0.00**			**$96.00**

Amount Allowed (45*) = Charges exceed your contracted/legislated fee arrangement
Amount Allowed (22*) = Patient has not yet met annual policy deductible ($6,000.00). All balances are patient's responsibility.
Amount Allowed (25*) = Requires Modifier 25 to be paid as a separate service

Source Document 7-3: Explanation of Benefits

MEDICARE CENGAGE

Medicare Cengage
P.O. Box 234434
San Francisco, CA 94137

Date: MM/DD/YYYY (Date charge entered in Activity 7-3)
Payment Number: 5644712
Payment Amount: $ 80.00

AMIR RAMAN, D.O.
Napa Valley Family Health Associates (NVFHA)
101 Vine Street
Napa, CA 94558

Account Number	**Patient Name**				**Subscriber Number**		**Claim Number**			
Dates of Service	**Description of Service**	**Amount Charged**	**Not Covered**	**Prov Adj Discount**	**Amount Allowed**	**Deduct/ Coins/ Copay**	**Paid to Provider**	**Adj Reason Code**	**Rmk Code**	**Patient Resp**
CARE1357	**Smith, Darryl**									
(Date charge entered in Activity 7-3)	G0180	$100.00	$0.00	$ 40.00	$ 60.00	$12.00	$48.00	45*		$12.00
(Date charge entered in Activity 7-3)	93000	$ 50.00	$0.00	$ 10.00	$ 40.00	$ 8.00	$32.00	45*		$ 8.00
TOTALS		**$150.00**	**$0.00**	**$50.00**	**$100.00**	**$20.00**	**$80.00**			**$20.00**

Amount Allowed (45*) = Charges exceed your contracted/legislated fee arrangement
Amount Allowed (20*) = Not a covered code

Source Document 7-4: Explanation of Benefits

BLUE CROSS BLUE SHIELD - CENGAGE

Blue Cross Blue Shield – Cengage
PO Box 32245
Los Angeles, CA 90002

Date: MM/DD/YYYY (Appt. date used in Activity 4-1)
Payment Number: 6444578
Payment Amount: $ 80.00

AMIR RAMAN, D.O.
Napa Valley Family Health Associates (NVFHA)
101 Vine Street
Napa, CA 94558

Account Number	**Patient Name**				**Subscriber Number**		**Claim Number**			
Dates of Service	**Description of Service**	**Amount Charged**	**Not Covered**	**Prov Adj Discount**	**Amount Allowed**	**Deduct/ Coins/ Copay**	**Paid to Provider**	**Adj Reason Code**	**Rmk Code**	**Patient Resp**
BCBS987	**Mcginness, Jim**									
(Appt. date used in Activity 4-1)	99213	$112.00	$0.00	$12.00	$ 100.00	$20.00	$80.00	45*		$20.00
TOTALS		**$112.00**	**$0.00**	**$12.00**	**$100.00**	**$20.00**	**$80.00**			**$20.00**

Amount Allowed (45*) = Charges exceed your contracted/legislated fee arrangement
Amount Allowed (20*) = Not a covered code

Source Document 9-1: Explanation of Benefits

CENTURY CENGAGE

CENTURY CENGAGE
P.O. Box 87542
San Jose, CA 95101

Date: MM/DD/YYYY (Appt. date used in Case Study 9-1)
Payment Number: 2344570
Payment Amount: $120.94

ANTHONY BROCKTON, M.D.
Napa Valley Family Health Associates (NVFHA)
101 Vine Street
Napa, CA 94558

Account Number	**Patient Name**				**Subscriber Number**		**Claim Number**			
Dates of Service	**Description of Service**	**Amount Charged**	**Not Covered**	**Prov Adj Discount**	**Amount Allowed**	**Deduct/ Coins/ Copay**	**Paid to Provider**	**Adj Reason Code**	**Rmk Code**	**Patient Resp**
9706416	**O'Toole, Gretchen**									
(Appt. date used in Case Study 9-1)	99213	$112.00	$0.00	$0.00	$112.00	$20.00	$57.00	45*		$20.00
(Appt. date used in Case Study 9-1)	99000	$0.00	$0.00	$0.00	$0.00	$0.00	$0.00	20*		$0.00
(Appt. date used in Case Study 9-1)	82962	$10.00	$0.00	$0.00	$10.00	$5.00	$5.00	45*		$5.00
(Appt. date used in Case Study 9-1)	80061	$37.44	$0.00	$0.00	$37.44	$20.00	$17.44	45*		$20.00
(Appt. date used in Case Study 9-1)	36415	$15.00	$0.00	$0.00	$15.00	$5.00	$10.00	45*		$5.00
(Appt. date used in Case Study 9-1)	93000	$46.50	$0.00	$0.00	$46.50	$15.00	$31.50	45*		$15.00
TOTALS		**$220.94**	**$0.00**	**$0.00**	**$220.94**	**$65.00**	**$120.94**			**$65.00**

Amount Allowed (45*) = Charges exceed your contracted/legislated fee arrangement
Amount Allowed (20*) = Not a covered code